ICD-10

The ICD-10 Classification of Mental and Behavioural Disorders

Clinical descriptions and diagnostic guidelines

World Health Organization
Geneva
1992

Reprinted 1993, 1994, 1995, 1998, 2000, 2002, 2004

WHO Library Cataloguing in Publication Data

The ICD-10 classification of mental and behavioural
    disorders : clinical descriptions and diagnostic guidelines.

    1.Mental disorders — classification   2.Mental disorders — diagnosis

    ISBN 92 4 154422 8   (NLM Classification: WM 15)

Printed in Switzerland

9057/9522/9928/10297/11833/12786/14450 — 33000
2003/15477 — Strategic — 2000

Contents

Preface

In the early 1960s, the Mental Health Programme of the World Health Organization (WHO) became actively engaged in a programme aiming to improve the diagnosis and classification of mental disorders. At that time, WHO convened a series of meetings to review knowledge, actively involving representatives of different disciplines, various schools of thought in psychiatry, and all parts of the world in the programme. It stimulated and conducted research on criteria for classification and for reliability of diagnosis, and produced and promulgated procedures for joint rating of videotaped interviews and other useful research methods. Numerous proposals to improve the classification of mental disorders resulted from the extensive consultation process, and these were used in drafting the Eighth Revision of the International Classification of Diseases (ICD-8). A glossary defining each category of mental disorder in ICD-8 was also developed. The programme activities also resulted in the establishment of a network of individuals and centres who continued to work on issues related to the improvement of psychiatric classification (*1, 2*).

The 1970s saw further growth of interest in improving psychiatric classification worldwide. Expansion of international contacts, the undertaking of several international collaborative studies, and the availability of new treatments all contributed to this trend. Several national psychiatric bodies encouraged the development of specific criteria for classification in order to improve diagnostic reliability. In particular, the American Psychiatric Association developed and promulgated its Third Revision of the Diagnostic and Statistical Manual, which incorporated operational criteria into its classification system.

In 1978, WHO entered into a long-term collaborative project with the Alcohol, Drug Abuse and Mental Health Administration (ADAMHA) in the USA, aiming to facilitate further improvements in the classification and diagnosis of mental disorders, and alcohol- and drug-related problems (*3*). A series of workshops brought together scientists from a number of different psychiatric traditions and cultures, reviewed knowledge in specified areas, and developed recommendations for future research. A major international conference on classification and diagnosis was held in Copenhagen, Denmark, in 1982 to review the recommendations that emerged from these workshops and to outline a research agenda and guidelines for future work (*4*).

Several major research efforts were undertaken to implement the recommendations of the Copenhagen conference. One of them, involving centres in 17 countries, had as its aim the development of the Composite International Diagnostic Interview, an instrument suitable for conducting epidemiological studies of mental disorders in general population groups in different countries (5). Another major project focused on developing an assessment instrument suitable for use by clinicians (Schedules for Clinical Assessment in Neuropsychiatry) (6). Still another study was initiated to develop an instrument for the assessment of personality disorders in different countries (the International Personality Disorder Examination) (7).

In addition, several lexicons have been, or are being, prepared to provide clear definitions of terms (8). A mutually beneficial relationship evolved between these projects and the work on definitions of mental and behavioural disorders in the Tenth Revision of the International Classification of Diseases and Related Health Problems (ICD-10) (9). Converting diagnostic criteria into diagnostic algorithms incorporated in the assessment instruments was useful in uncovering inconsistencies, ambiguities and overlap and allowing their removal. The work on refining the ICD-10 also helped to shape the assessment instruments. The final result was a clear set of criteria for ICD-10 and assessment instruments which can produce data necessary for the classification of disorders according to the criteria included in Chapter V(F) of ICD-10.

The Copenhagen conference also recommended that the viewpoints of the different psychiatric traditions be presented in publications describing the origins of the classification in the ICD-10. This resulted in several major publications, including a volume that contains a series of presentations highlighting the origins of classification in contemporary psychiatry (10).

The preparation and publication of this work, *Clinical descriptions and diagnostic guidelines*, are the culmination of the efforts of numerous people who have contributed to it over many years. The work has gone through several major drafts, each prepared after extensive consultation with panels of experts, national and international psychiatric societies, and individual consultants. The draft in use in 1987 was the basis of field trials conducted in some 40 countries, which constituted the largest ever research effort of its type designed to improve psychiatric diagnosis (11, 12). The results of the trials were used in finalizing these guidelines.

This work is the first of a series of publications developed from Chapter V(F) of ICD-10. Other texts will include diagnostic criteria for researchers, a version for use by general health care workers, a multiaxial presentation, and "crosswalks" — allowing cross-reference between corresponding terms in ICD-10, ICD-9 and ICD-8.

Use of this publication is described in the Introduction, and a subsequent section of the book provides notes on some of the frequently discussed difficulties of classification. The Acknowledgements section is of particular significance since it bears witness to the vast number of individual experts and institutions, all over the world, who actively participated in the production of the classification and the guidelines. All the major traditions and schools of psychiatry are represented, which gives this work its uniquely international character. The classification and the guidelines were produced and tested in many languages; it is hoped that the arduous process of ensuring equivalence of translations has resulted in improvements in the clarity, simplicity and logical structure of the texts in English and in other languages.

A classification is a way of seeing the world at a point in time. There is no doubt that scientific progress and experience with the use of these guidelines will ultimately require their revision and updating. I hope that such revisions will be the product of the same cordial and productive worldwide scientific collaboration as that which has produced the current text.

Norman Sartorius
Director, Division of Mental Health
World Health Organization

References

1. Kramer, M. et al. The ICD-9 classification of mental disorders: a review of its developments and contents. *Acta psychiatrica scandinavica,* **59**: 241 – 262 (1979).

2. Sartorius, N. Classification: an international perspective. *Psychiatric annals,* **6**: 22 – 35 (1976).

3. Jablensky, A. et al. Diagnosis and classification of mental disorders and alcohol- and drug-related problems: a research agenda for the 1980s. *Psychological medicine,* **13**: 907 – 921 (1983).

4. *Mental disorders, alcohol- and drug-related problems: international perspectives on their diagnosis and classification.* Amsterdam, Excerpta Medica, 1985 (International Congress Series, No. 669).

5. Robins, L. et al. The composite international diagnostic interview. *Archives of general psychiatry,* **45**: 1069 – 1077 (1989).

6. Wing, J.K. et al. SCAN: schedules for clinical assessment in neuropsychiatry. *Archives of general psychiatry,* **47**: 589 – 593 (1990).

7. Loranger, A.W. et al. The WHO/ADAMHA international pilot study of personality disorders: background and purpose. *Journal of personality disorders,* **5**(3): 296 – 306 (1991).

8. *Lexicon of psychiatric and mental health terms. Vol. 1.* Geneva, World Health Organization, 1989.

9. *International Statistical Classification of Diseases and Related Health Problems. Tenth Revision. Vol. 1: Tabular list,* 1992. *Vol. 2: Instruction Manual,* 1993. *Vol. 3: Index,* 1994. Geneva, World Health Organization.

10. Sartorius, N. et al. (ed.) *Sources and traditions in classification in psychiatry.* Toronto, Hogrefe and Huber, 1990.

11. Sartorius, N. et al. (ed.) *Psychiatric classification in an international perspective. British journal of psychiatry,* **152** (Suppl. 1) (1988).

12. Sartorius, N. et al. Progress towards achieving a common language in psychiatry: results from the field trials of the clinical guidelines accompanying the WHO Classification of Mental and Behavioural Disorders in ICD-10. *Archives of general psychiatry,* 1993, **50**: 115–124.

Acknowledgements

Many individuals and organizations have contributed to the production of the classification of mental and behavioural disorders in ICD-10 and to the development of the texts that accompany it. The field trials of the ICD-10 proposals, for example, involved researchers and clinicians in some 40 countries; it is clearly impossible to present a complete list of all those who participated in this effort. What follows is a mention of individuals and agencies whose contributions were central to the creation of the documents composing the ICD-10 family of classifications and guidelines.

The individuals who produced the initial drafts of the classification and guidelines are included in the list of principal investigators on pages 312 – 325: their names are marked by an asterisk. Dr A. Jablensky, then Senior Medical Officer in the Division of Mental Health of WHO, in Geneva, coordinated this part of the programme and thus made a major contribution to the proposals. Once the proposals for the classification were assembled and circulated for comment to WHO expert panels and many other individuals, including those listed below, an amended version of the classification was produced for field tests. These were conducted according to a protocol produced by WHO staff with the help of Dr J. Burke, Dr J.E. Cooper, and Dr J. Mezzich and involved a large number of centres, whose work was coordinated by Field Trial Coordinating Centres (FTCCs). The FTCCs (listed on pages xi – xii) also undertook the task of producing equivalent translations of the ICD in the languages used in their countries.

Dr N. Sartorius had overall responsibility for the work on the classification of mental and behavioural disorders in ICD-10 and for the production of accompanying documents.

Throughout the phase of field testing and subsequently, Dr J.E. Cooper acted as chief consultant to the project and provided invaluable guidance and help to the WHO coordinating team. Among the team members were Dr J. van Drimmelen, who has worked with WHO from the beginning of the process of developing ICD-10 proposals, and Mrs J. Wilson, who conscientiously and efficiently handled the innumerable administrative tasks linked to the field tests and other activities related to the projects. Mr A. L'Hours provided generous support, ensuring compliance between the ICD-10 development in general and the production of this classification, and Mr G. Gemert produced the index.

A number of other consultants, including in particular Dr A. Bertelsen, Dr H. Dilling, Dr J. López-Ibor, Dr C. Pull, Dr D. Regier, Dr M. Rutter and Dr N. Wig, were also closely involved in this work, functioning not only as heads of FTCCs for the field trials but also providing advice and guidance about issues in their area of expertise and relevant to the psychiatric traditions of the groups of countries about which they were particularly knowledgeable.

Among the agencies whose help was of vital importance were the Alcohol, Drug Abuse and Mental Health Administration in the USA, which provided generous support to the activities preparatory to the drafting of ICD-10, and which ensured effective and productive consultation between groups working on ICD-10 and those working on the fourth revision of the American Psychiatric Association's Diagnostic and Statistical Manual (DSM-IV) classification; the WHO Advisory Committee on ICD-10, chaired by Dr E. Strömgren; and the World Psychiatric Association which, through its President, Dr C. Stefanis, and the special committee on classification, assembled comments of numerous psychiatrists in its member associations and gave most valuable advice during both the field trials and the finalization of the proposals. Other nongovernmental organizations in official and working relations with WHO, including the World Federation for Mental Health, the World Association for Psychosocial Rehabilitation, the World Association of Social Psychiatry, the World Federation of Neurology, and the International Union of Psychological Societies, helped in many ways, as did the WHO Collaborating Centres for Research and Training in Mental Health, located in some 40 countries.

Governments of WHO Member States, including in particular Belgium, Germany, the Netherlands, Spain and the USA, also provided direct support to the process of developing the classification of mental and behavioural disorders, both through their designated contributions to WHO and through contributions and financial support to the centres that participated in this work.

The ICD-10 proposals are thus a product of collaboration, in the true sense of the word, between very many individuals and agencies in numerous countries. They were produced in the hope that they will serve as a strong support to the work of the many who are concerned with caring for the mentally ill and their families, worldwide.

No classification is ever perfect: further improvements and simplifications should become possible with increases in our knowledge and as experience with the classification accumulates. The task of collecting and digesting comments and results of tests of the classification will remain largely on the shoulders of the centres that collaborated with WHO in the development of the classification. Their addresses are listed below because it is hoped that they will continue to be involved in the improvement of the WHO classifications and associated materials in the future and to assist the Organization in this work as generously as they have so far.

Numerous publications have arisen from Field Trial Centres describing results of their studies in connection with ICD-10. A full list of these publications and reprints of the articles can be obtained from Division of Mental Health, World Health Organization, 1211 Geneva 27, Switzerland.

Field Trial Coordinating Centres and Directors

Dr A. Bertelsen, Institute of Psychiatric Demography, Psychiatric Hospital, University of Aarhus, Risskov, Denmark

Dr D. Caetano, Department of Psychiatry, State University of Campinas, Campinas, Brazil

Dr S. Channabasavanna, National Institute of Mental Health and Neurosciences, Bangalore, India

Dr H. Dilling, Psychiatric Clinic of the Medical School, Lübeck, Germany

Dr M. Gelder, Department of Psychiatry, Oxford University Hospital, Warneford Hospital, Headington, England

Dr D. Kemali, University of Naples, First Faculty of Medicine and Surgery, Institute of Medical Psychology and Psychiatry, Naples, Italy

Dr J.J. López-Ibor Jr, López-Ibor Clinic, Pierto de Hierro, Madrid, Spain

Dr G. Mellsop, The Wellington Clinical School, Wellington Hospital, Wellington, New Zealand

Dr Y. Nakane, Department of Neuropsychiatry, Nagasaki University, School of Medicine, Nagasaki, Japan

Dr A. Okasha, Department of Psychiatry, Ain-Shams University, Cairo, Egypt

Dr C. Pull, Department of Neuropsychiatry, Centre Hospitalier de Luxembourg, Luxembourg, Luxembourg

Dr D. Regier, Director, Division of Clinical Research, National Institute of Mental Health, Rockville, MD, USA

Dr S. Tzirkin, All Union Research Centre of Mental Health, Institute of Psychiatry, Academy of Medical Sciences, Moscow, Russian Federation

Dr Xu Tao-Yuan, Department of Psychiatry, Shanghai Psychiatric Hospital, Shanghai, China

Former directors of field trial centres

Dr J.E. Cooper, Department of Psychiatry, Queen's Medical Centre, Nottingham, England

Dr R. Takahashi, Department of Psychiatry, Tokyo Medical and Dental University, Tokyo, Japan

Dr N. Wig, Regional Adviser for Mental Health, World Health Organization, Regional Office for the Eastern Mediterranean, Alexandria, Egypt

Dr Yang De-sen, Hunan Medical College, Changsha, Hunan, China

Introduction

Chapter V, Mental and behavioural disorders, of ICD-10 is to be available in several different versions for different purposes. This version, *Clinical descriptions and diagnostic guidelines*, is intended for general clinical, educational and service use. *Diagnostic criteria for research* has been produced for research purposes and is designed to be used in conjunction with this book. The much shorter glossary provided by Chapter V(F) for ICD-10 itself is suitable for use by coders or clerical workers, and also serves as a reference point for compatibility with other classifications; it is not recommended for use by mental health professionals. Shorter and simpler versions of the classifications for use by primary health care workers are now in preparation, as is a multiaxial scheme. *Clinical descriptions and diagnostic guidelines* has been the starting point for the development of the different versions, and the utmost care has been taken to avoid problems of incompatibility between them.

Layout

It is important that users study this general introduction, and also read carefully the additional introductory and explanatory texts at the beginning of several of the individual categories. This is particularly important for F23. – (Acute and transient psychotic disorders), and for the block F30 – F39 (Mood [affective] disorders). Because of the long-standing and notoriously difficult problems associated with the description and classification of these disorders, special care has been taken to explain how the classification has been approached.

For each disorder, a description is provided of the main clinical features, and also of any important but less specific associated features. "Diagnostic guidelines" are then provided in most cases, indicating the number and balance of symptoms usually required before a confident diagnosis can be made. The guidelines are worded so that a degree of flexibility is retained for diagnostic decisions in clinical work, particularly in the situation where provisional diagnosis may have to be made before the clinical picture is entirely clear or information is complete. To avoid repetition, clinical descriptions and some

1

general diagnostic guidelines are provided for certain groups of disorders, in addition to those that relate only to individual disorders.

When the requirements laid down in the diagnostic guidelines are clearly fulfilled, the diagnosis can be regarded as "confident". When the requirements are only partially fulfilled, it is nevertheless useful to record a diagnosis for most purposes. It is then for the diagnostician and other users of the diagnostic statements to decide whether to record the lesser degrees of confidence (such as "provisional" if more information is yet to come, or "tentative" if more information is unlikely to become available) that are implied in these circumstances. Statements about the duration of symptoms are also intended as general guidelines rather than strict requirements; clinicians should use their own judgement about the appropriateness of choosing diagnoses when the duration of particular symptoms is slightly longer or shorter than that specified.

The diagnostic guidelines should also provide a useful stimulus for clinical teaching, since they serve as a reminder about points of clinical practice that can be found in a fuller form in most textbooks of psychiatry. They may also be suitable for some types of research projects, where the greater precision (and therefore restriction) of the diagnostic criteria for research are not required.

These descriptions and guidelines carry no theoretical implications, and they do not pretend to be comprehensive statements about the current state of knowledge of the disorders. They are simply a set of symptoms and comments that have been agreed, by a large number of advisors and consultants in many different countries, to be a reasonable basis for defining the limits of categories in the classification of mental disorders.

Principal differences between Chapter V(F) of ICD-10 and Chapter V of ICD-9

General principles of ICD-10

ICD-10 is much larger than ICD-9. Numeric codes (001 – 999) were used in ICD-9, whereas an alphanumeric coding scheme, based on codes with a single letter followed by two numbers at the three-character level (A00 – Z99), has been adopted in ICD-10. This has significantly enlarged the number of categories available for the classification. Further detail is then provided by means of decimal numeric subdivisions at the four-character level.

The chapter that dealt with mental disorders in ICD-9 had only 30 three-character categories (290 – 319); Chapter V(F) of ICD-10 has 100 such categories. A proportion of these categories has been left unused for the time being, so as to allow the introduction of changes into the classification without the need to redesign the entire system.

ICD-10 as a whole is designed to be a central ("core") classification for a family of disease- and health-related classifications. Some members of the family of classifications are derived by using a fifth or even sixth character to specify more detail. In others, the categories are condensed to give broad groups suitable for use, for instance, in primary health care or general medical practice. There is a multiaxial presentation of Chapter V(F) of ICD-10 and a version for child psychiatric practice and research. The "family" also includes classifications that cover information not contained in the ICD, but having important medical or health implications, e.g. the classification of impairments, disabilities and handicaps, the classification of procedures in medicine, and the classification of reasons for encounter between patients and health workers.

Neurosis and psychosis

The traditional division between neurosis and psychosis that was evident in ICD-9 (although deliberately left without any attempt to define these concepts) has not been used in ICD-10. However, the term "neurotic" is still retained for occasional use and occurs, for instance, in the heading of a major group (or block) of disorders F40 – F48, "Neurotic, stress-related and somatoform disorders". Except for depressive neurosis, most of the disorders regarded as neuroses by those who use the concept are to be found in this block, and the remainder are in the subsequent blocks. Instead of following the neurotic – psychotic dichotomy, the disorders are now arranged in groups according to major common themes or descriptive likenesses, which makes for increased convenience of use. For instance, cyclothymia (F34.0) is in the block F30 – F39, Mood [affective] disorders, rather than in F60 – F69, Disorders of adult personality and behaviour; similarly, all disorders associated with the use of psychoactive substances are grouped together in F10 – F19, regardless of their severity.

"Psychotic" has been retained as a convenient descriptive term, particularly in F23, Acute and transient psychotic disorders. Its use does not involve assumptions about psychodynamic mechanisms, but simply indicates the presence of hallucinations, delusions, or a limited number of severe abnormalities of

3

behaviour, such as gross excitement and overactivity, marked psychomotor retardation, and catatonic behaviour.

Other differences between ICD-9 and ICD-10

All disorders attributable to an organic cause are grouped together in the block F00 – F09, which makes the use of this part of the classification easier than the arrangement in the ICD-9.

The new arrangement of mental and behavioural disorders due to psychoactive substance use in the block F10 – F19 has also been found more useful than the earlier system. The third character indicates the substance used, the fourth and fifth characters the psychopathological syndrome, e.g. from acute intoxication and residual states; this allows the reporting of all disorders related to a substance even when only three-character categories are used.

The block that covers schizophrenia, schizotypal states and delusional disorders (F20 – F29) has been expanded by the introduction of new categories such as undifferentiated schizophrenia, postschizophrenic depression, and schizotypal disorder. The classification of acute short-lived psychoses, which are commonly seen in most developing countries, is considerably expanded compared with that in the ICD-9.

Classification of affective disorders has been particularly influenced by the adoption of the principle of grouping together disorders with a common theme. Terms such as ''neurotic depression'' and ''endogenous depression'' are not used, but their close equivalents can be found in the different types and severities of depression now specified (including dysthymia (F34.1)).

The behavioural syndromes and mental disorders associated with physiological dysfunction and hormonal changes, such as eating disorders, nonorganic sleep disorders, and sexual dysfunctions, have been brought together in F50 – F59 and described in greater detail than in ICD-9, because of the growing needs for such a classification in liaison psychiatry.

Block F60 – F69 contains a number of new disorders of adult behaviour such as pathological gambling, fire-setting, and stealing, as well as the more traditional disorders of personality. Disorders of sexual preference are clearly differentiated from disorders of gender identity, and homosexuality in itself is no longer included as a category.

4

Some further comments about changes between the provisions for the coding of disorders specific to childhood and mental retardation can be found on pages 18 – 20.

Problems of terminology

Disorder

The term "disorder" is used throughout the classification, so as to avoid even greater problems inherent in the use of terms such as "disease" and "illness". "Disorder" is not an exact term, but it is used here to imply the existence of a clinically recognizable set of symptoms or behaviour associated in most cases with distress and with interference with personal functions. Social deviance or conflict alone, without personal dysfunction, should not be included in mental disorder as defined here.

Psychogenic and psychosomatic

The term "psychogenic" has not been used in the titles of categories, in view of its different meanings in different languages and psychiatric traditions. It still occurs occasionally in the text, and should be taken to indicate that the diagnostician regards obvious life events or difficulties as playing an important role in the genesis of the disorder.

"Psychosomatic" is not used for similar reasons and also because use of this term might be taken to imply that psychological factors play no role in the occurrence, course and outcome of other diseases that are not so described. Disorders described as psychosomatic in other classifications can be found here in F45. – (somatoform disorders), F50. – (eating disorders), F52. – (sexual dysfunction), and F54. – (psychological or behavioural factors associated with disorders or diseases classified elsewhere). It is particularly important to note category F54. – (category 316 in ICD-9) and to remember to use it for specifying the association of physical disorders, coded elsewhere in ICD-10, with an emotional causation. A common example would be the recording of psychogenic asthma or eczema by means of both F54 from Chapter V(F) and the appropriate code for the physical condition from other chapters in ICD-10.

Impairment, disability, handicap and related terms

The terms "impairment", "disability" and "handicap" are used according to the recommendations of the system adopted by WHO.[1] Occasionally, where justified by clinical tradition, the terms are used in a broader sense. See also pages 8 and 9 regarding dementia and its relationships with impairment, disability and handicap.

Some specific points for users

Children and adolescents

Blocks F80–F89 (disorders of psychological development) and F90–F98 (behavioural and emotional disorders with onset usually occurring in childhood and adolescence) cover only those disorders that are specific to childhood and adolescence. A number of disorders placed in other categories can occur in persons of almost any age, and should be used for children and adolescents when required. Examples are disorders of eating (F50. –), sleeping (F51. –) and gender identity (F64. –). Some types of phobia occurring in children pose special problems for classification, as noted in the description of F93.1 (phobic anxiety disorder of childhood).

Recording more than one diagnosis

It is recommended that clinicians should follow the general rule of recording as many diagnoses as are necessary to cover the clinical picture. When recording more than one diagnosis, it is usually best to give one precedence over the others by specifying it as the main diagnosis, and to label any others as subsidiary or additional diagnoses. Precedence should be given to that diagnosis most relevant to the purpose for which the diagnoses are being collected; in clinical work this is often the disorder that gave rise to the consultation or contact with health services. In many cases it will be the disorder that necessitates admission to an inpatient, outpatient or day-care service. At other times, for example when reviewing the patient's whole career, the most important diagnosis may well be the "life-time" diagnosis, which could be different from the one

---

[1] *International classification of impairments, disabilities and handicaps.* Geneva, World Health Organization, 1980.

most relevant to the immediate consultation (for instance a patient with chronic schizophrenia presenting for an episode of care because of symptoms of acute anxiety). If there is any doubt about the order in which to record several diagnoses, or the diagnostician is uncertain of the purpose for which information will be used, a useful rule is to record the diagnoses in the numerical order in which they appear in the classification.

Recording diagnoses from other chapters of ICD-10

The use of other chapters of the ICD-10 system in addition to Chapter V(F) is strongly recommended. The categories most relevant to mental health services are listed in the Annex to this book.

7

Notes on selected categories in the classification of mental and behavioural disorders in ICD-10

In the course of preparation of the ICD-10 chapter on mental disorder, certain categories attracted considerable interest and debate before a reasonable level of consensus could be achieved among all concerned. Brief notes are presented here on some of the issues that were raised.

Dementia (F01 – F03) and its relationships with impairment, disability and handicap

Although a decline in cognitive abilities is essential for the diagnosis of dementia, no consequent interference with the performance of social roles, either within the family or with regard to employment, is used as a diagnostic guideline or criterion. This is a particular instance of a general principle that applies to the definitions of all the disorders in Chapter V(F) of ICD-10, adopted because of the wide variations between different cultures, religions, and nationalities in terms of work and social roles that are available, or regarded as appropriate. Nevertheless, once a diagnosis has been made using other information, the extent to which an individual's work, family, or leisure activities are hindered or even prevented is often a useful indicator of the severity of a disorder.

This is an opportune moment to refer to the general issue of the relationships between symptoms, diagnostic criteria, and the system adopted by WHO for describing impairment, disability, and handicap[1]. In terms of this system, *impairment* (i.e. a "loss or abnormality... of structure or function") is manifest psychologically by interference with mental functions such as memory, attention, and emotive functions. Many types of psychological impairment have always been recognized as psychiatric symptoms. To a lesser degree, some types of *disability* (defined in the WHO system as "a restriction or lack... of ability to perform an activity in the manner or within the range considered normal for a human being") have also conventionally been regarded as

---

[1] *International classification of impairments, disabilities and handicaps.* Geneva, World Health Organization, 1980.

psychiatric symptoms. Examples of disability at the personal level include the ordinary, and usually necessary, activities of daily life involved in personal care and survival related to washing, dressing, eating, and excretion. Interference with these activities is often a direct consequence of psychological impairment, and is influenced little, if at all, by culture. Personal disabilities can therefore legitimately appear among diagnostic guidelines and criteria, particularly for dementia.

In contrast, a *handicap* ("the disadvantage for an individual... that prevents or limits the performance of a role that is normal...for that individual") represents the effects of impairments or disabilities in a wide social context that may be heavily influenced by culture. Handicaps should therefore not be used as essential components of a diagnosis.

Duration of symptoms required for schizophrenia (F20. –)

Prodromal states

Before the appearance of typical schizophrenic symptoms, there is sometimes a period of weeks or months — particularly in young people — during which a prodrome of nonspecific symptoms appears (such as loss of interest, avoiding the company of others, staying away from work, being irritable and oversensitive). These symptoms are not diagnostic of any particular disorder, but neither are they typical of the healthy state of the individual. They are often just as distressing to the family and as incapacitating to the patient as the more clearly morbid symptoms, such as delusions and hallucinations, which develop later. Viewed retrospectively, such prodromal states seem to be an important part of the development of the disorder, but little systematic information is available as to whether similar prodromes are common in other psychiatric disorders, or whether similar states appear and disappear from time to time in individuals who never develop any diagnosable psychiatric disorder.

If a prodrome typical of and specific to schizophrenia could be identified, described reliably, and shown to be uncommon in those with other psychiatric disorders and those with no disorders at all, it would be justifiable to include a prodrome among the optional criteria for schizophrenia. For the purposes of ICD-10, it was considered that insufficient information is available on these points at present to justify the inclusion of a prodromal state as a contributor to this diagnosis. An additional, closely related, and still unsolved problem is the extent to which such prodromes can be distinguished from schizoid and paranoid personality disorders.

Separation of acute and transient psychotic disorders (F23. –) from schizophrenia (F20. –)

In ICD-10, the diagnosis of schizophrenia depends upon the presence of typical delusions, hallucinations or other symptoms (described on pages 86 – 89), and a minimum duration of 1 month is specified.

Strong clinical traditions in several countries, based on descriptive though not epidemiological studies, contribute towards the conclusion that, whatever the nature of the dementia praecox of Kraepelin and the schizophrenias of Bleuler, it, or they, are not the same as very acute psychoses that have an abrupt onset, a short course of a few weeks or even days, and a favourable outcome. Terms such as "bouffée délirante", "psychogenic psychosis", "schizophreniform psychosis", "cycloid psychosis" and "brief reactive psychosis" indicate the widespread but diverse opinion and traditions that have developed. Opinions and evidence also vary as to whether transient but typical schizophrenic symptoms may occur with these disorders, and whether they are usually or always associated with acute psychological stress (bouffée délirante, at least, was originally described as not usually associated with an obvious psychological precipitant).

Given the present lack of knowledge about both schizophrenia and these more acute disorders, it was considered that the best option for ICD-10 would be to allow sufficient time for the symptoms of the acute disorders to appear, be recognized, and largely subside, before a diagnosis of schizophrenia was made. Most clinical reports and authorities suggest that, in the large majority of patients with these acute psychoses, onset of psychotic symptoms occurs over a few days, or over 1 – 2 weeks at most, and that many patients recover with or without medication within 2 – 3 weeks. It therefore seems appropriate to specify 1 month as the transition point between the acute disorders in which symptoms of the schizophrenic type have been a feature and schizophrenia itself. For patients with psychotic, but non-schizophrenic, symptoms that persist beyond the 1-month point, there is no need to change the diagnosis until the duration requirement of delusional disorder (F22.0) is reached (3 months, as discussed below).

A similar duration suggests itself when acute symptomatic psychoses (amfetamine psychosis is the best example) are considered. Withdrawal of the toxic agent is usually followed by disappearance of the symptoms over 8 – 10 days, but since it often takes 7 – 10 days for the symptoms to become manifest and troublesome (and for the patient to present to the psychiatric services), the overall duration is often 20 days or more. About 30 days, or 1 month, would therefore seem an appropriate time to allow as an overall duration before calling the disorder schizophrenia, if the typical symptoms persist. To adopt a 1-month duration of typical psychotic symptoms as a necessary criterion for the diagnosis of schizophrenia rejects the assumption that schizophrenia must be of comparatively long duration. A duration of 6 months has been adopted in more than one national classification, but in the present state of ignorance there appear to be no advantages in restricting the diagnosis of schizophrenia in this way. In two large international collaborative studies on schizophrenia and related disorders[1], the second of which was epidemiologically based, a substantial proportion of patients were found whose clear and typical schizophrenic symptoms lasted for more than 1 month but less than 6 months, and who made good, if not complete, recoveries from the disorder. It therefore seems best for the purposes of ICD-10 to avoid any assumption about necessary chronicity for schizophrenia, and to regard the term as descriptive of a syndrome with a variety of causes (many of which are still unknown) and a variety of outcomes, depending upon the balance of genetic, physical, social, and cultural influences.

There has also been considerable debate about the most appropriate duration of symptoms to specify as necessary for the diagnosis of persistent delusional disorder (F22. –). Three months was finally chosen as being the least unsatisfactory, since to delay the decision point to 6 months or more makes it necessary to introduce another intermediate category between acute and transient psychotic disorders (F23. –) and persistent delusional disorder. The whole subject of the relationship between the disorders under discussion awaits more and better information than is at present available; a comparatively simple solution, which gives precedence to the acute and transient states, seemed the best option, and perhaps one that will stimulate research.

---

[1] *The international pilot study of schizophrenia.* Geneva, World Health Organization, 1973 (Offset Publication, No. 2).

Sartorius, N. et al. Early manifestations and first contact incidence of schizophrenia in different cultures. A preliminary report on the initial evaluation phase of the WHO Collaborative Study on Determinants of Outcome of Severe Mental Disorders. *Psychological medicine,* **16**: 909 – 928 (1986).

The principle of describing and classifying a disorder or group of disorders so as to display options rather than to use built-in assumptions, has been used for acute and transient psychotic disorders (F23. –); these and related points are discussed briefly in the introduction to that category (pages 97 – 99).

The term "schizophreniform" has not been used for a defined disorder in this classification. This is because it has been applied to several different clinical concepts over the last few decades, and associated with various mixtures of characteristics such as acute onset, comparatively brief duration, atypical symptoms or mixtures of symptoms, and a comparatively good outcome. There is no evidence to suggest a preferred choice for its usage, so the case for its inclusion as a diagnostic term was considered to be weak. Moreover, the need for an intermediate category of this type is obviated by the use of F23. – (acute and transient psychotic disorders) and its subdivisions, together with the requirement of 1 month of psychotic symptoms for a diagnosis of schizophrenia. As guidance for those who do use schizophreniform as a diagnostic term, it has been inserted in several places as an inclusion term relevant to those disorders that have the most overlap with the meanings it has acquired. These are: "schizophreniform attack or psychosis, NOS" in F20.8 (other schizophrenia), and "brief schizophreniform disorder or psychosis" in F23.2 (acute schizophrenia-like psychotic disorder).

Simple schizophrenia (F20.6)

This category has been retained because of its continued use in some countries, and because of the uncertainty about its nature and its relationships to schizoid personality disorder and schizotypal disorder, which will require additional information for resolution. The criteria proposed for its differentiation highlight the problems of defining the mutual boundaries of this whole group of disorders in practical terms.

Schizoaffective disorders (F25. –)

The evidence at present available as to whether schizoaffective disorders (F25. –) as defined in the ICD-10 should be placed in block F20 – F29 (schizophrenia, schizotypal and delusional disorders) or in F30 – F39 (mood [affective] disorders) is fairly evenly balanced. The final decision to place it in F20 – F29 was influenced by feedback from the field trials of the 1987 draft, and by comments resulting from the worldwide circulation of the same draft to member societies of the World Psychiatric Association. It is clear that widespread and strong clinical traditions exist that favour its retention among schizophrenia and delusional disorders. It is relevant to this discussion that, given a set of affective symptoms, the addition of only mood-incongruent delusions is not sufficient to change the diagnosis to a schizoaffective category. At least one typically schizophrenic symptom must be present with the affective symptoms during the same episode of the disorder.

Mood [affective] disorders (F30 – F39)

It seems likely that psychiatrists will continue to disagree about the classification of disorders of mood until methods of dividing the clinical syndromes are developed that rely at least in part upon physiological or biochemical measurement, rather than being limited as at present to clinical descriptions of emotions and behaviour. As long as this limitation persists, one of the major choices lies between a comparatively simple classification with only a few degrees of severity, and one with greater details and more subdivisions.

The 1987 draft of ICD-10 used in the field trials had the merit of simplicity, containing, for example, only mild and severe depressive episodes, no separation of hypomania from mania, and no recommendation to specify the presence or absence of familiarly clinical concepts, such as the "somatic" syndrome or affective hallucinations and delusions. However, feedback from many of the clinicians involved in the field trials, and other comments received from a variety of sources, indicated a widespread demand for opportunities to specify several grades of depression and the other features noted above. In addition, it is clear from the preliminary analysis of field trial data that in many centres the category of "mild depressive episode" often had a comparatively low inter-rater reliability.

It has also become evident that the views of clinicians on the required number of subdivisions of depression are strongly influenced by the types of patient they encounter most frequently. Those working in primary care, outpatient clinics and liaison settings need ways of describing patients with mild but clinically significant states of depression, whereas those whose work is mainly with inpatients frequently need to use the more extreme categories.

Further consultations with experts on affective disorders resulted in the present versions. Options for specifying several aspects of affective disorders have been included, which, although still some way from being scientifically respectable, are regarded by psychiatrists in many parts of the world as clinically useful. It is hoped that their inclusion will stimulate further discussion and research into their true clinical value.

Unsolved problems remain about how best to define and make diagnostic use of the incongruence of delusions with mood. There would seem to be both enough evidence and sufficient clinical demand for the inclusion of provisions for mood-congruent or mood-incongruent delusions to be included, at least as an "optional extra".

Recurrent brief depressive disorder

Since the introduction of ICD-9, sufficient evidence has accumulated to justify the provision of a special category for the brief episodes of depression that meet the severity criteria but not the duration criteria for depressive episode (F32. –). These recurrent states are of unclear nosological significance and the provision of a category for their recording should encourage the collection of information that will lead to a better understanding of their frequency and long-term course.

Agoraphobia and panic disorder

There has been considerable debate recently as to which of agoraphobia and panic disorder should be regarded as primary. From an international and cross-cultural perspective, the amount and type of evidence available does not appear to justify rejection of the still widely accepted notion that the phobic disorder is best regarded as the prime disorder, with attacks of panic usually indicating its severity.

Mixed categories of anxiety and depression

Psychiatrists and others, especially in developing countries, who see patients in primary health care services should find particular use for F41.2 (mixed anxiety and depressive disorder), F41.3 (other mixed disorders), the various subdivisions of F43.2 (adjustment disorder), and F44.7 (mixed dissociative [conversion] disorder). The purpose of these categories is to facilitate the description of disorders manifest by a mixture of symptoms for which a simpler and more traditional psychiatric label is not appropriate but which nevertheless represent significantly common, severe states of distress and interference with functioning. They also result in frequent referral to primary care, medical and psychiatric services. Difficulties in using these categories reliably may be encountered, but it is important to test them and — if necessary — improve their definition.

Dissociative and somatoform disorders, in relation to hysteria

The term "hysteria" has not been used in the title for any disorder in Chapter V(F) of ICD-10 because of its many and varied shades of meaning. Instead, "dissociative" has been preferred, to bring together disorders previously termed hysteria, of both dissociative and conversion types. This is largely because patients with the dissociative and conversion varieties often share a number of other characteristics, and in addition they frequently exhibit both varieties at the same or different times. It also seems reasonable to presume that the same (or very similar) psychological mechanisms are common to both types of symptoms.

There appears to be widespread international acceptance of the usefulness of grouping together several disorders with a predominantly physical or somatic mode of presentation under the term "somatoform". For the reasons already given, however, this new concept was not considered to be an adequate reason for separating amnesias and fugues from dissociative sensory and motor loss.

If multiple personality disorder (F44.81) does exist as something other than a culture-specific or even iatrogenic condition, then it is presumably best placed among the dissociative group.

Neurasthenia

Although omitted from some classification systems, neurasthenia has been retained as a category in ICD-10, since this diagnosis is still regularly and widely used in a number of countries. Research carried out in various settings has demonstrated that a significant proportion of cases diagnosed as neurasthenia can also be classified under depression or anxiety: there are, however, cases in which the clinical syndrome does not match the description of any other category but does meet all the criteria specified for a syndrome of neurasthenia. It is hoped that further research on neurasthenia will be stimulated by its inclusion as a separate category.

Culture-specific disorders

The need for a separate category for disorders such as latah, amok, koro, and a variety of other possibly culture-specific disorders has been expressed less often in recent years. Attempts to identify sound descriptive studies, preferably with an epidemiological basis, that would strengthen the case for these inclusions as disorders clinically distinguishable from others already in the classification have failed, so they have not been separately classified. Descriptions of these disorders currently available in the literature suggest that they may be regarded as local variants of anxiety, depression, somatoform disorder, or adjustment disorder; the nearest equivalent code should therefore be used if required, together with an additional note of which culture-specific disorder is involved. There may also be prominent elements of attention-seeking behaviour or adoption of the sick role akin to that described in F68.1 (intentional production or feigning of symptoms or disabilities), which can also be recorded.

Mental and behavioural disorders associated with the puerperium (F53. –)

This category is unusual and apparently paradoxical in carrying a recommendation that it should be used only when unavoidable. Its inclusion is a recognition of the very real practical problems in many developing countries that make the gathering of details about many cases of puerperal illness virtually impossible. However, even in the absence of sufficient information to allow a diagnosis of some variety of affective disorder (or, more rarely, schizophrenia), there will usually be enough known to allow diagnosis of a mild (F53.0) or severe (F53.1) disorder; this subdivision is useful for estimations of workload, and when decisions are to be made about provision of services.

The inclusion of this category should not be taken to imply that, given adequate information, a significant proportion of cases of postpartum mental illness cannot be classified in other categories. Most experts in this field are of the opinion that a clinical picture of puerperal psychosis is so rarely (if ever) reliably distinguishable from affective disorder or schizophrenia that a special category is not justified. Any psychiatrist who is of the minority opinion that special postpartum psychoses do indeed exist may use this category, but should be aware of its real purpose.

Disorders of adult personality (F60. –)

In all current psychiatric classifications, disorders of adult personality include a variety of severe problems, whose solution requires information that can come only from extensive and time-consuming investigations. The difference between observations and interpretation becomes particularly troublesome when attempts are made to write detailed guidelines or diagnostic criteria for these disorders; and the number of criteria that must be fulfilled before a diagnosis is regarded as confirmed remains an unsolved problem in the light of present knowledge. Nevertheless, the attempts that have been made to specify guidelines and criteria for this category may help to demonstrate that a new approach to the description of personality disorders is required.

After initial hesitation, a brief description of borderline personality disorder (F60.31) was finally included as a subcategory of emotionally unstable personality disorder (F60.3), again in the hope of stimulating investigations.

Other disorders of adult personality and behaviour (F68)

Two categories that have been included here but were not present in ICD-9 are F68.0, elaboration of physical symptoms for psychological reasons, and F68.1, intentional production or feigning of symptoms or disabilities, either physical or psychological [factitious disorder]. Since these are, strictly speaking, disorders of role or illness behaviour, it should be convenient for psychiatrists to have them grouped with other disorders of adult behaviour. Together with malingering (Z76.5), which has always been outside Chapter V of the ICD, the disorders from a trio of diagnoses often need to be considered together. The crucial difference between the first two and malingering is that the motivation for malingering is obvious and usually confined to situations where personal danger, criminal sentencing, or large sums of money are involved.

Mental retardation (F70 – F79)

The policy for Chapter V(F) of ICD-10 has always been to deal with mental retardation as briefly and as simply as possible, acknowledging that justice can be done to this topic only by means of a comprehensive, possibly multiaxial, system. Such a system needs to be developed separately, and work to produce appropriate proposals for international use is now in progress.

Disorders with onset specific to childhood

F80 – F89 Disorders of psychological development

Disorders of childhood such as infantile autism and disintegrative psychosis, classified in ICD-9 as psychoses, are now more appropriately contained in F84. – , pervasive developmental disorders. While some uncertainty remains about their nosological status, it has been considered that sufficient information is now available to justify the inclusion of the syndromes of Rett and Asperger in this group as specified disorders. Overactive disorder associated with mental retardation and stereotyped movements (F84.4) has been included in spite of its mixed nature, because evidence suggests that this may have considerable practical utility.

F90 – F98 Behavioural and emotional disorders with onset usually occurring in childhood and adolescence

Differences in international opinion about the broadness of the concept of hyperkinetic disorder have been a well-known problem for many years, and were discussed in detail at the meetings between WHO advisors and other experts held under the auspices of the WHO – ADAMHA joint project. Hyperkinetic disorder is now defined more broadly in ICD-10 than it was in ICD-9. The ICD-10 definition is also different in the relative emphasis given to the constituent symptoms of the overall hyperkinetic syndrome; since recent empirical research was used as the basis for the definition, there are good reasons for believing that the definition in ICD-10 represents a significant improvement.

Hyperkinetic conduct disorder (F90.1) is one of the few examples of a combination category remaining in ICD-10, Chapter V(F). The use of this diagnosis indicates that the criteria for both hyperkinetic disorder (F90. –) and conduct disorder (F91. –) are fulfilled. These few exceptions to the general rule were considered justified on the grounds of clinical convenience in view of the frequent coexistence of those disorders and the demonstrated later importance of the mixed syndrome. However, in *The ICD-10 Classification of Mental and Behavioural Disorders: Diagnostic criteria for research* (DCR-10) it is recommended that, for research purposes, individual cases in these categories be described in terms of hyperactivity, emotional disturbance, and severity of conduct disorder (in addition to the combination category being used as an overall diagnosis).

Oppositional defiant disorder (F91.3) was not in ICD-9, but has been included in ICD-10 because of evidence of its predictive potential for later conduct problems. There is, however, a cautionary note recommending its use mainly for younger children.

The ICD-9 category 313 (disturbances of emotion specific to childhood and adolescence) has been developed into two separate categories for ICD-10, namely emotional disorders with onset specific to childhood (F93. –) and disorders of social functioning with onset specific to childhood and adolescence (F94. –). This is because of the continuing need for a differentiation between children and adults with respect to various forms of morbid anxiety and related emotions. The frequency with which emotional disorders in childhood are followed by no significant similar disorder in adult life, and the frequent onset of neurotic disorders in adults are clear indicators of this need. The key defining criterion used in ICD-10 is the appropriateness to the developmental stage of the child of the emotion shown, plus an unusual degree of persistence with disturbance of function. In other words, these childhood disorders are significant exaggerations of emotional states and reactions that are regarded as normal for the age in question when occurring in only a mild form. If the content of the emotional state is unusual, or if it occurs at an unusual age, the general categories elsewhere in the classification should be used.

In spite of its name, the new category F94. – (disorders of social functioning with onset specific to childhood and adolescence) does not go against the general rule for ICD-10 of not using interference with social roles as a diagnostic criterion. The abnormalities of social functioning involved in F94. – are of a limited number and contained within the parent – child relationship and the immediate family; these relationships do not have the same connotations or show the same cultural variations as those formed in the context of work or of providing for the family, which are excluded from use as diagnostic criteria.

A number of categories that will be used frequently by child psychiatrists, such as eating disorders (F50. –), nonorganic sleep disorders (F51. –), and gender identity disorders (F64. –), are to be found in the general sections of the classifications because of their frequent onset and occurrence in adults as well as children. Nevertheless, clinical features specific to childhood were thought to justify the additional categories of feeding disorder of infancy (F98.2) and pica of infancy and childhood (F98.3).

Users of blocks F80 – F89 and F90 – F98 also need to be aware of the contents of the neurological chapter of ICD-10 (Chapter VI(G)). This contains syndromes with predominantly physical manifestations and clear "organic" etiology, of which the Kleine – Levin syndrome (G47.8) is of particular interest to child psychiatrists.

Unspecified mental disorder (F99)

There are practical reasons why a category for the recording of "unspecified mental disorder" is required in ICD-10, but the subdivision of the whole of the classificatory space available for Chapter V(F) into 10 blocks, each covering a specific area, posed a problem for this requirement. It was decided that the least unsatisfactory solution was to use the last category in the numerical order of the classification, i.e. F99.

Deletion of categories proposed for earlier drafts of ICD-10

The process of consultation and reviews of the literature that preceded the drafting of Chapter V(F) of ICD-10 resulted in numerous proposals for changes. Decisions on whether to accept or reject proposals were influenced by a number of factors. These included the results of the field tests of the classification, consultations with heads of WHO collaborative centres, results of collaboration with nongovernmental organizations, advice from members of WHO expert advisory panels, results of translations of the classification, and the constraints of the rules governing the structure of the ICD as a whole.

It was normally easy to reject proposals that were idiosyncratic and unsupported by evidence, and to accept others that were accompanied by sound justification. Some proposals, although reasonable when considered in isolation, could not be accepted because of the implications that even minor changes to one part of the classification would have for other parts. Some other proposals had clear merit, but more research would be necessary before they could be considered for international use. A number of these proposals included in early versions of the general classification were omitted from the final version, including "accentuation of personality traits" and "hazardous use of psychoactive substances". It is hoped that research into the status and usefulness of these and other innovative categories will continue.

List of categories

F00 – F09
Organic, including symptomatic, mental disorders

F00 Dementia in Alzheimer's disease
F00.0 Dementia in Alzheimer's disease with early onset
F00.1 Dementia in Alzheimer's disease with late onset
F00.2 Dementia in Alzheimer's disease, atypical or mixed type
F00.9 Dementia in Alzheimer's disease, unspecified

F01 Vascular dementia
F01.0 Vascular dementia of acute onset
F01.1 Multi-infarct dementia
F01.2 Subcortical vascular dementia
F01.3 Mixed cortical and subcortical vascular dementia
F01.8 Other vascular dementia
F01.9 Vascular dementia, unspecified

F02 Dementia in other diseases classified elsewhere
F02.0 Dementia in Pick's disease
F02.1 Dementia in Creutzfeldt – Jakob disease
F02.2 Dementia in Huntington's disease
F02.3 Dementia in Parkinson's disease
F02.4 Dementia in human immunodeficiency virus [HIV] disease
F02.8 Dementia in other specified diseases classified elsewhere

F03 Unspecified dementia

A fifth character may be added to specify dementia in F00 – F03, as follows:
    .x0 Without additional symptoms
    .x1 Other symptoms, predominantly delusional
    .x2 Other symptoms, predominantly hallucinatory
    .x3 Other symptoms, predominantly depressive
    .x4 Other mixed symptoms

F04 Organic amnesic syndrome, not induced by alcohol and other psychoactive substances

F05 Delirium, not induced by alcohol and other psychoactive substances
F05.0 Delirium, not superimposed on dementia, so described
F05.1 Delirium, superimposed on dementia
F05.8 Other delirium
F05.9 Delirium, unspecified

F06 Other mental disorders due to brain damage and dysfunction and to physical disease
F06.0 Organic hallucinosis
F06.1 Organic catatonic disorder
F06.2 Organic delusional [schizophrenia-like] disorder
F06.3 Organic mood [affective] disorders
    .30 Organic manic disorder
    .31 Organic bipolar affective disorder
    .32 Organic depressive disorder
    .33 Organic mixed affective disorder
F06.4 Organic anxiety disorder
F06.5 Organic dissociative disorder
F06.6 Organic emotionally labile [asthenic] disorder
F06.7 Mild cognitive disorder
F06.8 Other specified mental disorders due to brain damage and dysfunction and to physical disease
F06.9 Unspecified mental disorder due to brain damage and dysfunction and to physical disease

F07 Personality and behavioural disorders due to brain disease, damage and dysfunction
F07.0 Organic personality disorder
F07.1 Postencephalitic syndrome
F07.2 Postconcussional syndrome
F07.8 Other organic personality and behavioural disorders due to brain disease, damage and dysfunction
F07.9 Unspecified organic personality and behavioural disorder due to brain disease, damage and dysfunction

F09 Unspecified organic or symptomatic mental disorder

F10 – F19
Mental and behavioural disorders due to psychoactive substance use

F10. – Mental and behavioural disorders due to use of alcohol

F11. – Mental and behavioural disorders due to use of opioids

F12. – Mental and behavioural disorders due to use of cannabinoids

F13. – Mental and behavioural disorders due to use of sedatives or hypnotics

F14. – Mental and behavioural disorders due to use of cocaine

F15. – Mental and behavioural disorders due to use of other stimulants, including caffeine

F16. – Mental and behavioural disorders due to use of hallucinogens

F17. – Mental and behavioural disorders due to use of tobacco

F18. – Mental and behavioural disorders due to use of volatile solvents

F19. – Mental and behavioural disorders due to multiple drug use and use of other psychoactive substances

Four- and five-character categories may be used to specify the clinical conditions, as follows:

F1x.0 Acute intoxication
.00 Uncomplicated
.01 With trauma or other bodily injury
.02 With other medical complications
.03 With delirium
.04 With perceptual distortions
.05 With coma
.06 With convulsions
.07 Pathological intoxication

F1x.1 Harmful use

F1x.2 Dependence syndrome
    .20 Currently abstinent
    .21 Currently abstinent, but in a protected environment
    .22 Currently on a clinically supervised maintenance or replacement regime [controlled dependence]
    .23 Currently abstinent, but receiving treatment with aversive or blocking drugs
    .24 Currently using the substance [active dependence]
    .25 Continuous use
    .26 Episodic use [dipsomania]

F1x.3 Withdrawal state
    .30 Uncomplicated
    .31 With convulsions

F1x.4 Withdrawal state with delirium
    .40 Without convulsions
    .41 With convulsions

F1x.5 Psychotic disorder
    .50 Schizophrenia-like
    .51 Predominantly delusional
    .52 Predominantly hallucinatory
    .53 Predominantly polymorphic
    .54 Predominantly depressive symptoms
    .55 Predominantly manic symptoms
    .56 Mixed

F1x.6 Amnesic syndrome

F1x.7 Residual and late-onset psychotic disorder
    .70 Flashbacks
    .71 Personality or behaviour disorder
    .72 Residual affective disorder
    .73 Dementia
    .74 Other persisting cognitive impairment
    .75 Late-onset psychotic disorder

F1x.8 Other mental and behavioural disorders

F1x.9 Unspecified mental and behavioural disorder

F20-F29
Schizophrenia, schizotypal and delusional disorders

F20 Schizophrenia
F20.0 Paranoid schizophrenia
F20.1 Hebephrenic schizophrenia
F20.2 Catatonic schizophrenia
F20.3 Undifferentiated schizophrenia
F20.4 Post-schizophrenic depression
F20.5 Residual schizophrenia
F20.6 Simple schizophrenia
F20.8 Other schizophrenia
F20.9 Schizophrenia, unspecified

A fifth character may be used to classify course:
.x0 Continuous
.x1 Episodic with progressive deficit
.x2 Episodic with stable deficit
.x3 Episodic remittent
.x4 Incomplete remission
.x5 Complete remission
.x8 Other
.x9 Course uncertain, period of observation too short

F21 Schizotypal disorder

F22 Persistent delusional disorders
F22.0 Delusional disorder
F22.8 Other persistent delusional disorders
F22.9 Persistent delusional disorder, unspecified

F23 Acute and transient psychotic disorders
F23.0 Acute polymorphic psychotic disorder without symptoms of schizophrenia
F23.1 Acute polymorphic psychotic disorder with symptoms of schizophrenia
F23.2 Acute schizophrenia-like psychotic disorder
F23.3 Other acute predominantly delusional psychotic disorders
F23.8 Other acute and transient psychotic disorders
F23.9 Acute and transient psychotic disorders unspecified

A fifth character may be used to identify the presence or absence of associated acute stress:

> .x0 Without associated acute stress
> .x1 With associated acute stress

F24 Induced delusional disorder

F25 Schizoaffective disorders
F25.0 Schizoaffective disorder, manic type
F25.1 Schizoaffective disorder, depressive type
F25.2 Schizoaffective disorder, mixed type
F25.8 Other schizoaffective disorders
F25.9 Schizoaffective disorder, unspecified

F28 Other nonorganic psychotic disorders

F29 Unspecified nonorganic psychosis

F30 – F39
Mood [affective] disorders

F30 Manic episode
F30.0 Hypomania
F30.1 Mania without psychotic symptoms
F30.2 Mania with psychotic symptoms
F30.8 Other manic episodes
F30.9 Manic episode, unspecified

F31 Bipolar affective disorder
F31.0 Bipolar affective disorder, current episode hypomanic
F31.1 Bipolar affective disorder, current episode manic without psychotic symptoms
F31.2 Bipolar affective disorder, current episode manic with psychotic symptoms
F31.3 Bipolar affective disorder, current episode mild or moderate depression
    .30 Without somatic syndrome
    .31 With somatic syndrome
F31.4 Bipolar affective disorder, current episode severe depression without psychotic symptoms
F31.5 Bipolar affective disorder, current episode severe depression with psychotic symptoms
F31.6 Bipolar affective disorder, current episode mixed
F31.7 Bipolar affective disorder, currently in remission
F31.8 Other bipolar affective disorders
F31.9 Bipolar affective disorder, unspecified

F32 Depressive episode
F32.0 Mild depressive episode
    .00 Without somatic syndrome
    .01 With somatic syndrome
F32.1 Moderate depressive episode
    .10 Without somatic syndrome
    .11 With somatic syndrome
F32.2 Severe depressive episode without psychotic symptoms
F32.3 Severe depressive episode with psychotic symptoms
F32.8 Other depressive episodes
F32.9 Depressive episode, unspecified

F33 Recurrent depressive disorder

F33.0 Recurrent depressive disorder, current episode mild
.00 Without somatic syndrome
.01 With somatic syndrome
F33.1 Recurrent depressive disorder, current episode moderate
.10 Without somatic syndrome
.11 With somatic syndrome
F33.2 Recurrent depressive disorder, current episode severe without psychotic symptoms
F33.3 Recurrent depressive disorder, current episode severe with psychotic symptoms
F33.4 Recurrent depressive disorder, currently in remission
F33.8 Other recurrent depressive disorders
F33.9 Recurrent depressive disorder, unspecified

F34 Persistent mood [affective] disorders

F34.0 Cyclothymia
F34.1 Dysthymia
F34.8 Other persistent mood [affective] disorders
F34.9 Persistent mood [affective] disorder, unspecified

F38 Other mood [affective] disorders

F38.0 Other single mood [affective] disorders
.00 Mixed affective episode
F38.1 Other recurrent mood [affective] disorders
.10 Recurrent brief depressive disorder
F38.8 Other specified mood [affective] disorders

F39 Unspecified mood [affective] disorder

F40 – F48
Neurotic, stress-related and somatoform disorders

F40 Phobic anxiety disorders
F40.0 Agoraphobia
.00 Without panic disorder
.01 With panic disorder
F40.1 Social phobias
F40.2 Specific (isolated) phobias
F40.8 Other phobic anxiety disorders
F40.9 Phobic anxiety disorder, unspecified

F41 Other anxiety disorders
F41.0 Panic disorder [episodic paroxysmal anxiety]
F41.1 Generalized anxiety disorder
F41.2 Mixed anxiety and depressive disorder
F41.3 Other mixed anxiety disorders
F41.8 Other specified anxiety disorders
F41.9 Anxiety disorder, unspecified

F42 Obsessive – compulsive disorder
F42.0 Predominantly obsessional thoughts or ruminations
F42.1 Predominantly compulsive acts [obsessional rituals]
F42.2 Mixed obsessional thoughts and acts
F42.8 Other obsessive – compulsive disorders
F42.9 Obsessive – compulsive disorder, unspecified

F43 Reaction to severe stress, and adjustment disorders
F43.0 Acute stress reaction
F43.1 Post-traumatic stress disorder
F43.2 Adjustment disorders
.20 Brief depressive reaction
.21 Prolonged depressive reaction
.22 Mixed anxiety and depressive reaction
.23 With predominant disturbance of other emotions
.24 With predominant disturbance of conduct
.25 With mixed disturbance of emotions and conduct
.28 With other specified predominant symptoms
F43.8 Other reactions to severe stress
F43.9 Reaction to severe stress, unspecified

F44 Dissociative [conversion] disorders

F44.0 Dissociative amnesia

F44.1 Dissociative fugue

F44.2 Dissociative stupor

F44.3 Trance and possession disorders

F44.4 Dissociative motor disorders

F44.5 Dissociative convulsions

F44.6 Dissociative anaesthesia and sensory loss

F44.7 Mixed dissociative [conversion] disorders

F44.8 Other dissociative [conversion] disorders

    .80 Ganser's syndrome

    .81 Multiple personality disorder

    .82 Transient dissociative [conversion] disorders occurring in childhood and adolescence

    .88 Other specified dissociative [conversion] disorders

F44.9 Dissociative [conversion] disorder, unspecified

F45 Somatoform disorders

F45.0 Somatization disorder

F45.1 Undifferentiated somatoform disorder

F45.2 Hypochondriacal disorder

F45.3 Somatoform autonomic dysfunction

    .30 Heart and cardiovascular system

    .31 Upper gastrointestinal tract

    .32 Lower gastrointestinal tract

    .33 Respiratory system

    .34 Genitourinary system

    .38 Other organ or system

F45.4 Persistent somatoform pain disorder

F45.8 Other somatoform disorders

F45.9 Somatoform disorder, unspecified

F48 Other neurotic disorders

F48.0 Neurasthenia

F48.1 Depersonalization – derealization syndrome

F48.8 Other specified neurotic disorders

F48.9 Neurotic disorder, unspecified

F50 – F59
Behavioural syndromes associated with physiological disturbances and physical factors

F50 Eating disorders
F50.0 Anorexia nervosa

F50.1 Atypical anorexia nervosa

F50.2 Bulimia nervosa

F50.3 Atypical bulimia nervosa

F50.4 Overeating associated with other psychological disturbances

F50.5 Vomiting associated with other psychological disturbances

F50.8 Other eating disorders

F50.9 Eating disorder, unspecified

F51 Nonorganic sleep disorders
F51.0 Nonorganic insomnia

F51.1 Nonorganic hypersomnia

F51.2 Nonorganic disorder of the sleep-wake schedule

F51.3 Sleepwalking [somnambulism]

F51.4 Sleep terrors [night terrors]

F51.5 Nightmares

F51.8 Other nonorganic sleep disorders

F51.9 Nonorganic sleep disorder, unspecified

F52 Sexual dysfunction, not caused by organic disorder or disease
F52.0 Lack or loss of sexual desire

F52.1 Sexual aversion and lack of sexual enjoyment

    .10 Sexual aversion

    .11 Lack of sexual enjoyment

F52.2 Failure of genital response

F52.3 Orgasmic dysfunction

F52.4 Premature ejaculation

F52.5 Nonorganic vaginismus

F52.6 Nonorganic dyspareunia

F52.7 Excessive sexual drive

F52.8 Other sexual dysfunction, not caused by organic disorders or disease

F52.9 Unspecified sexual dysfunction, not caused by organic disorder or disease

F53 Mental and behavioural disorders associated with the puerperium, not elsewhere classified
> F53.0 Mild mental and behavioural disorders associated with the puerperium, not elsewhere classified
> F53.1 Severe mental and behavioural disorders associated with the puerperium, not elsewhere classified
> F53.8 Other mental and behavioural disorders associated with the puerperium, not elsewhere classified
> F53.9 Puerperal mental disorder, unspecified

F54 Psychological and behavioural factors associated with disorders or diseases classified elsewhere

F55 Abuse of non-dependence-producing substances
> F55.0 Antidepressants
> F55.1 Laxatives
> F55.2 Analgesics
> F55.3 Antacids
> F55.4 Vitamins
> F55.5 Steroids or hormones
> F55.6 Specific herbal or folk remedies
> F55.8 Other substances that do not produce dependence
> F55.9 Unspecified

F59 Unspecified behavioural syndromes associated with physiological disturbances and physical factors

F60 – F69
Disorders of adult personality and behaviour

F60 Specific personality disorders
F60.0 Paranoid personality disorder
F60.1 Schizoid personality disorder
F60.2 Dissocial personality disorder
F60.3 Emotionally unstable personality disorder
    .30 Impulsive type
    .31 Borderline type
F60.4 Histrionic personality disorder
F60.5 Anankastic personality disorder
F60.6 Anxious [avoidant] personality disorder
F60.7 Dependent personality disorder
F60.8 Other specific personality disorders
F60.9 Personality disorder, unspecified

F61 Mixed and other personality disorders
F61.0 Mixed personality disorders
F61.1 Troublesome personality changes

F62 Enduring personality changes, not attributable to brain damage and disease
F62.0 Enduring personality change after catastrophic experience
F62.1 Enduring personality change after psychiatric illness
F62.8 Other enduring personality changes
F62.9 Enduring personality change, unspecified

F63 Habit and impulse disorders
F63.0 Pathological gambling
F63.1 Pathological fire-setting [pyromania]
F63.2 Pathological stealing [kleptomania]
F63.3 Trichotillomania
F63.8 Other habit and impulse disorders
F63.9 Habit and impulse disorder, unspecified

F64 Gender identity disorders
F64.0 Transsexualism
F64.1 Dual-role transvestism
F64.2 Gender identity disorder of childhood

F64.8 Other gender identity disorders
F64.9 Gender identity disorder, unspecified

F65 Disorders of sexual preference

F65.0 Fetishism
F65.1 Fetishistic transvestism
F65.2 Exhibitionism
F65.3 Voyeurism
F65.4 Paedophilia
F65.5 Sadomasochism
F65.6 Multiple disorders of sexual preference
F65.8 Other disorders of sexual preference
F65.9 Disorder of sexual preference, unspecified

F66 Psychological and behavioural disorders associated with sexual development and orientation

F66.0 Sexual maturation disorder
F66.1 Egodystonic sexual orientation
F66.2 Sexual relationship disorder
F66.8 Other psychosexual development disorders
F66.9 Psychosexual development disorder, unspecified

A fifth character may be used to indicate association with:

        .x0 Heterosexuality
        .x1 Homosexuality
        .x2 Bisexuality
        .x8 Other, including prepubertal

F68 Other disorders of adult personality and behaviour

F68.0 Elaboration of physical symptoms for psychological reasons
F68.1 Intentional production or feigning of symptoms or disabilities, either physical or psychological [factitious disorder]
F68.8 Other specified disorders of adult personality and behaviour

F69 Unspecified disorder of adult personality and behaviour

F70 – F79
Mental retardation

F70 Mild mental retardation

F71 Moderate mental retardation

F72 Severe mental retardation

F73 Profound mental retardation

F78 Other mental retardation

F79 Unspecified mental retardation

A fourth character may be used to specify the extent of associated behaviowal impairment:

F7x.0 No, or minimal, impairment of behaviour
F7x.1 Significant impairment of behaviour requiring attention or treatment
F7x.8 Other impairments of behaviour
F7x.9 Without mention of impairment of behaviour

F80 – F89
Disorders of psychological development

F80 Specific developmental disorders of speech and language
F80.0 Specific speech articulation disorder
F80.1 Expressive language disorder
F80.2 Receptive language disorder
F80.3 Acquired aphasia with epilepsy [Landau – Kleffner syndrome]
F80.8 Other developmental disorders of speech and language
F80.9 Developmental disorder of speech and language, unspecified

F81 Specific developmental disorders of scholastic skills
F81.0 Specific reading disorder
F81.1 Specific spelling disorder
F81.2 Specific disorder of arithmetical skills
F81.3 Mixed disorder of scholastic skills
F81.8 Other developmental disorders of scholastic skills
F81.9 Developmental disorder of scholastic skills, unspecified

F82 Specific developmental disorder of motor function

F83 Mixed specific developmental disorders

F84 Pervasive developmental disorders
F84.0 Childhood autism
F84.1 Atypical autism
F84.2 Rett's syndrome
F84.3 Other childhood disintegrative disorder
F84.4 Overactive disorder associated with mental retardation and stereotyped movements
F84.5 Asperger's syndrome
F84.8 Other pervasive developmental disorders
F84.9 Pervasive developmental disorder, unspecified

F88 Other disorders of psychological development

F89 Unspecified disorder of psychological development

F90 – F98
Behavioural and emotional disorders with onset usually occurring in childhood and adolescence

F90 Hyperkinetic disorders
F90.0 Disturbance of activity and attention
F90.1 Hyperkinetic conduct disorder
F90.8 Other hyperkinetic disorders
F90.9 Hyperkinetic disorder, unspecified

F91 Conduct disorders
F91.0 Conduct disorder confined to the family context
F91.1 Unsocialized conduct disorder
F91.2 Socialized conduct disorder
F91.3 Oppositional defiant disorder
F91.8 Other conduct disorders
F91.9 Conduct disorder, unspecified

F92 Mixed disorders of conduct and emotions
F92.0 Depressive conduct disorder
F92.8 Other mixed disorders of conduct and emotions
F92.9 Mixed disorder of conduct and emotions, unspecified

F93 Emotional disorders with onset specific to childhood
F93.0 Separation anxiety disorder of childhood
F93.1 Phobic anxiety disorder of childhood
F93.2 Social anxiety disorder of childhood
F93.3 Sibling rivalry disorder
F93.8 Other childhood emotional disorders
F93.9 Childhood emotional disorder, unspecified

F94 Disorders of social functioning with onset specific to childhood and adolescence
F94.0 Elective mutism
F94.1 Reactive attachment disorder of childhood
F94.2 Disinhibited attachment disorder of childhood
F94.8 Other childhood disorders of social functioning
F94.9 Childhood disorders of social functioning, unspecified

F95 Tic disorders

F95.0 Transient tic disorder

F95.1 Chronic motor or vocal tic disorder

F95.2 Combined vocal and multiple motor tic disorder [de la Tourette's syndrome]

F95.8 Other tic disorders

F95.9 Tic disorder, unspecified

F98 Other behavioural and emotional disorders with onset usually occurring in childhood and adolescence

F98.0 Nonorganic enuresis

F98.1 Nonorganic encopresis

F98.2 Feeding disorder of infancy and childhood

F98.3 Pica of infancy and childhood

F98.4 Stereotyped movement disorders

F98.5 Stuttering [stammering]

F98.6 Cluttering

F98.8 Other specified behavioural and emotional disorders with onset usually occurring in childhood and adolescence

F98.9 Unspecified behavioural and emotional disorders with onset usually occurring in childhood and adolescence

F99
Unspecified mental disorder

F99 Mental disorder, not otherwise specified

Clinical descriptions
and
diagnostic guidelines

F00 – F09
Organic, including symptomatic, mental disorders

Overview of this block

F00 Dementia in Alzheimer's disease

F00.0 Dementia in Alzheimer's disease with early onset

F00.1 Dementia in Alzheimer's disease with late onset

F00.2 Dementia in Alzheimer's disease, atypical or mixed type

F00.9 Dementia in Alzheimer's disease, unspecified

F01 Vascular dementia

F01.0 Vascular dementia of acute onset

F01.1 Multi-infarct dementia

F01.2 Subcortical vascular dementia

F01.3 Mixed cortical and subcortical vascular dementia

F01.8 Other vascular dementia

F01.9 Vascular dementia, unspecified

F02 Dementia in other diseases classified elsewhere

F02.0 Dementia in Pick's disease

F02.1 Dementia in Creutzfeldt – Jakob disease

F02.2 Dementia in Huntington's disease

F02.3 Dementia in Parkinson's disease

F02.4 Dementia in human immunodeficiency virus [HIV] disease

F02.8 Dementia in other specified diseases classified elsewhere

F03 Unspecified dementia

A fifth character may be used to specifiy dementia in F00 – F03, as follows:

.x0 Without additional symptoms

.x1 Other symptoms, predominantly delusional

.x2 Other symptoms, predominantly hallucinatory

.x3 Other symptoms, predominantly depressive

.x4 Other mixed symptoms

F04 Organic amnesic syndrome, not induced by alcohol and other psychoactive substances

F05 Delirium, not induced by alcohol and other psychoactive substances

F05.0 Delirium, not superimposed on dementia, so described

F05.1 Delirium, superimposed on dementia

F05.8 Other delirium

F05.9 Delirium, unspecified

F06 Other mental disorders due to brain damage and dysfunction and to physical disease

F06.0 Organic hallucinosis

F06.1 Organic catatonic disorder

F06.2 Organic delusional [schizophrenia-like] disorder

F06.3 Organic mood [affective] disorders

.30 Organic manic disorder

.31 Organic bipolar affective disorder

.32 Organic depressive disorder

.33 Organic mixed affective disorder

F06.4 Organic anxiety disorder

F06.5 Organic dissociative disorder

F06.6 Organic emotionally labile [asthenic] disorder

F06.7 Mild cognitive disorder

F06.8 Other specified mental disorders due to brain damage and dysfunction and to physical disease

F06.9 Unspecified mental disorder due to brain damage and dysfunction and to physical disease

F07 Personality and behavioural disorders due to brain disease, damage and dysfunction

F07.0 Organic personality disorder

F07.1 Postencephalitic syndrome

F07.2 Postconcussional syndrome

F07.8 Other organic personality and behavioural disorders due to brain disease, damage and dysfunction

F07.9 Unspecified organic personality and behavioural disorders due to brain disease, damage and dysfunction

F09 Unspecified organic or symptomatic mental disorder

Introduction

This block comprises a range of mental disorders grouped together on the basis of their common, demonstrable etiology in cerebral disease, brain injury, or other insult leading to cerebral dysfunction. The dysfunction may be *primary,* as in diseases, injuries, and insults that affect the brain directly or with predilection; or *secondary,* as in systemic diseases and disorders that attack the brain only as one of the multiple organs or systems of the body involved. Alcohol- and drug-caused brain disorders, though logically belonging to this group, are classified under F10 – F19 because of practical advantages in keeping all disorders due to psychoactive substance use in a single block.

Although the spectrum of psychopathological manifestations of the conditions included here is broad, the essential features of the disorders form two main clusters. On the one hand, there are syndromes in which the invariable and most prominent features are either disturbances of cognitive functions, such as memory, intellect, and learning, or disturbances of the sensorium, such as disorders of consciousness and attention. On the other hand, there are syndromes of which the most conspicuous manifestations are in the areas of perception (hallucinations), thought contents (delusions), or mood and emotion (depression, elation, anxiety), or in the overall pattern of personality and behaviour, while cognitive or sensory dysfunction is minimal or difficult to ascerta in. The latter group of disorders has less secure footing in this block than the former because it contains many disorders that are symptomatically similar to conditions classified in other blocks (F20 – F29, F30 – F39, F40 – F49, F60 – F69) and are known to occur without gross cerebral pathological change or dysfunction. However, the growing evidence that a variety of cerebral and systemic diseases are causally related to the occurrence of such syndromes provides sufficient justification for their inclusion here in a clinically oriented classification.

The majority of the disorders in this block can, at least theoretically, have their onset at any age, except perhaps early childhood. In practice, most tend to start in adult life or old age. While some of these disorders are seemingly irreversible and progressive, others are transient or respond to currently available treatments.

Use of the term "organic" does not imply that conditions elsewhere in this classification are "nonorganic" in the sense of having no cerebral substrate. In the present context, the term "organic" means simply that the syndrome so classified can be attributed to an independently diagnosable cerebral or systemic disease or disorder. The term "symptomatic" is used for those organic mental disorders in which cerebral involvement is secondary to a systemic extracerebral disease or disorder.

It follows from the foregoing that, in the majority of cases, the recording of a diagnosis of any one of the disorders in this block will require the use of two codes: one for the psychopathological syndrome and another for the underlying disorder. The etiological code should be selected from the relevant chapter of the overall ICD-10 classification.

Dementia

A general description of dementia is given here, to indicate the minimum requirement for the diagnosis of dementia of any type, and is followed by the criteria that govern the diagnosis of more specific types.

Dementia is a syndrome due to disease of the brain, usually of a chronic or progressive nature, in which there is disturbance of multiple higher cortical functions, including memory, thinking, orientation, comprehension, calculation, learning capacity, language, and judgement. Consciousness is not clouded. Impairments of cognitive function are commonly accompanied, and occasionally preceded, by deterioration in emotional control, social behaviour, or motivation. This syndrome occurs in Alzheimer's disease, in cerebrovascular disease, and in other conditions primarily or secondarily affecting the brain.

In assessing the presence or absence of a dementia, special care should be taken to avoid false-positive identification: motivational or emotional factors, particularly depression, in addition to motor slowness and general physical frailty, rather than loss of intellectual capacity, may account for failure to perform.

Dementia produces an appreciable decline in intellectual functioning, and usually some interference with personal activities of daily living, such as washing, dressing, eating, personal hygiene, excretory and toilet activities. How such a decline manifests itself will depend largely on the social and cultural setting in which the patient lives. Changes in role performance, such as lowered ability to keep or find a job, should not be used as criteria of dementia because of the large cross-cultural differences that exist in what is appropriate, and because there may be frequent, externally imposed changes in the availability of work within a particular culture.

If depressive symptoms are present but the criteria for depressive episode (F32.0 – F32.3) are not fulfilled, they can be recorded by means of a fifth character. The presence of hallucinations or delusions may be treated similarly.

.x0 Without additional symptoms
.x1 Other symptoms, predominantly delusional
.x2 Other symptoms, predominantly hallucinatory
.x3 Other symptoms, predominantly depressive
.x4 Other mixed symptoms

Diagnostic guidelines

The primary requirement for diagnosis is evidence of a decline in both memory and thinking which is sufficient to impair personal activities of daily living, as described above. The impairment of memory typically affects the registration, storage, and retrieval of new information, but previously learned and familiar material may also be lost, particularly in the later stages. Dementia is more than dysmnesia: there is also impairment of thinking and of reasoning capacity, and a reduction in the flow of ideas. The processing of incoming information is impaired, in that the individual finds it increasingly difficult to attend to more than one stimulus at a time, such as taking part in a conversation with several persons, and to shift the focus of attention from one topic to another. If dementia is the sole diagnosis, evidence of clear consciousness is required. However, a double diagnosis of delirium superimposed upon dementia is common (F05.1). The above symptoms and impairments should have been evident *for at least 6 months* for a confident clinical diagnosis of dementia to be made.

Differential diagnosis. Consider: a depressive disorder (F30 – F39), which may exhibit many of the features of an early dementia, especially memory impairment, slowed thinking, and lack of spontaneity; delirium (F05); mild or moderate mental retardation (F70 – F71); states of subnormal cognitive functioning attributable to a severely impoverished social environment and limited education; iatrogenic mental disorders due to medication (F06. –).

Dementia may *follow* any other organic mental disorder classified in this block, or *coexist* with some of them, notably delirium (see F05.1).

F00 Dementia in Alzheimer's disease

Alzheimer's disease is a primary degenerative cerebral disease of unknown etiology, with characteristic neuropathological and neurochemical features. It is usually insidious in onset and develops slowly but steadily over a period of years. This period can be as short as 2 or 3 years, but can occasionally be considerably longer. The onset can be in middle adult life or even earlier (Alzheimer's disease with early onset), but the incidence is higher in later life (Alzheimer's disease with late onset). In cases with onset before the age of 65 – 70, there is the likelihood of a family history of a similar dementia, a more rapid course, and prominence of features of temporal and parietal lobe damage, including dysphasia or dyspraxia. In cases with a later onset, the course tends to be slower and to be characterized by more general impairment of higher cortical functions. Patients with Down's syndrome are at high risk of developing Alzheimer's disease.

There are characteristic changes in the brain: a marked reduction in the population of neurons, particularly in the hippocampus, substantia innominata, locus ceruleus, and temporoparietal and frontal cortex; appearance of neurofibrillary tangles made of paired helical filaments; neuritic (argentophil) plaques, which consist largely of amyloid and show a definite progression in their development (although plaques without amyloid are also known to exist); and granulovacuolar bodies. Neurochemical changes have also been found, including a marked reduction in the enzyme choline acetyltransferase, in acetylcholine itself, and in other neurotransmitters and neuromodulators.

As originally described, the clinical features are accompanied by the above brain changes. However, it now appears that the two do not always progress in parallel: one may be indisputably present with only minimal evidence of the other. Nevertheless, the clinical features of Alzheimer's disease are such that it is often possible to make a presumptive diagnosis on clinical grounds alone.

Dementia in Alzheimer's disease is at present irreversible.

Diagnostic guidelines

The following features are essential for a definite diagnosis:

(a) Presence of a dementia as described above.

(b) Insidious onset with slow deterioration. While the onset usually seems difficult to pinpoint in time, realization by others that the defects exist may come suddenly. An apparent plateau may occur in the progression.

(c) Absence of clinical evidence, or findings from special investigations, to suggest that the mental state may be due to other systemic or brain disease which can induce a dementia (e.g. hypothyroidism, hypercalcaemia, vitamin B_{12} deficiency, niacin deficiency, neurosyphilis, normal pressure hydrocephalus, or subdural haematoma).

(d) Absence of a sudden, apoplectic onset, or of neurological signs of focal damage such as hemiparesis, sensory loss, visual field defects, and incoordination occurring early in the illness (although these phenomena may be superimposed later).

In a certain proportion of cases, the features of Alzheimer's disease and vascular dementia may both be present. In such cases, double diagnosis (and coding) should be made. When the vascular dementia precedes the Alzheimer's disease, it may be impossible to diagnose the latter on clinical grounds.

Includes: primary degenerative dementia of the Alzheimer's type

Differential diagnosis. Consider: a depressive disorder (F30 – F39); delirium (F05. –); organic amnesic syndrome (F04); other primary dementias, such as in Pick's, Creutzfeldt–Jakob or Huntington's disease (F02. –); secondary dementias associated with a variety of physical diseases, toxic states, etc. (F02.8); mild, moderate or severe mental retardation (F70 – F72).

Dementia in Alzheimer's disease may coexist with vascular dementia (to be coded F00.2), as when cerebrovascular episodes (multi-infarct phenomena) are superimposed on a clinical picture and history suggesting Alzheimer's disease. Such episodes may result in sudden exacerbations of the manifestations of dementia. According to postmortem findings, both types may coexist in as many as 10 – 15% of all dementia cases.

F00.0 **Dementia in Alzheimer's disease with early onset**

Dementia in Alzheimer's disease beginning before the age of 65. There is relatively rapid deterioration, with marked multiple disorders of the higher cortical functions. Aphasia, agraphia, alexia, and apraxia occur relatively early in the course of the dementia in most cases.

Diagnostic guidelines

As for dementia, described above, with onset before the age of 65 years, and usually with rapid progression of symptoms. Family history of Alzheimer's disease is a contributory but not necessary factor for the diagnosis, as is a family history of Down's syndrome or of lymphoma.

Includes: Alzheimer's disease, type 2
presenile dementia, Alzheimer's type

F00.1 **Dementia in Alzheimer's disease with late onset**

Dementia in Alzheimer's disease where the clinically observable onset is after the age of 65 years and usually in the late 70s or thereafter, with a slow progression, and usually with memory impairment as the principal feature.

Diagnostic guidelines

As for dementia, described above, with attention to the presence or absence of features differentiating the disorder from the early-onset subtype (F00.0).

Includes: Alzheimer's disease, type 1
senile dementia, Alzheimer's type

F00.2 **Dementia in Alzheimer's disease, atypical or mixed type**

Dementias that do not fit the descriptions and guidelines for either F00.0 or F00.1 should be classified here; mixed Alzheimer's and vascular dementias are also included here.

F00.9 **Dementia in Alzheimer's disease, unspecified**

F01 Vascular dementia

Vascular (formerly arteriosclerotic) dementia, which includes multi-infarct dementia, is distinguished from dementia in Alzheimer's disease by its history of onset, clinical features, and subsequent course. Typically, there is a history of transient ischaemic attacks with brief impairment of consciousness, fleeting pareses, or visual loss. The dementia may also follow a succession of acute cerebrovascular accidents or, less commonly, a single major stroke. Some impairment of memory and thinking then becomes apparent. Onset, which is usually in later life, can be abrupt, following one particular ischaemic episode, or there may be more gradual emergence. The dementia is usually the result of infarction of the brain due to vascular diseases, including hypertensive cerebrovascular disease. The infarcts are usually small but cumulative in their effect.

Diagnostic guidelines

The diagnosis presupposes the presence of a dementia as described above. Impairment of cognitive function is commonly uneven, so that there may be memory loss, intellectual impairment, and focal neurological signs. Insight and judgement may be relatively well preserved. An abrupt onset or a stepwise deterioration, as well as the presence of focal neurological signs and symptoms, increases the probability of the diagnosis; in some cases, confirmation can be provided only by computerized axial tomography or, ultimately, neuropathological examination.

Associated features are: hypertension, carotid bruit, emotional lability with transient depressive mood, weeping or explosive laughter, and transient episodes of clouded consciousness or delirium, often provoked by further infarction. Personality is believed to be relatively well preserved, but personality changes may be evident in a proportion of cases with apathy, disinhibition, or accentuation of previous traits such as egocentricity, paranoid attitudes, or irritability.

Includes: arteriosclerotic dementia

Differential diagnosis. Consider: delirium (F05. –); other dementia, particularly in Alzheimer's disease (F00. –); mood [affective] disorders (F30 – F39); mild or moderate mental retardation (F70 – F71); subdural haemorrhage (traumatic (S06.5), nontraumatic (I62.0)).

Vascular dementia may coexist with dementia in Alzheimer's disease (to be coded F00.2), as when evidence of a vascular episode is superimposed on a clinical picture and history suggesting Alzheimer's disease.

F01.0 Vascular dementia of acute onset

Usually develops rapidly after a succession of strokes from cerebrovascular thrombosis, embolism, or haemorrhage. In rare cases, a single large infarction may be the cause.

F01.1 Multi-infarct dementia

This is more gradual in onset than the acute form, following a number of minor ischaemic episodes which produce an accumulation of infarcts in the cerebral parenchyma.

Includes: predominantly cortical dementia

F01.2 Subcortical vascular dementia

There may be a history of hypertension and foci of ischaemic destruction in the deep white matter of the cerebral hemispheres, which can be suspected on clinical grounds and demonstrated on computerized axial tomography scans. The cerebral cortex is usually preserved and this contrasts with the clinical picture, which may closely resemble that of dementia in Alzheimer's disease. (Where diffuse demyelination of white matter can be demonstrated, the term ''Binswanger's encephalopathy'' may be used.)

F01.3 Mixed cortical and subcortical vascular dementia

Mixed cortical and subcortical components of the vascular dementia may be suspected from the clinical features, the results of investigations (including autopsy), or both.

F01.8 Other vascular dementia

F01.9 Vascular dementia, unspecified

F02 Dementia in other diseases classified elsewhere

Cases of dementia due, or presumed to be due, to causes other than Alzheimer's disease or cerebrovascular disease. Onset may be at any time in life, though rarely in old age.

Diagnostic guidelines

Presence of a dementia as described above; presence of features characteristic of one of the specified syndromes, as set out in the following categories.

F02.0 Dementia in Pick's disease

A progressive dementia, commencing in middle life (usually between 50 and 60 years), characterized by slowly progressing changes of character and social deterioration, followed by impairment of intellect, memory, and language functions, with apathy, euphoria, and (occasionally) extrapyramidal phenomena. The neuropathological picture is one of selective atrophy of the frontal and temporal lobes, but without the occurrence of neuritic plaques and neurofibrillary tangles in excess of that seen in normal aging. Cases with early onset tend to exhibit a more malignant course. The social and behavioural manifestations often precede frank memory impairment.

Diagnostic guidelines

The following features are required for a definite diagnosis:

(a) a progressive dementia;
(b) a predominance of frontal lobe features with euphoria, emotional blunting, and coarsening of social behaviour, disinhibition, and either apathy or restlessness;
(c) behavioural manifestations, which commonly precede frank memory impairment.

Frontal lobe features are more marked than temporal and parietal, unlike Alzheimer's disease.

Differential diagnosis. Consider: dementia in Alzheimer's disease (F00); vascular dementia (F01); dementia secondary to other disorders such as neurosyphilis (F02.8); normal pressure hydrocephalus (characterized by extreme psychomotor slowing, and gait and sphincter disturbances) (G91.2); other neurological or metabolic disorders.

F02.1 Dementia in Creutzfeldt – Jakob disease

A progressive dementia with extensive neurological signs, due to specific neuropathological changes (subacute spongiform encephalopathy) that are presumed to be caused by a transmissible agent. Onset is usually in middle or later life, typically in the fifth decade, but may be at any adult age. The course is subacute, leading to death within 1 – 2 years.

Diagnostic guidelines

Creutzfeldt – Jakob disease should be suspected in all cases of a dementia that progresses fairly rapidly over months to 1 or 2 years and that is accompanied or followed by multiple neurological symptoms. In some cases, such as the so-called amyotrophic form, the neurological signs may precede the onset of the dementia.

There is usually a progressive spastic paralysis of the limbs, accompanied by extrapyramidal signs with tremor, rigidity, and choreoathetoid movements. Other variants may include ataxia, visual failure, or muscle fibrillation and atrophy of the upper motor neuron type. The triad consisting of
— rapidly progressing, devastating dementia,
— pyramidal and extrapyramidal disease with myoclonus, and
— a characteristic (triphasic) electroencephalogram
is thought to be highly suggestive of this disease.

Differential diagnosis. Consider: Alzheimer's disease (F00. –) or Pick's disease (F02.0); Parkinson's disease (F02.3); postencephalitic parkinsonism (G21.3).

The rapid course and early motor involvement should suggest Creutzfeldt – Jakob disease.

F02.2   Dementia in Huntington's disease

A dementia occurring as part of a widespread degeneration of the brain. Huntington's disease is transmitted by a single autosomal dominant gene. Symptoms typically emerge in the third and fourth decade, and the sex incidence is probably equal. In a proportion of cases, the earliest symptoms may be depression, anxiety, or frank paranoid illness, accompanied by a personality change. Progression is slow, leading to death usually within 10 to 15 years.

Diagnostic guidelines

The association of choreiform movement disorder, dementia, and family history of Huntington's disease is highly suggestive of the diagnosis, though sporadic cases undoubtedly occur.

Involuntary choreiform movements, typically of the face, hands, and shoulders, or in the gait, are early manifestations. They usually precede the dementia and only rarely remain absent until the dementia is very advanced. Other motor phenomena may predominate when the onset is at an unusually young age (e.g. striatal rigidity) or at a late age (e.g. intention tremor).

The dementia is characterized by the predominant involvement of frontal lobe functions in the early stage, with relative preservation of memory until later.

Includes: dementia in Huntington's chorea

Differential diagnosis. Consider: other cases of choreic movements; Alzheimer's, Pick's or Creutzfeldt – Jakob disease (F00. – , F02.0, F02.1).

F02.3 Dementia in Parkinson's disease

A dementia developing in the course of established Parkinson's disease (especially its severe forms). No particular distinguishing clinical features have yet been demonstrated. The dementia may be different from that in either Alzheimer's disease or vascular dementia; however, there is also evidence that it may be the manifestation of a co-occurrence of one of these conditions with Parkinson's disease. This justifies the identification of cases of Parkinson's disease with dementia for research until the issue is resolved.

Diagnostic guidelines

Dementia developing in an individual with advanced, usually severe, Parkinson's disease.

Includes: dementia in paralysis agitans
dementia in parkinsonism

Differential diagnosis. Consider: other secondary dementias (F02.8); multi-infarct dementia (F01.1) associated with hypertensive or diabetic vascular disease; brain tumour (C70 – C72); normal pressure hydrocephalus (G91.2).

F02.4 Dementia in human immunodeficiency virus [HIV] disease

A disorder characterized by cognitive deficits meeting the clinical diagnostic criteria for dementia, in the absence of a concurrent illness or condition other than HIV infection that could explain the findings.

HIV dementia typically presents with complaints of forgetfulness, slowness, poor concentration, and difficulties with problem-solving and reading. Apathy, reduced spontaneity, and social withdrawal are common, and in a significant minority of affected individuals the illness may present atypically as an affective disorder, psychosis, or seizures. Physical examination often reveals tremor, impaired rapid repetitive movements, imbalance, ataxia, hypertonia, generalized hyperreflexia, positive frontal release signs, and impaired pursuit and saccadic eye movements.

Children also develop an HIV-associated neurodevelopmental disorder characterized by developmental delay, hypertonia, microcephaly, and basal ganglia calcification. The neurological involvement most often occurs in the absence of opportunistic infections and neoplasms, which is not the case for adults.

HIV dementia generally, but not invariably, progresses quickly (over weeks or months) to severe global dementia, mutism, and death.

Includes: AIDS – dementia complex
HIV encephalopathy or subacute encephalitis

F02.8 Dementia in other specified diseases classified elsewhere

Dementia can occur as a manifestation or consequence of a variety of cerebral and somatic conditions. To specify the etiology, the ICD-10 code for the underlying condition should be added.

Parkinsonism – dementia complex of Guam should also be coded here (identified by a fifth character, if necessary). It is a rapidly progressing dementia followed by extrapyramidal dysfunction and, in some cases, amyotrophic lateral sclerosis. The disease was originally described on the island of Guam where it occurs with high frequency in the indigenous population, affecting twice as many males as females; it is now known to occur also in Papua New Guinea and Japan.

Includes: dementia in:
  carbon monoxide poisoning (T58)
  cerebral lipidosis (E75. –)
  epilepsy (G40. –)
  general paralysis of the insane (A52.1)
  hepatolenticular degeneration (Wilson's disease) (E83.0)
  hypercalcaemia (E83.5)
  hypothyroidism, acquired (E00. – , E02)
  intoxications (T36 – T65)
  multiple sclerosis (G35)
  neurosyphilis (A52.1)
  niacin deficiency [pellagra] (E52)
  polyarteritis nodosa (M30.0)
  systemic lupus erythematosus (M32. –)
  trypanosomiasis (African B56. – , American B57. –)
  vitamin B_{12} deficiency (E53.8)

F03 Unspecified dementia

This category should be used when the general criteria for the diagnosis of dementia are satisfied, but when it is not possible to identify one of the specific types (F00.0 – F02.9).

Includes: presenile or senile dementia NOS
  presenile or senile psychosis NOS
  primary degenerative dementia NOS

F04 Organic amnesic syndrome, not induced by alcohol and other psychoactive substances

A syndrome of prominent impairment of recent and remote memory. While immediate recall is preserved, the ability to learn new material is markedly reduced and this results in anterograde amnesia and disorientation in time. Retrograde amnesia of varying intensity is also present but its extent may lessen over time if the underlying lesion or pathological process has a tendency to recover. Confabulation may be a marked feature but is not invariably present. Perception and other cognitive functions, including the intellect, are usually intact and provide a background against which the memory disturbance appears as particularly striking. The prognosis depends on the course of the underlying lesion (which typically affects the hypothalamic – diencephalic system or the hippocampal region); almost complete recovery is, in principle, possible.

Diagnostic guidelines

For a definitive diagnosis it is necessary to establish:

(a) presence of a memory impairment manifest in a defect of recent memory (impaired learning of new material); anterograde and retrograde amnesia, and a reduced ability to recall past experiences in reverse order of their occurrence;

(b) history or objective evidence of an insult to, or a disease of, the brain (especially with bilateral involvement of the diencephalic and medial temporal structures);

(c) absence of a defect in immediate recall (as tested, for example, by the digit span), of disturbances of attention and consciousness, and of global intellectual impairment.

Confabulations, lack of insight, and emotional changes (apathy, lack of initiative) are additional, though not in every case necessary, pointers to the diagnosis.

Includes: Korsakov's syndrome or psychosis, nonalcoholic

Differential diagnosis. This disorder should be distinguished from other organic syndromes in which memory impairment is prominent (e.g. dementia or delirium), from dissociative amnesia (F44.0), from impaired memory function in depressive disorders (F30 – F39), and from malingering presenting with a complaint of memory loss (Z76.5). Korsakov's syndrome induced by alcohol or drugs should not be coded here but in the appropriate section (F1x.6).

F05 Delirium, not induced by alcohol and other psychoactive substances

An etiologically nonspecific syndrome characterized by concurrent disturbances of consciousness and attention, perception, thinking, memory, psychomotor behaviour, emotion, and the sleep – wake cycle. It may occur at any age but is most common after the age of 60 years. The delirious state is transient and of fluctuating

57

intensity; most cases recover within 4 weeks or less. However, delirium lasting, with fluctuations, for up to 6 months is not uncommon, especially when arising in the course of chronic liver disease, carcinoma, or subacute bacterial endocarditis. The distinction that is sometimes made between acute and subacute delirium is of little clinical relevance; the condition should be seen as a unitary syndrome of variable duration and severity ranging from mild to very severe. A delirious state may be superimposed on, or progress into, dementia.

This category should *not* be used for states of delirium associated with the use of psychoactive drugs specified in F10 – F19. Delirious states due to prescribed medication (such as acute confusional states in elderly patients due to antidepressants) should be coded here. In such cases, the medication concerned should also be recorded by means of an additional T code from Chapter XIX of ICD-10.

Diagnostic guidelines

For a definite diagnosis, symptoms, mild or severe, should be present *in each one* of the following areas:

(a) impairment of consciousness and attention (on a continuum from clouding to coma; reduced ability to direct, focus, sustain, and shift attention);

(b) global disturbance of cognition (perceptual distortions, illusions and hallucinations — most often visual; impairment of abstract thinking and comprehension, with or without transient delusions, but typically with some degree of incoherence; impairment of immediate recall and of recent memory but with relatively intact remote memory; disorientation for time as well as, in more severe cases, for place and person);

(c) psychomotor disturbances (hypo- or hyperactivity and unpredictable shifts from one to the other; increased reaction time; increased or decreased flow of speech; enhanced startle reaction);

(d) disturbance of the sleep – wake cycle (insomnia or, in severe cases, total sleep loss or reversal of the sleep – wake cycle; daytime drowsiness; nocturnal worsening of symptoms; disturbing dreams or nightmares, which may continue as hallucinations after awakening);

(e) emotional disturbances, e.g. depression, anxiety or fear, irritability, euphoria, apathy, or wondering perplexity.

The onset is usually rapid, the course diurnally fluctuating, and the total duration of the condition less than 6 months. The above clinical picture is so characteristic that a fairly confident diagnosis of delirium can be made even if the underlying cause is not clearly established. In addition to a history of an underlying physical or brain disease, evidence of cerebral dysfunction (e.g. an abnormal electroencephalogram, usually but not invariably showing a slowing of the background activity) may be required if the diagnosis is in doubt.

Includes: acute brain syndrome
acute confusional state (nonalcoholic)
acute infective psychosis
acute organic reaction
acute psycho-organic syndrome

Differential diagnosis. Delirium should be distinguished from other organic syndromes, especially dementia (F00 – F03), from acute and transient psychotic disorders (F23. –), and from acute states in schizophrenia (F20. –) or mood [affective] disorders (F30 – F39) in which confusional features may be present. Delirium, induced by alcohol and other psychoactive substances, should be coded in the appropriate section (F1x.4).

F05.0   Delirium, not superimposed on dementia, so described
This code should be used for delirium that is not superimposed upon pre-existing dementia.

F05.1   Delirium, superimposed on dementia
This code should be used for conditions meeting the above criteria but developing in the course of a dementia (F00 – F03).

F05.8   Other delirium

Includes: delirium of mixed origin
subacute confusional state or delirium

F05.9   Delirium, unspecified

F06 Other mental disorders due to brain damage and dysfunction and to physical disease

This category includes miscellaneous conditions causally related to brain dysfunction due to primary cerebral disease, to systemic disease affecting the brain secondarily, to endocrine disorders such as Cushing's syndrome or other somatic illnesses, and to some exogenous toxic substances (but excluding alcohol and drugs classified under F10–F19) or hormones. These conditions have in common clinical features that do not by themselves allow a presumptive diagnosis of an organic mental disorder, such as dementia or delirium. Rather, the clinical manifestations resemble, or are identical with, those of disorders not regarded as "organic" in the specific sense restricted to this block of the classification. Their inclusion here is based on the hypothesis that they are directly caused by cerebral disease or dysfunction rather than resulting from either a fortuitous association with such disease or dysfunction, or a psychological reaction to its symptoms, such as schizophrenia-like disorders associated with long-standing epilepsy.

The decision to classify a clinical syndrome here is supported by the following:

(a) evidence of cerebral disease, damage or dysfunction, or of systemic physical disease, known to be associated with one of the listed syndromes;

(b) a temporal relationship (weeks or a few months) between the development of the underlying disease and the onset of the mental syndrome;

(c) recovery from the mental disorder following removal or improvement of the underlying presumed cause;

(d) absence of evidence to suggest an alternative cause of the mental syndrome (such as a strong family history or precipitating stress).

Conditions (a) and (b) justify a provisional diagnosis; if all four are present, the certainty of diagnostic classification is significantly increased.

The following are among the conditions known to increase the relative risk for the syndromes classified here: epilepsy; limbic encephalitis; Huntington's disease; head trauma; brain neoplasms; extracranial neoplasms with remote CNS effects (especially carcinoma of the pancreas); vascular cerebral disease, lesions, or malformations; lupus erythematosus and other collagen diseases; endocrine disease (especially hypo- and hyperthyroidism, Cushing's disease); metabolic disorders (e.g. hypoglycaemia, porphyria, hypoxia); tropical infectious and parasitic diseases (e.g. trypanosomiasis); toxic effects of nonpsychotropic drugs (propranolol, levodopa, methyldopa, steroids, antihypertensives, antimalarials).

Excludes: mental disorders associated with delirium (F05. –)
mental disorders associated with dementia as classified in F00 – F03

F06.0 Organic hallucinosis

A disorder of persistent or recurrent hallucinations, usually visual or auditory, that occur in clear consciousness and may or may not be recognized by the subject as such. Delusional elaboration of the hallucinations may occur, but insight is not infrequently preserved.

Diagnostic guidelines

In addition to the general criteria in the introduction to F06 above, there should be evidence of persistent or recurrent hallucinations in any modality; no clouding of consciousness; no significant intellectual decline; no predominant disturbance of mood; and no predominance of delusions.

Includes: Dermatozoenwahn
organic hallucinatory state (nonalcoholic)

Excludes: alcoholic hallucinosis (F10.52)
schizophrenia (F20. –)

F06.1 Organic catatonic disorder

A disorder of diminished (stupor) or increased (excitement) psychomotor activity associated with catatonic symptoms. The extremes of psychomotor disturbance may alternate. It is not known whether the full range of catatonic disturbances described in schizophrenia occurs in such organic states, nor has it been conclusively determined whether an organic catatonic state may occur in clear consciousness or whether it is always a manifestation of delirium, with subsequent partial or total amnesia. This calls for caution in making this diagnosis and for a careful delimitation of the condition from delirium. Encephalitis and carbon monoxide poisoning are presumed to be associated with this syndrome more often than other organic causes.

Diagnostic guidelines

The general criteria for assuming organic etiology, laid down in the introduction to F06, must be met. In addition, there should be one of the following:

(a) stupor (diminution or complete absence of spontaneous movement with partial or complete mutism, negativism, and rigid posturing);
(b) excitement (gross hypermotility with or without a tendency to assaultiveness);
(c) both (shifting rapidly and unpredictably from hypo- to hyperactivity).

Other catatonic phenomena that increase confidence in the diagnosis are: stereotypies, waxy flexibility, and impulsive acts.

Excludes: catatonic schizophrenia (20.2)
dissociative stupor (F44.2)
stupor NOS (R40.1)

F06.2 Organic delusional [schizophrenia-like] disorder

A disorder in which persistent or recurrent delusions dominate the clinical picture. The delusions may be accompanied by hallucinations but are not confined to their content. Features suggestive of schizophrenia, such as bizarre delusions, hallucinations, or thought disorder, may also be present.

Diagnostic guidelines

The general criteria for assuming an organic etiology, laid down in the introduction to F06, must be met. In addition, there should be delusions (persecutory, of bodily change, jealousy, disease, or death of the subject or another person). Hallucinations, thought disorder, or isolated catatonic phenomena may be present. Consciousness and memory must not be affected. This diagnosis should not be made if the presumed evidence of organic causation is nonspecific or limited to findings such as enlarged cerebral ventricles (visualized on computerized axial tomography) or "soft" neurological signs.

Includes: paranoid and paranoid-hallucinatory organic states
schizophrenia-like psychosis in epilepsy

Excludes: acute and transient psychotic disorders (F23. –)
drug-induced psychotic disorders (F1x.5)
persistent delusional disorder (F22. –)
schizophrenia (F20. –)

F06.3   Organic mood [affective] disorders

Disorders characterized by a change in mood or affect, usually
accompanied by a change in the overall level of activity. The only
criterion for inclusion of these disorders in this block is their presumed
direct causation by a cerebral or other physical disorder whose
presence must either be demonstrated independently (e.g. by means
of appropriate physical and laboratory investigations) or assumed
on the basis of adequate history information. The affective disorder
must follow the presumed organic factor and be judged not to
represent an emotional response to the patient's knowledge of
having, or having the symptoms of, a concurrent brain disorder.

Postinfective depression (e.g. following influenza) is a common
example and should be coded here. Persistent mild euphoria not
amounting to hypomania (which is sometimes seen, for instance,
in association with steroid therapy or antidepressants) should not
be coded here but under F06.8.

Diagnostic guidelines

In addition to the general criteria for assuming organic etiology,
laid down in the introduction to F06, the condition must meet
the requirements for a diagnosis of one of the disorders listed
under F30 – F33.

Excludes: mood [affective] disorders, nonorganic or unspecified
(F30 – F39)
right hemispheric affective disorder (F07.8)

The following five-character codes might be used to specify the clinical
disorder:

F06.30 Organic manic disorder

F06.31 Organic bipolar affective disorder

F06.32 Organic depressive disorder

F06.33 Organic mixed affective disorder

F06.4   Organic anxiety disorder

A disorder characterized by the essential descriptive features of a generalized anxiety disorder (F41.1), a panic disorder (F41.0), or a combination of both, but arising as a consequence of an organic disorder capable of causing cerebral dysfunction (e.g. temporal lobe epilepsy, thyrotoxicosis, or phaechromocytoma).

Excludes: anxiety disorders, nonorganic or unspecified (F41. –)

F06.5   Organic dissociative disorder

A disorder that meets the requirements for one of the disorders in F44. – (dissociative [conversion] disorder) and for which the general criteria for organic etiology are also fulfilled (as described in the introduction to this block).

Excludes: dissociative [conversion] disorders, nonorganic or
            unspecified (F44. –)

F06.6   Organic emotionally labile [asthenic] disorder

A disorder characterized by marked and persistent emotional incontinence or lability, fatiguability, or a variety of unpleasant physical sensations (e.g. dizziness) and pains regarded as being due to the presence of an organic disorder. This disorder is thought to occur in association with cerebrovascular disease or hypertension more often than with other causes.

Excludes: somatoform disorders, nonorganic or unspecified (F45. –)

F06.7   Mild cognitive disorder

This disorder may precede, accompany, or follow a wide variety of infections and physical disorders, both cerebral and systemic (including HIV infection). Direct neurological evidence of cerebral involvement is not necessarily present, but there may nevertheless be distress and interference with usual activities. The boundaries of this category are still to be firmly established. When associated with a physical disorder from which the patient recovers, mild cognitive disorder does not last for more than a few additional weeks. This diagnosis should not be made if the condition is clearly attributable to a mental or behavioural disorder classified in any of the remaining blocks in this book.

Diagnostic guidelines

The main feature is a decline in cognitive performance. This may include memory impairment, learning or concentration difficulties. Objective tests usually indicate abnormality. The symptoms are such that a diagnosis of dementia (F00 – F03), organic amnesic syndrome (F04) or delirium (F05. –) cannot be made.

Differential diagnosis. The disorder can be differentiated from postencephalitic syndrome (F07.1) and postconcussional syndrome (F07.2) by its different etiology, more restricted range of generally milder symptoms, and usually shorter duration.

F06.8   Other specified mental disorders due to brain damage and dysfunction and to physical disease
Examples are abnormal mood states occurring during treatment with steroids or antidepressants.

Includes: epileptic psychosis NOS

F06.9   Unspecified mental disorder due to brain damage and dysfunction and to physical disease

F07   Personality and behavioural disorders due to brain disease, damage and dysfunction

Alteration of personality and behaviour can be a residual or concomitant disorder of brain disease, damage, or dysfunction. In some instances, differences in the manifestation of such residual or concomitant personality and behavioural syndromes may be suggestive of the type and/or localization of the intracerebral problem, but the reliability of this kind of diagnostic inference should not be overestimated. Thus the underlying etiology should always be sought by independent means and, if known, recorded.

F07.0 Organic personality disorder

This disorder is characterized by a significant alteration of the habitual patterns of premorbid behaviour. The expression of emotions, needs, and impulses is particularly affected. Cognitive functions may be defective mainly or even exclusively in the areas of planning and anticipating the likely personal and social consequences, as in the so-called frontal lobe syndrome. However, it is now known that this syndrome occurs not only with frontal lobe lesions but also with lesions to other circumscribed areas of the brain.

Diagnostic guidelines

In addition to an established history or other evidence of brain disease, damage, or dysfunction, a definitive diagnosis requires the presence of two or more of the following features:

(a) consistently reduced ability to persevere with goal-directed activities, especially those involving longer periods of time and postponed gratification;

(b) altered emotional behaviour, characterized by emotional lability, shallow and unwarranted cheerfulness (euphoria, inappropriate jocularity), and easy change to irritability or short-lived outbursts of anger and aggression; in some instances apathy may be a more prominent feature;

(c) expression of needs and impulses without consideration of consequences or social convention (the patient may engage in dissocial acts, such as stealing, inappropriate sexual advances, or voracious eating, or may exhibit disregard for personal hygiene);

(d) cognitive disturbances, in the form of suspiciousness or paranoid ideation, and/or excessive preoccupation with a single, usually abstract, theme (e.g. religion, "right" and "wrong");

(e) marked alteration of the rate and flow of language production, with features such as circumstantiality, over-inclusiveness, viscosity, and hypergraphia;

(f) altered sexual behaviour (hyposexuality or change of sexual preference).

Includes: frontal lobe syndrome
limbic epilepsy personality syndrome
lobotomy syndrome
organic pseudopsychopathic personality
organic pseudoretarded personality
postleucotomy syndrome

Excludes: enduring personality change after catastrophic experience (F62.0)

enduring personality change after psychiatric illness (F62.1)

postconcussional syndrome (F07.2)

postencephalitic syndrome (F07.1)

specific personality disorder (F60. –)

F07.1 Postencephalitic syndrome

The syndrome includes residual behavioural change following recovery from either viral or bacterial encephalitis. Symptoms are nonspecific and vary from individual to individual, from one infectious agent to another, and, most consistently, with the age of the individual at the time of infection. The principal difference between this disorder and the organic personality disorders is that it is often reversible.

Diagnostic guidelines

The manifestations may include general malaise, apathy or irritability, some lowering of cognitive functioning (learning difficulties), altered sleep and eating patterns, and changes in sexuality and in social judgement. There may be a variety of residual neurological dysfunctions such as paralysis, deafness, aphasia, constructional apraxia, and acalculia.

Excludes: organic personality disorder (F07.0)

F07.2 Postconcussional syndrome

The syndrome occurs following head trauma (usually sufficiently severe to result in loss of consciousness) and includes a number of disparate symptoms such as headache, dizziness (usually lacking the features of true vertigo), fatigue, irritability, difficulty in concentrating and performing mental tasks, impairment of memory, insomnia, and reduced tolerance to stress, emotional excitement, or alcohol. These symptoms may be accompanied by feelings of depression or anxiety, resulting from some loss of self-esteem and fear of permanent brain damage. Such feelings enhance the original symptoms and a vicious circle results. Some patients become hypochondriacal, embark on a search for diagnosis and cure, and may adopt a permanent sick role. The etiology of these symptoms is not always clear, and both organic and psychological factors have been proposed to account for them. The nosological status of this condition is thus somewhat uncertain. There is little doubt, however, that this syndrome is common and distressing to the patient.

67

Diagnostic guidelines

At least three of the features described above should be present for a definite diagnosis. Careful evaluation with laboratory techniques (electroencephalography, brain stem evoked potentials, brain imaging, oculonystagmography) may yield objective evidence to substantiate the symptoms but results are often negative. The complaints are not necessarily associated with compensation motives.

Includes: postcontusional syndrome (encephalopathy)
post-traumatic brain syndrome, nonpsychotic

F07.8 Other organic personality and behavioural disorders due to brain disease, damage and dysfunction

Brain disease, damage, or dysfunction may produce a variety of cognitive, emotional, personality, and behavioural disorders, not all of which are classifiable under the preceding rubrics. However, since the nosological status of the tentative syndromes in this area is uncertain, they should be coded as "other". A fifth character may be added, if necessary, to identify presumptive individual entities such as:

Right hemispheric organic affective disorder (changes in the ability to express or comprehend emotion in individuals with right hemisphere disorder). Although the patient may superficially appear to be depressed, depression is not usually present: it is the expression of emotion that is restricted.

Also code here:

(a) any other specified but presumptive syndromes of personality or behavioural change due to brain disease, damage, or dysfunction other than those listed under F07.0 – F07.2; and

(b) conditions with mild degrees of cognitive impairment not yet amounting to dementia in progressive mental disorders such as Alzheimer's disease, Parkinson's disease, etc. The diagnosis should be changed when the criteria for dementia are fulfilled.

Excludes: delirium (F05. –)

F07.9 **Unspecified organic personality and behavioural disorder due to brain disease, damage and dysfunction**

Includes: organic psychosyndrome

F09 Unspecified organic or symptomatic mental disorder

This category should only be used for recording mental disorders of known organic etiology.

Includes: organic psychosis NOS
symptomatic psychosis NOS

Excludes: psychosis NOS (F29)

F10 – F19
Mental and behavioural disorders due to psychoactive substance use

Overview of this block

F10. – **Mental and behavioural disorders due to use of alcohol**

F11. – **Mental and behavioural disorders due to use of opioids**

F12. – **Mental and behavioural disorders due to use of cannabinoids**

F13. – **Mental and behavioural disorders due to use of sedatives or hypnotics**

F14. – **Mental and behavioural disorders due to use of cocaine**

F15. – **Mental and behavioural disorders due to use of other stimulants, including caffeine**

F16. – **Mental and behavioural disorders due to use of hallucinogens**

F17. – **Mental and behavioural disorders due to use of tobacco**

F18. – **Mental and behavioural disorders due to use of volatile solvents**

F19. – **Mental and behavioural disorders due to multiple drug use and use of other psychoactive substances**

Four- and five-character codes may be used to specify the clinical conditions, as follows:

F1x.0   Acute intoxication
.00 Uncomplicated
.01 With trauma or other bodily injury
.02 With other medical complications
.03 With delirium
.04 With perceptual distortions
.05 With coma
.06 With convulsions
.07 Pathological intoxication

F1x.1   Harmful use

F1x.2   Dependence syndrome
.20 Currently abstinent
.21 Currently abstinent, but in a protected environment
.22 Currently on a clinically supervised maintenance or replacement regime [controlled dependence]

.23 Currently abstinent, but receiving treatment with aversive or blocking drugs

.24 Currently using the substance [active dependence]

.25 Continuous use

.26 Episodic use [dipsomania]

F1x.3 Withdrawal state

.30 Uncomplicated

.31 With convulsions

F1x.4 Withdrawal state with delirium

.40 Without convulsions

.41 With convulsions

F1x.5 Psychotic disorder

.50 Schizophrenia-like

.51 Predominantly delusional

.52 Predominantly hallucinatory

.53 Predominantly polymorphic

.54 Predominantly depressive symptoms

.55 Predominantly manic symptoms

.56 Mixed

F1x.6 Amnesic syndrome

F1x.7 Residual and late-onset psychotic disorder

.70 Flashbacks

.71 Personality or behaviour disorder

.72 Residual affective disorder

.73 Dementia

.74 Other persisting cognitive impairment

.75 Late-onset psychotic disorder

F1x.8 Other mental and behavioural disorders

F1x.9 Unspecified mental and behavioural disorder

Introduction

This block contains a wide variety of disorders that differ in severity (from uncomplicated intoxication and harmful use to obvious psychotic disorders and dementia), but that are all attributable to the use of one or more psychoactive substances (which may or may not have been medically prescribed).

The substance involved is indicated by means of the second and third characters (i.e. the first two digits after the letter F), and the fourth and fifth characters specify the clinical states. To save space, all the psychoactive substances are listed first, followed by the four-character codes; these should be used, as required, for each substance specified, but it should be noted that not all four-character codes are applicable to all substances.

Diagnostic guidelines

Identification of the psychoactive substance used may be made on the basis of self-report data, objective analysis of specimens of urine, blood, etc., or other evidence (presence of drug samples in the patient's possession, clinical signs and symptoms, or reports from informed third parties). It is always advisable to seek corroboration from more than one source of evidence relating to substance use.

Objective analyses provide the most compelling evidence of present or recent use, though these data have limitations with regard to past use and current levels of use.

Many drug users take more than one type of drug, but the diagnosis of the disorder should be classified, whenever possible, according to the most important single substance (or class of substances) used. This may usually be done with regard to the particular drug, or type of drug, causing the presenting disorder. When in doubt, code the drug or type of drug most frequently misused, particularly in those cases involving continuous or daily use.

Only in cases in which patterns of psychoactive substance taking are chaotic and indiscriminate, or in which the contributions of different drugs are inextricably mixed, should code F19. – be used (disorders resulting from multiple drug use).

Misuse of other than psychoactive substances, such as laxatives or aspirin, should be coded by means of F55. – (abuse of non-dependence-producing substances), with a fourth character to specify the type of substance involved.

Cases in which mental disorders (particularly delirium in the elderly) are due to psychoactive substances, but without the presence of one of the disorders in this block (e.g. harmful use or dependence syndrome), should be coded in F00 – F09. Where a state of delirium is superimposed upon such a disorder in this block, it should be coded by means of F1x.3 or F1x.4.

The level of alcohol involvement can be indicated by means of a supplementary code from Chapter XX of ICD-10: Y90. – (evidence of alcohol involvement determined by blood alcohol content) or Y91. – (evidence of alcohol involvement determined by level of intoxication).

F1x.0   Acute intoxication

A transient condition following the administration of alcohol or other psychoactive substance, resulting in disturbances in level of consciousness, cognition, perception, affect or behaviour, or other psychophysiological functions and responses.

This should be a main diagnosis only in cases where intoxication occurs without more persistent alcohol- or drug-related problems being concomitantly present. Where there are such problems, precedence should be given to diagnoses of harmful use (F1x.1), dependence syndrome (F1x.2), or psychotic disorder (F1x.5).

Diagnostic guidelines

Acute intoxication is usually closely related to dose levels (see ICD-10, Chapter XX). Exceptions to this may occur in individuals with certain underlying organic conditions (e.g. renal or hepatic insufficiency) in whom small doses of a substance may produce a disproportionately severe intoxicating effect. Disinhibition due to social context should also be taken into account (e.g. behavioural disinhibition at parties or carnivals). Acute intoxication is a transient phenomenon. Intensity of intoxication lessens with time, and effects eventually disappear in the absence of further use of the substance. Recovery is therefore complete except where tissue damage or another complication has arisen.

Symptoms of intoxication need not always reflect primary actions of the substance: for instance, depressant drugs may lead to symptoms of agitation or hyperactivity, and stimulant drugs may lead to socially withdrawn and introverted behaviour. Effects of substances such as cannabis and hallucinogens may be particularly unpredictable. Moreover, many psychoactive substances are capable of producing different types of effect at different dose levels. For example, alcohol may have apparently stimulant effects on behaviour at lower dose levels, lead to agitation and aggression with increasing dose levels, and produce clear sedation at very high levels.

Includes: acute drunkenness in alcoholism
"bad trips" (due to hallucinogenic drugs)
drunkenness NOS

Differential diagnosis. Consider acute head injury and hypoglycaemia. Consider also the possibilities of intoxication as the result of mixed substance use.

The following five-character codes may be used to indicate whether the acute intoxication was associated with any complications:

F1*x*.00 Uncomplicated
Symptoms of varying severity, usually dose-dependent, particularly at high dose levels.

F1*x*.01 With trauma or other bodily injury

F1*x*.02 With other medical complications
Complications such as haematemesis, inhalation of vomitus.

F1*x*.03 With delirium

F1*x*.04 With perceptual distortions

F1*x*.05 With coma

F1*x*.06 With convulsions

F1*x*.07 Pathological intoxication
Applies only to alcohol. Sudden onset of aggression and often violent behaviour that is not typical of the individual when sober, very soon after drinking amounts of alcohol that would not produce intoxication in most people.

F1*x*.1   Harmful use
A pattern of psychoactive substance use that is causing damage to health. The damage may be physical (as in cases of hepatitis from

Includes: chronic alcoholism
dipsomania
drug addiction

The diagnosis of the dependence syndrome may be further specified by the following five-character codes:

F1x.20 Currently abstinent

F1x.21 Currently abstinent, but in a protected environment
(e.g. in hospital, in a therapeutic community, in prison, etc.)

F1x.22 Currently on a clinically supervised maintenance or replacement regime [controlled dependence]
(e.g. with methadone; nicotine gum or nicotine patch)

F1x.23 Currently abstinent, but receiving treatment with aversive or blocking drugs
(e.g. naltrexone or disulfiram)

F1x.24 Currently using the substance [active dependence]

F1x.25 Continuous use

F1x.26 Episodic use [dipsomania]

F1x.3   Withdrawal state

A group of symptoms of variable clustering and severity occurring on absolute or relative withdrawal of a substance after repeated, and usually prolonged and/or high-dose, use of that substance. Onset and course of the withdrawal state are time-limited and are related to the type of substance and the dose being used immediately before abstinence. The withdrawal state may be complicated by convulsions.

Diagnostic guidelines

Withdrawal state is one of the indicators of dependence syndrome (see F1x.2) and this latter diagnosis should also be considered.

Withdrawal state should be coded as the main diagnosis if it is the reason for referral and sufficiently severe to require medical attention in its own right.

Physical symptoms vary according to the substance being used. Psychological disturbances (e.g. anxiety, depression, and sleep disorders) are also common features of withdrawal. Typically, the patient is likely to report that withdrawal symptoms are relieved by further substance use.

It should be remembered that withdrawal symptoms can be induced by conditioned/learned stimuli in the absence of immediately preceding substance use. In such cases a diagnosis of withdrawal state should be made only if it is warranted in terms of severity.

Differential diagnosis. Many symptoms present in drug withdrawal state may also be caused by other psychiatric conditions, e.g. anxiety states and depressive disorders. Simple "hangover" or tremor due to other conditions should not be confused with the symptoms of a withdrawal state.

The diagnosis of withdrawal state may be further specified by using the following five-character codes:

F1x.30 Uncomplicated

F1x.31 With convulsions

F1x.4 Withdrawal state with delirium

A condition in which the withdrawal state (see F1x.3) is complicated by delirium (see criteria for F05. –).

Alcohol-induced *delirium tremens* should be coded here. *Delirium tremens* is a short-lived, but occasionally life-threatening, toxic-confusional state with accompanying somatic disturbances. It is usually a consequence of absolute or relative withdrawal of alcohol in severely dependent users with a long history of use. Onset usually occurs after withdrawal of alcohol. In some cases the disorder appears during an episode of heavy drinking, in which case it should be coded here.

Prodromal symptoms typically include insomnia, tremulousness, and fear. Onset may also be preceded by withdrawal convulsions. The classical triad of symptoms includes clouding of consciousness and confusion, vivid hallucinations and illusions affecting any sensory modality, and marked tremor. Delusions, agitation, insomnia or sleep-cycle reversal, and autonomic overactivity are usually also present.

Excludes: delirium, not induced by drugs and alcohol (F05. –)

The diagnosis of withdrawal state with delirium may be further specified by using the following five-character codes:

F1x.40 Without convulsions

F1x.41 With convulsions

F1x.5   Psychotic disorder

A cluster of psychotic phenomena that occur during or immediately after psychoactive substance use and are characterized by vivid hallucinations (typically auditory, but often in more than one sensory modality), misidentifications, delusions and/or ideas of reference (often of a paranoid or persecutory nature), psychomotor disturbances (excitement or stupor), and an abnormal affect, which may range from intense fear to ecstasy. The sensorium is usually clear but some degree of clouding of consciousness, though not severe confusion, may be present. The disorder typically resolves at least partially within 1 month and fully within 6 months.

Diagnostic guidelines

A psychotic disorder occurring during or immediately after drug use (usually within 48 hours) should be recorded here provided that it is not a manifestation of drug withdrawal state with delirium (see F1x.4) or of late onset. Late-onset psychotic disorders (with onset more than 2 weeks after substance use) may occur, but should be coded as F1x.75.

Psychoactive substance-induced psychotic disorders may present with varying patterns of symptoms. These variations will be influenced by the type of substance involved and the personality of the user. For stimulant drugs such as cocaine and amfetamines, drug-induced psychotic disorders are generally closely related to high dose levels and/or prolonged use of the substance.

A diagnosis of a psychotic disorder should not be made merely on the basis of perceptual distortions or hallucinatory experiences when substances having primary hallucinogenic effects (e.g. lysergide (LSD),

79

mescaline, cannabis at high doses) have been taken. In such cases, and also for confusional states, a possible diagnosis of acute intoxication (F1x.0) should be considered.

Particular care should also be taken to avoid mistakenly diagnosing a more serious condition (e.g. schizophrenia) when a diagnosis of psychoactive substance-induced psychosis is appropriate. Many psychoactive substance-induced psychotic states are of short duration provided that no further amounts of the drug are taken (as in the case of amfetamine and cocaine psychoses). False diagnosis in such cases may have distressing and costly implications for the patient and for the health services.

Includes: alcoholic hallucinosis
alcoholic jealousy
alcoholic paranoia
alcoholic psychosis NOS

Differential diagnosis. Consider the possibility of another mental disorder being aggravated or precipitated by psychoactive substance use (e.g. schizophrenia (F20. −); mood [affective] disorder (F30 − F39); paranoid or schizoid personality disorder (F60.0, F60.1)). In such cases, a diagnosis of psychoactive substance-induced psychotic state may be inappropriate.

The diagnosis of psychotic state may be further specified by the following five-character codes:

F1x.50 Schizophrenia-like

F1x.51 Predominantly delusional

F1x.52 Predominantly hallucinatory
(includes alcoholic hallucinosis)

F1x.53 Predominantly polymorphic

F1x.54 Predominantly depressive symptoms

F1x.55 Predominantly manic symptoms

F1x.56 Mixed

F1x.6 Amnesic syndrome

A syndrome associated with chronic prominent impairment of recent memory; remote memory is sometimes impaired, while immediate recall is preserved. Disturbances of time sense and ordering of events are usually evident, as are difficulties in learning new material. Confabulation may be marked but is not invariably present. Other cognitive functions are usually relatively well preserved and amnesic defects are out of proportion to other disturbances.

Diagnostic guidelines

Amnesic syndrome induced by alcohol or other psychoactive substances coded here should meet the general criteria for organic amnesic syndrome (see F04). The primary requirements for this diagnosis are:

(a) memory impairment as shown in impairment of recent memory (learning of new material); disturbances of time sense (rearrangements of chronological sequence, telescoping of repeated events into one, etc.);
(b) absence of defect in immediate recall, of impairment of consciousness, and of generalized cognitive impairment;
(c) history or objective evidence of chronic (and particularly high-dose) use of alcohol or drugs.

Personality changes, often with apparent apathy and loss of initiative, and a tendency towards self-neglect may also be present, but should not be regarded as necessary conditions for diagnosis.

Although confabulation may be marked it should not be regarded as a necessary prerequisite for diagnosis.

Includes: Korsakov's psychosis or syndrome, alcohol- or other psychoactive substance-induced

Differential diagnosis. Consider: organic amnesic syndrome (nonalcoholic) (see F04); other organic syndromes involving marked impairment of memory (e.g. dementia or delirium) (F00 – F03; F05. –); a depressive disorder (F31 – F33).

81

F1x.7 Residual and late-onset psychotic disorder

A disorder in which alcohol- or psychoactive substance-induced changes of cognition, affect, personality, or behaviour persist beyond the period during which a direct psychoactive substance-related effect might reasonably be assumed to be operating.

Diagnostic guidelines

Onset of the disorder should be directly related to the use of alcohol or a psychoactive substance. Cases in which initial onset occurs later than episode(s) of substance use should be coded here only where clear and strong evidence is available to attribute the state to the residual effect of the substance. The disorder should represent a change from or marked exaggeration of prior and normal state of functioning.

The disorder should persist beyond any period of time during which direct effects of the psychoactive substance might be assumed to be operative (see F1x.0, acute intoxication). Alcohol- or psychoactive substance-induced dementia is not always irreversible; after an extended period of total abstinence, intellectual functions and memory may improve.

The disorder should be carefully distinguished from withdrawal-related conditions (see F1x.3 and F1x.4). It should be remembered that, under certain conditions and for certain substances, withdrawal state phenomena may be present for a period of many days or weeks after discontinuation of the substance.

Conditions induced by a psychoactive substance, persisting after its use, and meeting the criteria for diagnosis of psychotic disorder should not be diagnosed here (use F1x.5, psychotic disorder). Patients who show the chronic end-state of Korsakov's syndrome should be coded under F1x.6.

Differential diagnosis. Consider: pre-existing mental disorder masked by substance use and re-emerging as psychoactive substance-related effects fade (for example, phobic anxiety, a depressive disorder, schizophrenia, or schizotypal disorder). In the case of flashbacks, consider acute and transient psychotic disorders (F23. –). Consider also organic injury and mild or moderate mental retardation (F70 – F71), which may coexist with psychoactive substance misuse.

This diagnostic rubric may be further subdivided by using the following five-character codes:

F1x.70 Flashbacks

May be distinguished from psychotic disorders partly by their episodic nature, frequently of very short duration (seconds or minutes) and by their duplication (sometimes exact) of previous drug-related experiences.

F1x.71 Personality or behaviour disorder

Meeting the criteria for organic personality disorder (F07.0).

F1x.72 Residual affective disorder

Meeting the criteria for organic mood [affective] disorders (F06.3).

F1x.73 Dementia

Meeting the general criteria for dementia as outlined in the introduction to F00 – F09.

F1x.74 Other persisting cognitive impairment

A residual category for disorders with persisting cognitive impairment, which do not meet the criteria for psychoactive substance-induced amnesic syndrome (F1x.6) or dementia (F1x.73).

F1x.75 Late-onset psychotic disorder

F1x.8   Other mental and behavioural disorders

Code here any other disorder in which the use of a substance can be identified as contributing directly to the condition, but which does not meet the criteria for inclusion in any of the above disorders.

F1x.9   Unspecified mental and behavioural disorder

F20 – F29
Schizophrenia, schizotypal and delusional disorders

Overview of this block

F20 Schizophrenia
    F20.0 Paranoid schizophrenia
    F20.1 Hebephrenic schizophrenia
    F20.2 Catatonic schizophrenia
    F20.3 Undifferentiated schizophrenia
    F20.4 Post-schizophrenic depression
    F20.5 Residual schizophrenia
    F20.6 Simple schizophrenia
    F20.8 Other schizophrenia
    F20.9 Schizophrenia, unspecified

A fifth character may be used to classify course:
    F20.x0 Continuous
    F20.x1 Episodic with progressive deficit
    F20.x2 Episodic with stable deficit
    F20.x3 Episodic remittent
    F20.x4 Incomplete remission
    F20.x5 Complete remission
    F20.x8 Other
    F20.x9 Course uncertain, period of observation too short

F21 Schizotypal disorder

F22 Persistent delusional disorders
    F22.0 Delusional disorder
    F22.8 Other persistent delusional disorders
    F22.9 Persistent delusional disorder, unspecified

F23 Acute and transient psychotic disorders
    F23.0 Acute polymorphic psychotic disorder without symptoms of schizophrenia
    F23.1 Acute polymorphic psychotic disorder with symptoms of schizophrenia
    F23.2 Acute schizophrenia-like psychotic disorder
    F23.3 Other acute predominantly delusional psychotic disorder

F23.8   Other acute and transient psychotic disorders

F23.9   Acute and transient psychotic disorder, unspecified

A fifth character may be used to identify the presence or absence of associated acute stress:

F23.x0 Without associated acute stress

F23.x1 With associated acute stress

F24 Induced delusional disorder

F25 Schizoaffective disorders

F25.0   Schizoaffective disorder, manic type

F25.1   Schizoaffective disorder, depressive type

F25.2   Schizoaffective disorder, mixed type

F25.8   Other schizoaffective disorders

F25.9   Schizoaffective disorder, unspecified

F28 Other nonorganic psychotic disorders

F29 Unspecified nonorganic psychosis

Introduction

Schizophrenia is the commonest and most important disorder of this group. Schizotypal disorder possesses many of the characteristic features of schizophrenic disorders and is probably genetically related to them; however, the hallucinations, delusions, and gross behavioural disturbances of schizophrenia itself are absent and so this disorder does not always come to medical attention. Most of the delusional disorders are probably unrelated to schizophrenia, although they may be difficult to distinguish clinically, particularly in their early stages. They form a heterogeneous and poorly understood collection of disorders, which can conveniently be divided according to their typical duration into a group of persistent delusional disorders and a larger group of acute and transient psychotic disorders. The latter appear to be particularly common in developing countries. The subdivisions listed here should be regarded as provisional. Schizoaffective disorders have been retained in this section in spite of their controversial nature.

F20 Schizophrenia

The schizophrenic disorders are characterized in general by fundamental and characteristic distortions of thinking and perception, and by inappropriate or blunted affect. Clear consciousness and intellectual capacity are usually maintained, although certain cognitive deficits may evolve in the course of time. The disturbance involves the most basic functions that give the normal person a feeling of individuality, uniqueness, and self-direction. The most intimate thoughts, feelings, and acts are often felt to be known to or shared by others, and explanatory delusions may develop, to the effect that natural or supernatural forces are at work to influence the afflicted individual's thoughts and actions in ways that are often bizarre. The individual may see himself or herself as the pivot of all that happens. Hallucinations, especially auditory, are common and may comment on the individual's behaviour or thoughts. Perception is frequently disturbed in other ways: colours or sounds may seem unduly vivid or altered in quality, and irrelevant features of ordinary things may appear more important than the whole object or situation. Perplexity is also common early on and frequently leads to a belief that everyday situations possess a special, usually sinister, meaning intended uniquely for the individual. In the characteristic schizophrenic disturbance of thinking, peripheral and irrelevant features of a total concept, which are inhibited in normal directed mental activity, are brought to the fore and utilized in place of those that are relevant and appropriate to the situation. Thus thinking becomes vague, elliptical, and obscure, and its expression in speech sometimes incomprehensible. Breaks and interpolations in the train of thought are frequent, and thoughts may seem to be withdrawn by some outside agency. Mood is characteristically shallow, capricious, or incongruous. Ambivalence and disturbance of volition may appear as inertia, negativism, or stupor. Catatonia may be present. The onset may be acute, with seriously disturbed behaviour, or insidious, with a gradual development of odd ideas and conduct. The course of the disorder shows equally great variation and is by no means inevitably chronic or deteriorating (the course is specified by five-character categories). In a proportion of cases, which may vary in different cultures and populations, the outcome is complete, or nearly complete, recovery. The sexes are approximately equally affected but the onset tends to be later in women.

Although no strictly pathognomonic symptoms can be identified, for practical purposes it is useful to divide the above symptoms into groups that have special importance for the diagnosis and often occur together, such as:

(a) thought echo, thought insertion or withdrawal, and thought broadcasting;

(b) delusions of control, influence, or passivity, clearly referred to body or limb movements or specific thoughts, actions, or sensations; delusional perception;

(c) hallucinatory voices giving a running commentary on the patient's behaviour, or discussing the patient among themselves, or other types of hallucinatory voices coming from some part of the body;

(d) persistent delusions of other kinds that are culturally inappropriate and completely impossible, such as religious or political identity, or superhuman powers and abilities (e.g. being able to control the weather, or being in communication with aliens from another world);

(e) persistent hallucinations in any modality, when accompanied either by fleeting or half-formed delusions without clear affective content, or by persistent over-valued ideas, or when occurring every day for weeks or months on end;

(f) breaks or interpolations in the train of thought, resulting in incoherence or irrelevant speech, or neologisms;

(g) catatonic behaviour, such as excitement, posturing, or waxy flexibility, negativism, mutism, and stupor;

(h) "negative" symptoms such as marked apathy, paucity of speech, and blunting or incongruity of emotional responses, usually resulting in social withdrawal and lowering of social performance; it must be clear that these are not due to depression or to neuroleptic medication;

(i) a significant and consistent change in the overall quality of some aspects of personal behaviour, manifest as loss of interest, aimlessness, idleness, a self-absorbed attitude, and social withdrawal.

Diagnostic guidelines

The normal requirement for a diagnosis of schizophrenia is that a minimum of one very clear symptom (and usually two or more if less clear-cut) belonging to any one of the groups listed as (a) to (d) above, or symptoms from at least two of the groups referred to as (e) to (h), should have been clearly present for most of the time *during a period of 1 month or more.* Conditions meeting such symptomatic requirements but of duration less than 1 month (whether treated or not) should be diagnosed in the first instance as acute schizophrenia-like psychotic disorder (F23.2) and reclassified as schizophrenia if the symptoms persist for longer periods. Symptom (i) in the above list applies only to a diagnosis of simple schizophrenia (F20.6), and a duration of at least one year is required.

Viewed retrospectively, it may be clear that a prodromal phase in which symptoms and behaviour, such as loss of interest in work, social activities, and personal appearance and hygiene, together with generalized anxiety and mild degrees of depression and preoccupation, preceded the onset of psychotic symptoms by weeks or even months. Because of the difficulty in timing onset, the 1-month duration criterion applies only to the specific symptoms listed above and not to any prodromal nonpsychotic phase.

The diagnosis of schizophrenia should not be made in the presence of extensive depressive or manic symptoms unless it is clear that schizophrenic symptoms antedated the affective disturbance. If both schizophrenic and affective symptoms develop together and are evenly balanced, the diagnosis of schizoaffective disorder (F25. –) should be made, even if the schizophrenic symptoms by themselves would have justified the diagnosis of schizophrenia. Schizophrenia should not be diagnosed in the presence of overt brain disease or during states of drug intoxication or withdrawal. Similar disorders developing in the presence of epilepsy or other brain disease should be coded under F06.2 and those induced by drugs under F1*x*.5.

Pattern of course

The course of schizophrenic disorders can be classified by using the following five-character codes:

F20.*x*0 Continuous
F20.*x*1 Episodic with progressive deficit
F20.*x*2 Episodic with stable deficit
F20.*x*3 Episodic remittent
F20.*x*4 Incomplete remission
F20.*x*5 Complete remission
F20.*x*8 Other
F20.*x*9 Course uncertain, period of observation too short

F20.0 Paranoid schizophrenia

This is the commonest type of schizophrenia in most parts of the world. The clinical picture is dominated by relatively stable, often paranoid, delusions, usually accompanied by hallucinations, particularly of the auditory variety, and perceptual disturbances. Disturbances of affect, volition, and speech, and catatonic symptoms, are not prominent.

Examples of the most common paranoid symptoms are:

(a) delusions of persecution, reference, exalted birth, special mission, bodily change, or jealousy;
(b) hallucinatory voices that threaten the patient or give commands, or auditory hallucinations without verbal form, such as whistling, humming, or laughing;
(c) hallucinations of smell or taste, or of sexual or other bodily sensations; visual hallucinations may occur but are rarely predominant.

Thought disorder may be obvious in acute states, but if so it does not prevent the typical delusions or hallucinations from being described clearly. Affect is usually less blunted than in other varieties of schizophrenia, but a minor degree of incongruity is common, as are mood disturbances such as irritability, sudden anger, fearfulness, and suspicion. "Negative" symptoms such as blunting of affect and impaired volition are often present but do not dominate the clinical picture.

The course of paranoid schizophrenia may be episodic, with partial or complete remissions, or chronic. In chronic cases, the florid symptoms persist over years and it is difficult to distinguish discrete episodes. The onset tends to be later than in the hebephrenic and catatonic forms.

Diagnostic guidelines

The general criteria for a diagnosis of schizophrenia (see introduction to F20 above) must be satisfied. In addition, hallucinations and/or delusions must be prominent, and disturbances of affect, volition and speech, and catatonic symptoms must be relatively inconspicuous. The hallucinations will usually be of the kind described in (b) and (c) above. Delusions can be of almost any kind but delusions of control, influence, or passivity, and persecutory beliefs of various kinds are the most characteristic.

Includes: paraphrenic schizophrenia

Differential diagnosis. It is important to exclude epileptic and drug-induced psychoses, and to remember that persecutory delusions might carry little diagnostic weight in people from certain countries or cultures.

Excludes: involutional paranoid state (F22.8)
paranoia (F22.0)

F20.1 Hebephrenic schizophrenia

A form of schizophrenia in which affective changes are prominent, delusions and hallucinations fleeting and fragmentary, behaviour irresponsible and unpredictable, and mannerisms common. The mood is shallow and inappropriate and often accompanied by giggling or self-satisfied, self-absorbed smiling, or by a lofty manner, grimaces, mannerisms, pranks, hypochondriacal complaints, and reiterated phrases. Thought is disorganized and speech rambling and incoherent. There is a tendency to remain solitary, and behaviour seems empty of purpose and feeling. This form of schizophrenia usually starts between the ages of 15 and 25 years and tends to have a poor prognosis because of the rapid development of "negative" symptoms, particularly flattening of affect and loss of volition.

In addition, disturbances of affect and volition, and thought disorder are usually prominent. Hallucinations and delusions may be present but are not usually prominent. Drive and determination are lost and goals abandoned, so that the patient's behaviour becomes characteristically aimless and empty of purpose. A superficial and manneristic preoccupation with religion, philosophy, and other abstract themes may add to the listener's difficulty in following the train of thought.

Diagnostic guidelines

The general criteria for a diagnosis of schizophrenia (see introduction to F20 above) must be satisfied. Hebephrenia should normally be diagnosed for the first time only in adolescents or young adults. The premorbid personality is characteristically, but not necessarily, rather shy and solitary. For a confident diagnosis of hebephrenia, a period of 2 or 3 months of continuous observation is usually necessary, in order to ensure that the characteristic behaviours described above are sustained.

Includes: disorganized schizophrenia
hebephrenia

F20.2   Catatonic schizophrenia
Prominent psychomotor disturbances are essential and dominant features and may alternate between extremes such as hyperkinesis and stupor, or automatic obedience and negativism. Constrained attitudes and postures may be maintained for long periods. Episodes of violent excitement may be a striking feature of the condition.

For reasons that are poorly understood, catatonic schizophrenia is now rarely seen in industrial countries, though it remains common elsewhere. These catatonic phenomena may be combined with a dream-like (oneiroid) state with vivid scenic hallucinations.

Diagnostic guidelines

The general criteria for a diagnosis of schizophrenia (see introduction to F20 above) must be satisfied. Transitory and isolated catatonic symptoms may occur in the context of any other subtype of schizophrenia, but for a diagnosis of catatonic schizophrenia one or more of the following behaviours should dominate the clinical picture:

(a) stupor (marked decrease in reactivity to the environment and in spontaneous movements and activity) or mutism;

(b) excitement (apparently purposeless motor activity, not influenced by external stimuli);

(c) posturing (voluntary assumption and maintenance of inappropriate or bizarre postures);

(d) negativism (an apparently motiveless resistance to all instructions or attempts to be moved, or movement in the opposite direction);

(e) rigidity (maintenance of a rigid posture against efforts to be moved);

(f) waxy flexibility (maintenance of limbs and body in externally imposed positions); and

(g) other symptoms such as command automatism (automatic compliance with instructions), and perseveration of words and phrases.

In uncommunicative patients with behavioural manifestations of catatonic disorder, the diagnosis of schizophrenia may have to be provisional until adequate evidence of the presence of other symptoms is obtained. It is also vital to appreciate that catatonic symptoms are not diagnostic of schizophrenia. A catatonic symptom or symptoms may also be provoked by brain disease, metabolic disturbances, or alcohol and drugs, and may also occur in mood disorders.

Includes: catatonic stupor
schizophrenic catalepsy
schizophrenic catatonia
schizophrenic flexibilitas cerea

F20.3   Undifferentiated schizophrenia

Conditions meeting the general diagnostic criteria for schizophrenia (see introduction to F20 above) but not conforming to any of the above subtypes (F20.0 – F20.2), or exhibiting the features of more than one of them without a clear predominance of a particular set of diagnostic characteristics. This rubric should be used only for psychotic conditions (i.e. residual schizophrenia, F20.5, and post-schizophrenic depression, F20.4, are excluded) and after an attempt has been made to classify the condition into one of the three preceding categories.

Diagnostic guidelines

This category should be reserved for disorders that:

(a) meet the general criteria for schizophrenia;
(b) are either without sufficient symptoms to meet the criteria for only one of the subtypes F20.1, F20.2, F20.4, or F20.5, or with so many symptoms that more than one of the paranoid (F20.0), hebephrenic (F20.1), or catatonic (F20.4) subtypes are met.

Includes: atypical schizophrenia

F20.4 Post-schizophrenic depression

A depressive episode, which may be prolonged, arising in the aftermath of a schizophrenic illness. Some schizophrenic symptoms must still be present but no longer dominate the clinical picture. These persisting schizophrenic symptoms may be "positive" or "negative", though the latter are more common. It is uncertain, and immaterial to the diagnosis, to what extent the depressive symptoms have merely been uncovered by the resolution of earlier psychotic symptoms (rather than being a new development) or are an intrinsic part of schizophrenia rather than a psychological reaction to it. They are rarely sufficiently severe or extensive to meet criteria for a severe depressive episode (F32.2 and F32.3), and it is often difficult to decide which of the patient's symptoms are due to depression and which to neuroleptic medication or to the impaired volition and affective flattening of schizophrenia itself. This depressive disorder is associated with an increased risk of suicide.

Diagnostic guidelines

The diagnosis should be made only if:

(a) the patient has had a schizophrenic illness meeting the general criteria for schizophrenia (see introduction to F20 above) within the past 12 months;
(b) some schizophrenic symptoms are still present; and
(c) the depressive symptoms are prominent and distressing, fulfilling at least the criteria for a depressive episode (F32. –), and have been present for at least 2 weeks.

If the patient no longer has any schizophrenic symptoms, a depressive episode should be diagnosed (F32. –). If schizophrenic symptoms are still florid and prominent, the diagnosis should remain that of the appropriate schizophrenic subtype (F20.0, F20.1, F20.2, or F20.3).

F20.5 Residual schizophrenia

A chronic stage in the development of a schizophrenic disorder in which there has been a clear progression from an early stage (comprising one or more episodes with psychotic symptoms meeting the general criteria for schizophrenia described above) to a later stage characterized by long-term, though not necessarily irreversible, "negative" symptoms.

Diagnostic guidelines

For a confident diagnosis, the following requirements should be met:

(a) prominent "negative" schizophrenic symptoms, i.e. psychomotor slowing, underactivity, blunting of affect, passivity and lack of initiative, poverty of quantity or content of speech, poor nonverbal communication by facial expression, eye contact, voice modulation, and posture, poor self-care and social performance;

(b) evidence in the past of at least one clear-cut psychotic episode meeting the diagnostic criteria for schizophrenia;

(c) a period of *at least 1 year* during which the intensity and frequency of florid symptoms such as delusions and hallucinations have been minimal or substantially reduced *and* the "negative" schizophrenic syndrome has been present;

(d) absence of dementia or other organic brain disease or disorder, and of chronic depression or institutionalism sufficient to explain the negative impairments.

If adequate information about the patient's previous history cannot be obtained, and it therefore cannot be established that criteria for schizophrenia have been met at some time in the past, it may be necessary to make a provisional diagnosis of residual schizophrenia.

Includes: chronic undifferentiated schizophrenia
"Restzustand"
schizophrenic residual state

F20.6   Simple schizophrenia

An uncommon disorder in which there is an insidious but progressive development of oddities of conduct, inability to meet the demands of society, and decline in total performance. Delusions and hallucinations are not evident, and the disorder is less obviously psychotic than the hebephrenic, paranoid, and catatonic subtypes of schizophrenia. The characteristic ''negative'' features of residual schizophrenia (e.g. blunting of affect, loss of volition) develop without being preceded by any overt psychotic symptoms. With increasing social impoverishment, vagrancy may ensue and the individual may then become self-absorbed, idle, and aimless.

Diagnostic guidelines

Simple schizophrenia is a difficult diagnosis to make with any confidence because it depends on establishing the slowly progressive development of the characteristic ''negative'' symptoms of residual schizophrenia (see F20.5 above) without any history of hallucinations, delusions, or other manifestations of an earlier psychotic episode, and with significant changes in personal behaviour, manifest as a marked loss of interest, idleness, and social withdrawal over a period of at least one year.

Includes: schizophrenia simplex

F20.8   Other schizophrenia

Includes: cenesthopathic schizophrenia
            schizophreniform disorder NOS

Excludes: acute schizophrenia-like disorder (F23.2)
            cyclic schizophrenia (F25.2)
            latent schizophrenia (F23.2)

F20.9   Schizophrenia, unspecified

F21   Schizotypal disorder

A disorder characterized by eccentric behaviour and anomalies of thinking and affect which resemble those seen in schizophrenia, though no definite and characteristic schizophrenic anomalies have occurred at any stage. There is no dominant or typical disturbance, but any of the following may be present:

(a) inappropriate or constricted affect (the individual appears cold and aloof);
(b) behaviour or appearance that is odd, eccentric, or peculiar;
(c) poor rapport with others and a tendency to social withdrawal;
(d) odd beliefs or magical thinking, influencing behaviour and inconsistent with subcultural norms;
(e) suspiciousness or paranoid ideas;
(f) obsessive ruminations without inner resistance, often with dysmorphophobic, sexual or aggressive contents;
(g) unusual perceptual experiences including somatosensory (bodily) or other illusions, depersonalization or derealization;
(h) vague, circumstantial, metaphorical, overelaborate, or stereotyped thinking, manifested by odd speech or in other ways, without gross incoherence;
(i) occasional transient quasi-psychotic episodes with intense illusions, auditory or other hallucinations, and delusion-like ideas, usually occurring without external provocation.

The disorder runs a chronic course with fluctuations of intensity. Occasionally it evolves into overt schizophrenia. There is no definite onset and its evolution and course are usually those of a personality disorder. It is more common in individuals related to schizophrenics and is believed to be part of the genetic "spectrum" of schizophrenia.

Diagnostic guidelines

This diagnostic rubric is not recommended for general use because it is not clearly demarcated either from simple schizophrenia or from schizoid or paranoid personality disorders. If the term is used, three or four of the typical features listed above should have been present, continuously or episodically, for *at least 2 years*. The individual must never have met criteria for schizophrenia itself. A history of schizophrenia in a first-degree relative gives additional weight to the diagnosis but is not a prerequisite.

Includes: borderline schizophrenia
latent schizophrenia
latent schizophrenic reaction
prepsychotic schizophrenia
prodromal schizophrenia
pseudoneurotic schizophrenia

pseudopsychopathic schizophrenia
schizotypal personality disorder

Excludes: Asperger's syndrome (F84.5)
schizoid personality disorder (F60.1)

F22 Persistent delusional disorders

This group includes a variety of disorders in which long-standing delusions constitute the only, or the most conspicuous, clinical characteristic and which cannot be classified as organic, schizophrenic, or affective. They are probably heterogeneous, and have uncertain relationships to schizophrenia. The relative importance of genetic factors, personality characteristics, and life circumstances in their genesis is uncertain and probably variable.

F22.0 Delusional disorder

This group of disorders is characterized by the development either of a single delusion or of a set of related delusions which are usually persistent and sometimes lifelong. The delusions are highly variable in content. Often they are persecutory, hypochondriacal, or grandiose, but they may be concerned with litigation or jealousy, or express a conviction that the individual's body is misshapen, or that others think that he or she smells or is homosexual. Other psychopathology is characteristically absent, but depressive symptoms may be present intermittently, and olfactory and tactile hallucinations may develop in some cases. Clear and persistent auditory hallucinations (voices), schizophrenic symptoms such as delusions of control and marked blunting of affect, and definite evidence of brain disease are all incompatible with this diagnosis. However, occasional or transitory auditory hallucinations, particularly in elderly patients, do not rule out this diagnosis, provided that they are not typically schizophrenic and form only a small part of the overall clinical picture. Onset is commonly in middle age but sometimes, particularly in the case of beliefs about having a misshapen body, in early adult life. The content of the delusion, and the timing of its emergence, can often be related to the individual's life situation, e.g. persecutory delusions in members of minorities. Apart from actions and attitudes directly related to the delusion or delusional system, affect, speech, and behaviour are normal.

97

Diagnostic guidelines

Delusions constitute the most conspicuous or the only clinical characteristic. They must be present for at least 3 months and be clearly personal rather than subcultural. Depressive symptoms or even a full-blown depressive episode (F32. –) may be present intermittently, provided that the delusions persist at times when there is no disturbance of mood. There must be no evidence of brain disease, no or only occasional auditory hallucinations, and no history of schizophrenic symptoms (delusions of control, thought broadcasting, etc.).

Includes: paranoia
paranoid psychosis
paranoid state
paraphrenia (late)
sensitiver Beziehungswahn

Excludes: paranoid personality disorder (F60.0)
psychogenic paranoid psychosis (F23.3)
paranoid reaction (F23.3)
paranoid schizophrenia (F20.0)

F22.8   Other persistent delusional disorders

This is a residual category for persistent delusional disorders that do not meet the criteria for delusional disorder (F22.0). Disorders in which delusions are accompanied by persistent hallucinatory voices or by schizophrenic symptoms that are insufficient to meet criteria for schizophrenia (F20. –) should be coded here. Delusional disorders that have lasted for less than 3 months should, however, be coded, at least temporarily, under F23. – .

Includes: delusional dysmorphophobia
involutional paranoid state
paranoia querulans

F22.9   Persistent delusional disorder, unspecified

F23   Acute and transient psychotic disorders

Systematic clinical information that would provide definitive guidance on the classification of acute psychotic disorders is not yet available, and the limited data and clinical tradition that must therefore be used instead do not give rise to concepts that can be clearly defined and separated from each other. In the absence of a tried and tested multiaxial system, the method used here to avoid diagnostic confusion is to construct a diagnostic sequence that reflects the order of priority given to selected key features of the disorder. The order of priority used here is:

(a) an acute onset (within 2 weeks) as the defining feature of the whole group;
(b) the presence of typical syndromes;
(c) the presence of associated acute stress.

The classification is nevertheless arranged so that those who do not agree with this order of priority can still identify acute psychotic disorders with each of these specified features.

It is also recommended that whenever possible a further subdivision of onset be used, if applicable, for all the disorders of this group. *Acute onset* is defined as a change from a state without psychotic features to a clearly abnormal psychotic state, within a period of 2 weeks or less. There is some evidence that acute onset is associated with a good outcome, and it may be that the more abrupt the onset, the better the outcome. It is therefore recommended that, whenever appropriate, *abrupt onset* (within 48 hours or less) be specified.

The *typical syndromes* that have been selected are first, the rapidly changing and variable state, called here "polymorphic", that has been given prominence in acute psychotic states in several countries, and second, the presence of typical schizophrenic symptoms.

Associated acute stress can also be specified, with a fifth character if desired, in view of its traditional linkage with acute psychosis. The limited evidence available, however, indicates that a substantial proportion of acute psychotic disorders arise without associated stress, and provision has therefore been made for the presence or the absence of stress to be recorded. Associated acute stress is taken to mean

99

that the first psychotic symptoms occur within about 2 weeks of one or more events that would be regarded as stressful to most people in similar circumstances, within the culture of the person concerned. Typical events would be bereavement, unexpected loss of partner or job, marriage, or the psychological trauma of combat, terrorism, and torture. Long-standing difficulties or problems should not be included as a source of stress in this context.

Complete recovery usually occurs within 2 to 3 months, often within a few weeks or even days, and only a small proportion of patients with these disorders develop persistent and disabling states. Unfortunately, the present state of knowledge does not allow the early prediction of that small proportion of patients who will not recover rapidly.

These clinical descriptions and diagnostic guidelines are written on the assumption that they will be used by clinicians who may need to make a diagnosis when having to assess and treat patients within a few days or weeks of the onset of the disorder, not knowing how long the disorder will last. A number of reminders about the time limits and transition from one disorder to another have therefore been included, so as to alert those recording the diagnosis to the need to keep them up to date.

The nomenclature of these acute disorders is as uncertain as their nosological status, but an attempt has been made to use simple and familiar terms. "Psychotic disorder" is used as a term of convenience for all the members of this group (psychotic is defined in the general introduction, page 3) with an additional qualifying term indicating the major defining feature of each separate type as it appears in the sequence noted above.

Diagnostic guidelines

None of the disorders in the group satisfies the criteria for either manic (F30. −) or depressive (F32. −) episodes, although emotional changes and individual affective symptoms may be prominent from time to time.

These disorders are also defined by the absence of organic causation, such as states of concussion, delirium, or dementia. Perplexity, preoccupation, and inattention to the immediate conversation are

100

often present, but if they are so marked or persistent as to suggest delirium or dementia of organic cause, the diagnosis should be delayed until investigation or observation has clarified this point. Similarly, disorders in F23. – should not be diagnosed in the presence of obvious intoxication by drugs or alcohol. However, a recent minor increase in the consumption of, for instance, alcohol or marijuana, with no evidence of severe intoxication or disorientation, should not rule out the diagnosis of one of these acute psychotic disorders.

It is important to note that the 48-hour and the 2-week criteria are not put forward as the times of maximum severity and disturbance, but as times by which the psychotic symptoms have become obvious and disruptive of at least some aspects of daily life and work. The peak disturbance may be reached later in both instances; the symptoms and disturbance have only to be obvious by the stated times, in the sense that they will usually have brought the patient into contact with some form of helping or medical agency. Prodromal periods of anxiety, depression, social withdrawal, or mildly abnormal behaviour do not qualify for inclusion in these periods of time.

A fifth character may be used to indicate whether or nor the acute psychotic disorder is associated with acute stress:

F23.x0 Without associated acute stress

F23.x1 With associated acute stress

F23.0 Acute polymorphic psychotic disorder without symptoms of schizophrenia

An acute psychotic disorder in which hallucinations, delusions, and perceptual disturbances are obvious but markedly variable, changing from day to day or even from hour to hour. Emotional turmoil, with intense transient feelings of happiness and ecstasy or anxieties and irritability, is also frequently present. This polymorphic and unstable, changing clinical picture is characteristic, and even though individual affective or psychotic symptoms may at times be present, the criteria for manic episode (F30. –), depressive episode (F32. –), or schizophrenia (F20. –) are not fulfilled. This disorder is particularly likely to have an abrupt onset (within 48 hours) and a rapid resolution of symptoms; in a large proportion of cases there is no obvious precipitating stress.

If the symptoms persist for more than 3 months, the diagnosis should be changed. (Persistent delusional disorder (F22. –) or other nonorganic psychotic disorder (F28) is likely to be the most appropriate.)

Diagnostic guidelines

For a definite diagnosis:

(a) the onset must be acute (from a nonpsychotic state to a clearly psychotic state within 2 weeks or less);

(b) there must be several types of hallucination or delusion, changing in both type and intensity from day to day or within the same day;

(c) there should be a similarly varying emotional state; and

(d) in spite of the variety of symptoms, none should be present with sufficient consistency to fulfil the criteria for schizophrenia (F20. –) or for manic or depressive episode (F30. – or F32. –).

Includes: bouffée délirante without symptoms of schizophrenia or unspecified
cycloid psychosis without symptoms of schizophrenia or unspecified

F23.1 Acute polymorphic psychotic disorder with symptoms of schizophrenia

An acute psychotic disorder which meets the descriptive criteria for acute polymorphic psychotic disorder (F23.0) but in which typically schizophrenic symptoms are also consistently present.

Diagnostic guidelines

For a definite diagnosis, criteria (a), (b), and (c) specified for acute polymorphic psychotic disorder (F23.0) must be fulfilled; in addition, symptoms that fulfil the criteria for schizophrenia (F20. –) must have been present for the majority of the time since the establishment of an obviously psychotic clinical picture.

If the schizophrenic symptoms persist for more than 1 month, the diagnosis should be changed to schizophrenia (F20. –).

Includes: bouffée délirante with symptoms of schizophrenia
cycloid psychosis with symptoms of schizophrenia

F23.2 Acute schizophrenia-like psychotic disorder

An acute psychotic disorder in which the psychotic symptoms are comparatively stable and fulfil the criteria for schizophrenia (F20. –) but have lasted for less than 1 month. Some degree of emotional variability or instability may be present, but not to the extent described in acute polymorphic psychotic disorder (F23.0).

Diagnostic guidelines

For a definite diagnosis:

(a) the onset of psychotic symptoms must be acute (2 weeks or less from a nonpsychotic to a clearly psychotic state);

(b) symptoms that fulfil the criteria for schizophrenia (F20. –) must have been present for the majority of the time since the establishment of an obviously psychotic clinical picture;

(c) the criteria for acute polymorphic psychotic disorder are not fulfilled.

If the schizophrenic symptoms last for more than 1 month, the diagnosis should be changed to schizophrenia (F20. –).

Includes: acute (undifferentiated) schizophrenia
brief schizophreniform disorder
brief schizophreniform psychosis
oneirophrenia
schizophrenic reaction

Excludes: organic delusional [schizophrenia-like] disorder (F06.2)
schizophreniform disorder NOS (F20.8)

F23.3 Other acute predominantly delusional psychotic disorders

Acute psychotic disorders in which comparatively stable delusions or hallucinations are the main clinical features, but do not fulfil the criteria for schizophrenia (F20. –). Delusions of persecution or reference are common, and hallucinations are usually auditory (voices talking directly to the patient).

Diagnostic guidelines

For a definite diagnosis:

(a) the onset of psychotic symptoms must be acute (2 weeks or less from a nonpsychotic to a clearly psychotic state);

(b) delusions or hallucinations must have been present for the majority of the time since the establishment of an obviously psychotic state; and

(c) the criteria for neither schizophrenia (F20. –) nor acute polymorphic psychotic disorder (F23.0) are fulfilled.

If delusions persist for more than 3 months, the diagnosis should be changed to persistent delusional disorder (F22. –). If only hallucinations persist for more than 3 months, the diagnosis should be changed to other nonorganic psychotic disorder (F28).

Includes: paranoid reaction
psychogenic paranoid psychosis

F23.8 Other acute and transient psychotic disorders

Any other acute psychotic disorders that are unclassifiable under any other category in F23 (such as acute psychotic states in which definite delusions or hallucinations occur but persist for only small proportions of the time) should be coded here. States of undifferentiated excitement should also be coded here if more detailed information about the patient's mental state is not available, provided that there is no evidence of an organic cause.

F23.9 Acute and transient psychotic disorder, unspecified

Includes: (brief) reactive psychosis NOS

F24 Induced delusional disorder

A rare delusional disorder shared by two or occasionally more people with close emotional links. Only one person suffers from a genuine psychotic disorder; the delusions are induced in the other(s) and usually disappear when the people are separated. The psychotic illness of the dominant person is most commonly schizophrenic, but this is not necessarily or invariably so. Both the original delusions in the dominant person and the induced delusions are usually chronic and either persecutory or grandiose in nature. Delusional beliefs are transmitted this way only in uncommon circumstances. Almost invariably, the people concerned have an unusually close relationship and are isolated from others by language, culture, or geography. The individual in whom the delusions are induced is usually dependent on or subservient to the person with the genuine psychosis.

Diagnostic guidelines

A diagnosis of induced delusional disorder should be made only if:

(a) two or more people share the same delusion or delusional system and support one another in this belief;

(b) they have an unusually close relationship of the kind described above;

(c) there is temporal or other contextual evidence that the delusion was induced in the passive member(s) of the pair or group by contact with the active member.

Induced hallucinations are unusual but do not negate the diagnosis. However, if there are reasons for believing that two people living together have independent psychotic disorders neither should be coded here, even if some of the delusions are shared.

Includes: folie à deux
induced paranoid or psychotic disorder
symbiotic psychosis

Excludes: folie simultanée

F25 Schizoaffective disorders

These are episodic disorders in which both affective and schizophrenic symptoms are prominent within the same episode of illness, preferably simultaneously, but at least within a few days of each other. Their relationship to typical mood [affective] disorders (F30 – F39) and to schizophrenic disorders (F20 – F24) is uncertain. They are given a separate category because they are too common to be ignored. Other conditions in which affective symptoms are superimposed upon or form part of a pre-existing schizophrenic illness, or in which they coexist or alternate with other types of persistent delusional disorders, are classified under the appropriate category in F20 – F29. Mood-incongruent delusions or hallucinations in affective disorders (F30.2, F31.2, F31.5, F32.3, or F33.3) do not by themselves justify a diagnosis of schizoaffective disorder.

Patients who suffer from recurrent schizoaffective episodes, particularly those whose symptoms are of the manic rather than the depressive type, usually make a full recovery and only rarely develop a defect state.

Diagnostic guidelines

A diagnosis of schizoaffective disorder should be made only when *both* definite schizophrenic and definite affective symptoms are prominent *simultaneously*, or within a few days of each other, within the same episode of illness, and when, as a consequence of this, the episode of illness does not meet criteria for either schizophrenia or a depressive or manic episode. The term should not be applied to patients who exhibit schizophrenic symptoms and affective symptoms only in different episodes of illness. It is common, for example, for a schizophrenic patient to present with depressive symptoms in the aftermath of a psychotic episode (see post-schizophrenic depression (F20.4)). Some patients have recurrent schizoaffective episodes, which may be of the manic or depressive type or a mixture of the two. Others have one or two schizoaffective episodes interspersed between typical episodes of mania or depression. In the former case, schizoaffective disorder is the appropriate diagnosis. In the latter, the occurrence of an occasional schizoaffective episode does not invalidate a diagnosis of bipolar affective disorder or recurrent depressive disorder if the clinical picture is typical in other respects.

F25.0 Schizoaffective disorder, manic type

A disorder in which schizophrenic and manic symptoms are both prominent in the same episode of illness. The abnormality of mood usually takes the form of elation, accompanied by increased self-esteem and grandiose ideas, but sometimes excitement or irritability are more obvious and accompanied by aggressive behaviour and persecutory ideas. In both cases there is increased energy, overactivity, impaired concentration, and a loss of normal social inhibition. Delusions of reference, grandeur, or persecution may be present, but other more typically schizophrenic symptoms are required to establish the diagnosis. People may insist, for example, that their thoughts are being broadcast or interfered with, or that alien forces are trying to control them, or they may report hearing voices of varied kinds or express bizarre delusional ideas that are not merely grandiose or persecutory. Careful questioning is often required to establish that an individual really is experiencing these morbid phenomena, and not merely joking or talking in metaphors.

Schizoaffective disorders, manic type, are usually florid psychoses with an acute onset; although behaviour is often grossly disturbed, full recovery generally occurs within a few weeks.

Diagnostic guidelines

There must be a prominent elevation of mood, or a less obvious elevation of mood combined with increased irritability or excitement. Within the same episode, at least one and preferably two typically schizophrenic symptoms (as specified for schizophrenia (F20. –), diagnostic guidelines (a) – (d)) should be clearly present.

This category should be used both for a single schizoaffective episode of the manic type and for a recurrent disorder in which the majority of episodes are schizoaffective, manic type.

Includes: schizoaffective psychosis, manic type
schizophreniform psychosis, manic type

F25.1   Schizoaffective disorder, depressive type

A disorder in which schizophrenic and depressive symptoms are both prominent in the same episode of illness. Depression of mood is usually accompanied by several characteristic depressive symptoms or behavioural abnormalities such as retardation, insomnia, loss of energy, appetite or weight, reduction of normal interests, impairment of concentration, guilt, feelings of hopelessness, and suicidal thoughts. At the same time, or within the same episode, other more typically schizophrenic symptoms are present; patients may insist, for example, that their thoughts are being broadcast or interfered with, or that alien forces are trying to control them. They may be convinced that they are being spied upon or plotted against and this is not justified by their own behaviour. Voices may be heard that are not merely disparaging or condemnatory but that talk of killing the patient or discuss this behaviour between themselves. Schizoaffective episodes of the depressive type are usually less florid and alarming than schizoaffective episodes of the manic type, but they tend to last longer and the prognosis is less favourable. Although the majority of patients recover completely, some eventually develop a schizophrenic defect.

Diagnostic guidelines

There must be prominent depression, accompanied by at least two characteristic depressive symptoms or associated behavioural abnormalities as listed for depressive episode (F32. –); within the same episode, at least one and preferably two typically schizophrenic symptoms (as specified for schizophrenia (F20. –), diagnostic guidelines (a) – (d)) should be clearly present.

This category should be used both for a single schizoaffective episode, depressive type, and for a recurrent disorder in which the majority of episodes are schizoaffective, depressive type.

Includes: schizoaffective psychosis, depressive type
schizophreniform psychosis, depressive type

F25.2   Schizoaffective disorder, mixed type
Disorders in which symptoms of schizophrenia (F20. –) coexist with those of a mixed bipolar affective disorder (F31.6) should be coded here.

Includes: cyclic schizophrenia
mixed schizophrenic and affective psychosis

F25.8   Other schizoaffective disorders

F25.9   Schizoaffective disorder, unspecified

Includes: schizoaffective psychosis NOS

F28   Other nonorganic psychotic disorders

Psychotic disorders that do not meet the criteria for schizophrenia (F20. –) or for psychotic types of mood [affective] disorders (F30 – F39), and psychotic disorders that do not meet the symptomatic criteria for persistent delusional disorder (F22. –) should be coded here.

Includes: chronic hallucinatory psychosis NOS

F29   Unspecified nonorganic psychosis

This category should also be used for psychosis of unknown etiology.

Includes: psychosis NOS

Excludes: mental disorder NOS (F99)
            organic or symptomatic psychosis NOS (F09)

F30 – F39
Mood [affective] disorders

Overview of this block

F30 Manic episode
   F30.0 Hypomania
   F30.1 Mania without psychotic symptoms
   F30.2 Mania with psychotic symptoms
   F30.8 Other manic episodes
   F30.9 Manic episode, unspecified

F31 Bipolar affective disorder
   F31.0 Bipolar affective disorder, current episode hypomanic
   F31.1 Bipolar affective disorder, current episode manic without psychotic
        symptoms
   F31.2 Bipolar affective disorder, current episode manic with psychotic
        symptoms
   F31.3 Bipolar affective disorder, current episode mild or moderate
        depression
        .30 Without somatic syndrome
        .31 With somatic syndrome
   F31.4 Bipolar affective disorder, current episode severe depression without
        psychotic symptoms
   F31.5 Bipolar affective disorder, current episode severe depression with
        psychotic symptoms
   F31.6 Bipolar affective disorder, current episode mixed
   F31.7 Bipolar affective disorder, currently in remission
   F31.8 Other bipolar affective disorders
   F31.9 Bipolar affective disorder, unspecified

F32 Depressive episode
   F32.0 Mild depressive episode
        .00 Without somatic syndrome
        .01 With somatic syndrome
   F32.1 Moderate depressive episode
        .10 Without somatic syndrome
        .11 With somatic syndrome
   F32.2 Severe depressive episode without psychotic symptoms
   F32.3 Severe depressive episode with psychotic symptoms

110

F32.8 Other depressive episodes

F32.9 Depressive episode, unspecified

F33 Recurrent depressive disorder

F33.0 Recurrent depressive disorder, current episode mild

.00 Without somatic syndrome

.01 With somatic syndrome

F33.1 Recurrent depressive disorder, current episode moderate

.10 Without somatic syndrome

.11 With somatic syndrome

F33.2 Recurrent depressive disorder, current episode severe without psychotic symptoms

F33.3 Recurrent depressive disorder, current episode severe with psychotic symptoms

F33.4 Recurrent depressive disorder, currently in remission

F33.8 Other recurrent depressive disorders

F33.9 Recurrent depressive disorder, unspecified

F34 Persistent mood [affective] disorders

F34.0 Cyclothymia

F34.1 Dysthymia

F34.8 Other persistent mood [affective] disorders

F34.9 Persistent mood [affective] disorder, unspecified

F38 Other mood [affective] disorders

F38.0 Other single mood [affective] disorders

.00 Mixed affective episode

F38.1 Other recurrent mood [affective] disorders

.10 Recurrent brief depressive disorder

F38.8 Other specified mood [affective] disorders

F39 Unspecified mood [affective] disorder

Introduction

The relationship between etiology, symptoms, underlying biochemical processes, response to treatment, and outcome of mood [affective] disorders is not yet sufficiently well understood to allow their classification in a way that is likely to meet with universal approval. Nevertheless, a classification must be attempted, and that presented here is put forward in the hope that it will at least be acceptable, since it is the result of widespread consultation.

In these disorders, the fundamental disturbance is a change in mood or affect, usually to depression (with or without associated anxiety) or to elation. This mood change is normally accompanied by a change in the overall level of activity, and most other symptoms are either secondary to, or easily understood in the context of, such changes. Most of these disorders tend to be recurrent, and the onset of individual episodes is often related to stressful events or situations. This block deals with mood disorders in all age groups; those arising in childhood and adolescence should therefore be coded here.

The main criteria by which the affective disorders have been classified have been chosen for practical reasons, in that they allow common clinical disorders to be easily identified. Single episodes have been distinguished from bipolar and other multiple episode disorders because substantial proportions of patients have only one episode of illness, and severity is given prominence because of implications for treatment and for provision of different levels of service. It is acknowledged that the symptoms referred to here as "somatic" could also have been called "melancholic", "vital", "biological", or "endogeno-morphic", and that the scientific status of this syndrome is in any case somewhat questionable. It is to be hoped that the result of its inclusion here will be widespread critical appraisal of the usefulness of its separate identification. The classification is arranged so that this somatic syndrome can be recorded by those who so wish, but can also be ignored without loss of any other information.

Distinguishing between different grades of severity remains a problem; the three grades of mild, moderate, and severe have been specified here because many clinicians wish to have them available.

The terms "mania" and "severe depression" are used in this classification to denote the opposite ends of the affective spectrum; "hypomania" is used to denote an intermediate state without delusions, hallucinations, or complete disruption of normal activities, which is often (but not exclusively) seen as patients develop or recover from mania.

F30 Manic episode

Three degrees of severity are specified here, sharing the common underlying characteristics of elevated mood, and an increase in the quantity and speed of physical and mental activity. All the subdivisions of this category should be used only for a single manic episode. If previous or subsequent affective episodes (depressive, manic, or hypomanic), the disorder should be coded under bipolar affective disorder (F31. –).

Includes: bipolar disorder, single manic episode

F30.0 Hypomania

Hypomania is a lesser degree of mania (F30.1), in which abnormalities of mood and behaviour are too persistent and marked to be included under cyclothymia (F34.0) but are not accompanied by hallucinations or delusions. There is a persistent mild elevation of mood (for at least several days on end), increased energy and activity, and usually marked feelings of well-being and both physical and mental efficiency. Increased sociability, talkativeness, overfamiliarity, increased sexual energy, and a decreased need for sleep are often present but not to the extent that they lead to severe disruption of work or result in social rejection. Irritability, conceit, and boorish behaviour may take the place of the more usual euphoric sociability.

Concentration and attention may be impaired, thus diminishing the ability to settle down to work or to relaxation and leisure, but this may not prevent the appearance of interests in quite new ventures and activities, or mild over-spending.

Diagnostic guidelines

Several of the features mentioned above, consistent with elevated or changed mood and increased activity, should be present for at least several days on end, to a degree and with a persistence greater than described for cyclothymia (F34.0). Considerable interference with work or social activity is consistent with a diagnosis of hypomania, but if disruption of these is severe or complete, mania (F30.1 or F30.2) should be diagnosed.

Differential diagnosis. Hypomania covers the range of disorders of mood and level of activities between cyclothymia (F34.0) and mania

113

(F30.1 and F30.2). The increased activity and restlessness (and often weight loss) must be distinguished from the same symptoms occurring in hyperthyroidism and anorexia nervosa; early states of "agitated depression", particularly in late middle-age, may bear a superficial resemblance to hypomania of the irritable variety. Patients with severe obsessional symptoms may be active part of the night completing their domestic cleaning rituals, but their affect will usually be the opposite of that described here.

When a short period of hypomania occurs as a prelude to or aftermath of mania (F30.1 and F30.2), it is usually not worth specifying the hypomania separately.

F30.1　Mania without psychotic symptoms

Mood is elevated out of keeping with the individual's circumstances and may vary from carefree joviality to almost uncontrollable excitement. Elation is accompanied by increased energy, resulting in overactivity, pressure of speech, and a decreased need for sleep. Normal social inhibitions are lost, attention cannot be sustained, and there is often marked distractability. Self-esteem is inflated, and grandiose or over-optimistic ideas are freely expressed.

Perceptual disorders may occur, such as the appreciation of colours as especially vivid (and usually beautiful), a preoccupation with fine details of surfaces or textures, and subjective hyperacusis. The individual may embark on extravagant and impractical schemes, spend money recklessly, or become aggressive, amorous, or facetious in inappropriate circumstances. In some manic episodes the mood is irritable and suspicious rather than elated. The first attack occurs most commonly between the ages of 15 and 30 years, but may occur at any age from late childhood to the seventh or eighth decade.

Diagnostic guidelines

The episode should last for at least 1 week and should be severe enough to disrupt ordinary work and social activities more or less completely. The mood change should be accompanied by increased energy and several of the symptoms referred to above (particularly pressure of speech, decreased need for sleep, grandiosity, and excessive optimism).

F30.2   Mania with psychotic symptoms

The clinical picture is that of a more severe form of mania as described in F30.1. Inflated self-esteem and grandiose ideas may develop into delusions, and irritability and suspiciousness into delusions of persecution. In severe cases, grandiose or religious delusions of identity or role may be prominent, and flight of ideas and pressure of speech may result in the individual becoming incomprehensible. Severe and sustained physical activity and excitement may result in aggression or violence, and neglect of eating, drinking, and personal hygiene may result in dangerous states of dehydration and self-neglect. If required, delusions or hallucinations can be specified as congruent or incongruent with the mood. "Incongruent" should be taken as including affectively neutral delusions and hallucinations; for example, delusions of reference with no guilty or accusatory content, or voices speaking to the individual about events that have no special emotional significance.

Differential diagnosis. One of the commonest problems is differentiation of this disorder from schizophrenia, particularly if the stages of development through hypomania have been missed and the patient is seen only at the height of the illness when widespread delusions, incomprehensible speech, and violent excitement may obscure the basic disturbance of affect. Patients with mania that is responding to neuroleptic medication may present a similar diagnostic problem at the stage when they have returned to normal levels of physical and mental activity but still have delusions or hallucinations. Occasional hallucinations or delusions as specified for schizophrenia (F20. –) may also be classed as mood-incongruent, but if these symptoms are prominent and persistent, the diagnosis of schizoaffective disorder (F25. –) is more likely to be appropriate (see also page 14).

Includes: manic stupor

F30.8   Other manic episodes

F30.9   Manic episode, unspecified

Includes: mania NOS

F31   Bipolar affective disorder

This disorder is characterized by repeated (i.e. at least two) episodes in which the patient's mood and activity levels are significantly disturbed, this disturbance consisting on some occasions of an elevation of mood and increased energy and activity (mania or hypomania), and on others of a lowering of mood and decreased energy and activity (depression). Characteristically, recovery is usually complete between episodes, and the incidence in the two sexes is more nearly equal than in other mood disorders. As patients who suffer only from repeated episodes of mania are comparatively rare, and resemble (in their family history, premorbid personality, age of onset, and long-term prognosis) those who also have at least occasional episodes of depression, such patients are classified as bipolar.

Manic episodes usually begin abruptly and last for between 2 weeks and 4 – 5 months (median duration about 4 months). Depressions tend to last longer (median length about 6 months), though rarely for more than a year, except in the elderly. Episodes of both kinds often follow stressful life events or other mental trauma, but the presence of such stress is not essential for the diagnosis. The first episode may occur at any age from childhood to old age. The frequency of episodes and the pattern of remissions and relapses are both very variable, though remissions tend to get shorter as time goes on and depressions to become commoner and longer lasting after middle age.

Although the original concept of "manic – depressive psychosis" also included patients who suffered only from depression, the term "manic – depressive disorder or psychosis" is now used mainly as a synonym for bipolar disorder.

Includes: manic – depressive illness, psychosis or reaction

Excludes: bipolar disorder, single manic episode (F30. –)
cyclothymia (F34.0)

116

F31.0   Bipolar affective disorder, current episode hypomanic

Diagnostic guidelines

For a definite diagnosis:

(a) the current episode must fulfil the criteria for hypomania (F30.0); and

(b) there must have been at least one other affective episode (hypomanic, manic, depressive, or mixed) in the past.

F31.1   Bipolar affective disorder, current episode manic without psychotic symptoms

Diagnostic guidelines

For a definite diagnosis:

(a) the current episode must fulfil the criteria for mania without psychotic symptoms (F30.1); and

(b) there must have been at least one other affective episode (hypomanic, manic, depressive, or mixed) in the past.

F31.2   Bipolar affective disorder, current episode manic with psychotic symptoms

Diagnostic guidelines

For a definite diagnosis:

(a) the current episode must fulfil the criteria for mania with psychotic symptoms (F30.2); and

(b) there must have been at least one other affective episode (hypomanic, manic, depressive, or mixed) in the past.

If required, delusions or hallucinations may be specified as congruent or incongruent with mood (see F30.2).

F31.3   Bipolar affective disorder, current episode mild or moderate depression

Diagnostic guidelines

For a definite diagnosis:

(a) the current episode must fulfil the criteria for a depressive episode of either mild (F32.0) or moderate (F32.1) severity; and

(b) there must have been at least one hypomanic, manic, or mixed affective episode in the past.

A fifth character may be used to specify the presence or absence of a somatic syndrome in the current episode of depression:

F31.30 Without somatic syndrome

F31.31 With somatic syndrome

F31.4 Bipolar affective disorder, current episode severe depression without psychotic symptoms

Diagnostic guidelines

For a definite diagnosis:

(a) the current episode must fulfil the criteria for a severe depressive episode without psychotic symptoms (F32.2); and

(b) there must have been at least one hypomanic, manic, or mixed affective episode in the past.

F31.5 Bipolar affective disorder, current episode severe depression with psychotic symptoms

Diagnostic guidelines

For a definite diagnosis:

(a) the current episode must fulfil the criteria for a severe depressive episode with psychotic symptoms (F32.3); and

(b) there must have been at least one hypomanic, manic, or mixed affective episode in the past.

If required, delusions or hallucinations may be specified as congruent or incongruent with mood (see F30.2).

F31.6 Bipolar affective disorder, current episode mixed

The patient has had at least one manic, hypomanic, or mixed affective episode in the past and currently exhibits either a mixture or a rapid alternation of manic, hypomanic, and depressive symptoms.

Diagnostic guidelines

Although the most typical form of bipolar disorder consists of alternating manic and depressive episodes separated by periods of normal mood, it is not uncommon for depressive mood to be accompanied for days or weeks on end by overactivity and pressure of speech, or for a manic mood and grandiosity to be accompanied by agitation and loss of energy and libido. Depressive symptoms and symptoms of hypomania or mania may also alternate rapidly, from day to day or even from hour to hour. A diagnosis of mixed bipolar affective disorder should be made only if the two sets of symptoms are both prominent for the greater part of the current episode of illness, and if that episode has lasted for at least 2 weeks.

Excludes: single mixed affective episode (F38.0)

F31.7 Bipolar affective disorder, currently in remission

The patient has had at least one manic, hypomanic, or mixed affective episode in the past and in addition at least one other affective episode of hypomanic, manic, depressive, or mixed type, but is not currently suffering from any significant mood disturbance, and has not done so for several months. The patient may, however, be receiving treatment to reduce the risk of future episodes.

F31.8 Other bipolar affective disorders

Includes: bipolar II disorder
        recurrent manic episodes NOS

F31.9 Bipolar affective disorder, unspecified

F32 Depressive episode

In typical depressive episodes of all three varieties described below (mild (F32.0), moderate (F32.1), and severe (F32.2 and F32.3)), the individual usually suffers from depressed mood, loss of interest and enjoyment, and reduced energy leading to increased fatiguability and diminished activity. Marked tiredness after only slight effort is common. Other common symptoms are:

(a) reduced concentration and attention;
(b) reduced self-esteem and self-confidence;
(c) ideas of guilt and unworthiness (even in a mild type of episode);
(d) bleak and pessimistic views of the future;
(e) ideas or acts of self-harm or suicide;
(f) disturbed sleep;
(g) diminished appetite.

The lowered mood varies little from day to day, and is often unresponsive to circumstances, yet may show a characteristic diurnal variation as the day goes on. As with manic episodes, the clinical presentation shows marked individual variations, and atypical presentations are particularly common in adolescence. In some cases, anxiety, distress, and motor agitation may be more prominent at times than the depression, and the mood change may also be masked by added features such as irritability, excessive consumption of alcohol, histrionic behaviour, and exacerbation of pre-existing phobic or obsessional symptoms, or by hypochondriacal preoccupations. For depressive episodes of all three grades of severity, a duration of at least 2 weeks is usually required for diagnosis, but shorter periods may be reasonable if symptoms are unusually severe and of rapid onset.

Some of the above symptoms may be marked and develop characteristic features that are widely regarded as having special clinical significance. The most typical examples of these "somatic" symptoms (see introduction to this block, page 112) are: loss of interest or pleasure in activities that are normally enjoyable; lack of emotional reactivity to normally pleasurable surroundings and events; waking in the morning 2 hours or more before the usual time; depression worse in the morning; objective evidence of definite psychomotor retardation or agitation (remarked on or reported by other people); marked loss of appetite; weight loss (often defined as 5% or more of body weight in the past month); marked loss of libido. Usually, this somatic syndrome is not regarded as present unless about four of these symptoms are definitely present.

The categories of mild (F32.0), moderate (F32.1) and severe (F32.2 and F32.3) depressive episodes described in more detail below should be used only for a single (first) depressive episode. Further depressive episodes should be classified under one of the subdivisions of recurrent depressive disorder (F33. −).

These grades of severity are specified to cover a wide range of clinical states that are encountered in different types of psychiatric practice. Individuals with mild depressive episodes are common in primary care and general medical settings, whereas psychiatric inpatient units deal largely with patients suffering from the severe grades.

Acts of self-harm associated with mood [affective] disorders, most commonly self-poisoning by prescribed medication, should be recorded by means of an additional code from Chapter XX of ICD-10 (X60 – X84). These codes do not involve differentiation between attempted suicide and "parasuicide", since both are included in the general category of self-harm.

Differentiation between mild, moderate, and severe depressive episodes rests upon a complicated clinical judgement that involves the number, type, and severity of symptoms present. The extent of ordinary social and work activities is often a useful general guide to the likely degree of severity of the episode, but individual, social, and cultural influences that disrupt a smooth relationship between severity of symptoms and social performance are sufficiently common and powerful to make it unwise to include social performance amongst the essential criteria of severity.

The presence of dementia (F00 – F03) or mental retardation (F70 – F79) does not rule out the diagnosis of a treatable depressive episode, but communication difficulties are likely to make it necessary to rely more than usual for the diagnosis upon objectively observed somatic symptoms, such as psychomotor retardation, loss of appetite and weight, and sleep disturbance.

Includes: single episodes of depressive reaction, major depression (without psychotic symptoms), psychogenic depression or reactive depression (F32.0, F32.1 or F32.2)

F32.0   Mild depressive episode

Diagnostic guidelines

Depressed mood, loss of interest and enjoyment, and increased fatiguability are usually regarded as the most typical symptoms of depression, and at least two of these, plus at least two of the other symptoms described on page 119 (for F32. –) should usually be present for a definite diagnosis. None of the symptoms should be present to an intense degree. Minimum duration of the whole episode is about 2 weeks.

An individual with a mild depressive episode is usually distressed by the symptoms and has some difficulty in continuing with ordinary work and social activities, but will probably not cease to function completely.

A fifth character may be used to specify the presence of a somatic syndrome:

F32.00 Without somatic syndrome
The criteria for mild depressive episode are fulfilled, and there are few or none of the somatic symptoms present.

F32.01 With somatic syndrome
The criteria for mild depressive episode are fulfilled, and four or more of the somatic symptoms are also present. (If only two or three somatic symptoms are present but they are unusually severe, use of this category may be justified.)

F32.1 Moderate depressive episode

Diagnostic guidelines

At least two of the three most typical symptoms noted for mild depressive episode (F32.0) should be present, plus at least three (and preferably four) of the other symptoms. Several symptoms are likely to be present to a marked degree, but this is not essential if a particularly wide variety of symptoms is present overall. Minimum duration of the whole episode is about 2 weeks.

An individual with a moderately severe depressive episode will usually have considerable difficulty in continuing with social, work or domestic activities.

A fifth character may be used to specify the occurrence of a somatic syndrome:

F32.10 Without somatic syndrome
The criteria for moderate depressive episode are fulfilled, and few if any of the somatic symptoms are present.

F32.11 With somatic syndrome
The criteria for moderate depressive episode are fulfilled, and four or more or the somatic symptoms are present. (If only two or three somatic symptoms are present but they are unusually severe, use of this category may be justified.)

F32.2 Severe depressive episode without psychotic symptoms

In a severe depressive episode, the sufferer usually shows considerable distress or agitation, unless retardation is a marked feature. Loss of self-esteem or feelings of uselessness or guilt are likely to be prominent, and suicide is a distinct danger in particularly severe cases. It is presumed here that the somatic syndrome will almost always be present in a severe depressive episode.

Diagnostic guidelines

All three of the typical symptoms noted for mild and moderate depressive episodes (F32.0, F32.1) should be present, plus at least four other symptoms, some of which should be of severe intensity. However, if important symptoms such as agitation or retardation are marked, the patient may be unwilling or unable to describe many symptoms in detail. An overall grading of severe episode may still be justified in such instances. The depressive episode should usually last at least 2 weeks, but if the symptoms are particularly severe and of very rapid onset, it may be justified to make this diagnosis after less than 2 weeks.

During a severe depressive episode it is very unlikely that the sufferer will be able to continue with social, work, or domestic activities, except to a very limited extent.

This category should be used only for single episodes of severe depression without psychotic symptoms; for further episodes, a subcategory of recurrent depressive disorder (F33. –) should be used.

Includes: single episodes of agitated depression
melancholia or vital depression without psychotic symptoms

F32.3   Severe depressive episode with psychotic symptoms

Diagnostic guidelines

A severe depressive episode which meets the criteria given for F32.2 above and in which delusions, hallucinations, or depressive stupor are present. The delusions usually involve ideas of sin, poverty, or imminent disasters, responsibility for which may be assumed by the patient. Auditory or olfactory hallucinations are usually of defamatory or accusatory voices or of rotting filth or decomposing flesh. Severe psychomotor retardation may progress to stupor. If required, delusions or hallucinations may be specified as mood-congruent or mood-incongruent (see F30.2).

Differential diagnosis. Depressive stupor must be differentiated from catatonic schizophrenia (F20.2), from dissociative stupor (F44.2), and from organic forms of stupor. This category should be used only for single episodes of severe depression with psychotic symptoms; for further episodes a subcategory of recurrent depressive disorder (F33. –) should be used.

Includes: single episodes of major depression with psychotic symptoms, psychotic depression, psychogenic depressive psychosis, reactive depressive psychosis

F32.8 Other depressive episodes

Episodes should be included here which do not fit the descriptions given for depressive episodes described in F32.0 – F32.3, but for which the overall diagnostic impression indicates that they are depressive in nature. Examples include fluctuating mixtures of depressive symptoms (particularly the somatic variety) with non-diagnostic symptoms such as tension, worry, and distress, and mixtures of somatic depressive symptoms with persistent pain or fatigue not due to organic causes (as sometimes seen in general hospital services).

Includes: atypical depression
single episodes of "masked" depression NOS

F32.9 Depressive episode, unspecified

Includes: depression NOS
depressive disorder NOS

F33 Recurrent depressive disorder

The disorder is characterized by repeated episodes of depression as specified in depressive episode (mild (F32.0), moderate (F32.1)), or severe (F32.2 and F32.3)), without any history of independent episodes of mood elevation and overactivity that fulfil the criteria of mania (F30.1 and F30.2). However, the category should still be used if there is evidence of brief episodes of mild mood elevation and overactivity which fulfil the criteria of hypomania (F30.0) immediately after a depressive episode (sometimes apparently precipitated by treatment of a depression). The age of onset and the severity, duration, and frequency of the episodes of depression are all highly variable. In general, the first episode occurs later than in bipolar disorder, with a mean age of onset in the fifth decade. Individual episodes also last between 3 and 12 months (median duration about 6 months) but recur less frequently. Recovery is usually complete between episodes, but a minority of patients may develop a persistent depression, mainly in old age (for which this category should still be used). Individual episodes of any severity are often precipitated by stressful life events; in many cultures, both individual episodes and persistent depression are twice as common in women as in men.

The risk that a patient with recurrent depressive disorder will have an episode of mania never disappears completely, however many depressive episodes he or she has experienced. If a manic episode does occur, the diagnosis should change to bipolar affective disorder.

Recurrent depressive episode may be subdivided, as below, by specifying first the type of the current episode and then (if sufficient information is available) the type that predominates in all the episodes.

Includes: recurrent episodes of depressive reaction, psychogenic depression, reactive depression, seasonal affective disorder (F33.0 or F33.1)
recurrent episodes of endogenous depression, major depression, manic depressive psychosis (depressed type), psychogenic or reactive depressive psychosis, psychotic depression, vital depression (F33.2 or F33.3)

Excludes: recurrent brief depressive episodes (F38.1)

F33.0 Recurrent depressive disorder, current episode mild

Diagnostic guidelines

For a definite diagnosis:

(a) the criteria for recurrent depressive disorder (F33. –) should be fulfilled, and the current episode should fulfil the criteria for depressive episode, mild severity (F32.0); and

(b) at least two episodes should have lasted a minimum of 2 weeks and should have been separated by several months without significant mood disturbance.

Otherwise, the diagnosis should be other recurrent mood [affective] disorder (F38.1).

A fifth character may be used to specify the presence of a somatic syndrome in the current episode:

F33.00 Without somatic syndrome
(see F32.00)

F33.01 With somatic syndrome
(see F32.01)

If required, the predominant type of previous episodes (mild or moderate, severe, uncertain) may be specified.

F33.1 Recurrent depressive disorder, current episode moderate

Diagnostic guidelines

For a definite diagnosis:

(a) the criteria for recurrent depressive disorder (F33. –) should be fulfilled, and the current episode should fulfil the criteria for depressive episode, moderate severity (F32.1); and
(b) at least two episodes should have lasted a minimum of 2 weeks and should have been separated by several months without significant mood disturbance.

Otherwise the diagnosis should be other recurrent mood [affective] disorder (F38.1).

A fifth character may be used to specify the presence of a somatic syndrome in the current episode:

F33.10 Without somatic syndrome
(see F32.10)

F33.11 With somatic syndrome
(see F32.11)

If required, the predominant type of previous episodes (mild, moderate, severe, uncertain) may be specified.

F33.2   Recurrent depressive disorder, current episode severe without psychotic symptoms

Diagnostic guidelines

For a definite diagnosis:

(a) the criteria for recurrent depressive disorder (F32. –) should be fulfilled, and the current episode should fulfil the criteria for severe depressive episode without psychotic symptoms (F32.2); and

(b) at least two episodes should have lasted a minimum of 2 weeks and should have been separated by several months without significant mood disturbance.

Otherwise the diagnosis should be other recurrent mood [affective] disorder (F38.1).

If required, the predominant type of previous episodes (mild, moderate, severe, uncertain) may be specified.

F33.3   Recurrent depressive disorder, current episode severe with psychotic symptoms

Diagnostic guidelines

For a definite diagnosis:

(a) the criteria for recurrent depressive disorder (F33. –) should be fulfilled, and the current episode should fulfil the criteria for severe depressive episode with psychotic symptoms (F32.3); and

(b) at least two episodes should have lasted a minimum of 2 weeks and should have been separated by several months without significant mood disturbance.

Otherwise the diagnosis should be other recurrent mood [affective] disorder (F38.1).

If required, delusions or hallucinations may be specified as mood-congruent or mood-incongruent (see F30.2).

If required, the predominant type of previous episodes (mild, moderate, severe, uncertain) may be specified.

127

F33.4 Recurrent depressive disorder, currently in remission

Diagnostic guidelines

For a definite diagnosis:

(a) the criteria for recurrent depressive disorder (F33. –) should have been fulfilled in the past, but the current state should not fulfil the criteria for depressive episode of any degree of severity or for any other disorder in F30 – F39; and

(b) at least two episodes should have lasted a minimum of 2 weeks and should have been separated by several months without significant mood disturbance.

Otherwise the diagnosis should be other recurrent mood [affective] disorder (F38.1).

This category can still be used if the patient is receiving treatment to reduce the risk of further episodes.

F33.8 Other recurrent depressive disorders

F33.9 Recurrent depressive disorder, unspecified

Includes: monopolar depression NOS

F34 Persistent mood [affective] disorders

These are persistent and usually fluctuating disorders of mood in which individual episodes are rarely if ever sufficiently severe to warrant being described as hypomanic or even mild depressive episodes. Because they last for years at a time, and sometimes for the greater part of the individual's adult life, they involve considerable subjective distress and disability. In some instances, however, recurrent or single episodes of manic disorder, or mild or severe depressive disorder, may become superimposed on a persistent affective disorder. The persistent affective disorders are classified here rather than with the personality disorders because of evidence from family studies that they are genetically related to the mood disorders, and because they are sometimes amenable to the same treatments as mood disorders. Both early- and late-onset varieties of cyclothymia and dysthymia are described, and should be specified as such if required.

F34.0   Cyclothymia

A persistent instability of mood, involving numerous periods of mild depression and mild elation. This instability usually develops early in adult life and pursues a chronic course, although at times the mood may be normal and stable for months at a time. The mood swings are usually perceived by the individual as being unrelated to life events. The diagnosis is difficult to establish without a prolonged period of observation or an unusually good account of the individual's past behaviour. Because the mood swings are relatively mild and the periods of mood elevation may be enjoyable, cyclothymia frequently fails to come to medical attention. In some cases this may be because the mood change, although present, is less prominent than cyclical changes in activity, self-confidence, sociability, or appetitive behaviour. If required, age of onset may be specified as early (in late teenage or the twenties) or late.

Diagnostic guidelines

The essential feature is a persistent instability of mood, involving numerous periods of mild depression and mild elation, none of which has been sufficiently severe or prolonged to fulfil the criteria for bipolar affective disorder (F31. –) or recurrent depressive disorder (F33. –). This implies that individual episodes of mood swings do not fulfil the criteria for any of the categories described under manic episode (F30. –) or depressive episode (F32. –).

Includes: affective personality disorder
            cycloid personality
            cyclothymic personality

Differential diagnosis. This disorder is common in the relatives of patients with bipolar affective disorder (F31. –) and some individuals with cyclothymia eventually develop bipolar affective disorder themselves. It may persist throughout adult life, cease temporarily or permanently, or develop into more severe mood swings meeting the criteria for bipolar affective disorder (F31. –) or recurrent depressive disorder (F33. –)

F34.1   Dysthymia

A chronic depression of mood which does not currently fulfil the criteria for recurrent depressive disorder, mild or moderate severity (F33.0 or F33.1), in terms of either severity or duration of individual

129

episodes, although the criteria for mild depressive episode may have been fulfilled in the past, particularly at the onset of the disorder. The balance between individual phases of mild depression and intervening periods of comparative normality is very variable. Sufferers usually have periods of days or weeks when they describe themselves as well, but most of the time (often for months at a time) they feel tired and depressed; everything is an effort and nothing is enjoyed. They brood and complain, sleep badly and feel inadequate, but are usually able to cope with the basic demands of everyday life. Dysthymia therefore has much in common with the concepts of depressive neurosis and neurotic depression. If required, age of onset may be specified as early (in late teenage or the twenties) or late.

Diagnostic guidelines

The essential feature is a very long-standing depression of mood which is never, or only very rarely, severe enough to fulfil the criteria for recurrent depressive disorder, mild or moderate severity (F33.0 or F33.1). It usually begins early in adult life and lasts for at least several years, sometimes indefinitely. When the onset is later in life, the disorder is often the aftermath of a discrete depressive episode (F32. –) and associated with bereavement or other obvious stress.

Includes: depressive neurosis
depressive personality disorder
neurotic depression (with more than 2 years' duration)
persistent anxiety depression

Excludes: anxiety depression (mild or not persistent) (F41.2)
bereavement reaction, lasting less than 2 years (F43.21,
prolonged depressive reaction)
residual schizophrenia (F20.5)

F34.8 Other persistent mood [affective] disorders

A residual category for persistent affective disorders that are not sufficiently severe or long-lasting to fulfil the criteria for cyclothymia (F34.0) or dysthymia (F34.1) but that are nevertheless clinically significant. Some types of depression previously called "neurotic" are included here, provided that they do not meet the criteria for either cyclothymia (F34.0) or dysthymia (F34.1) or for depressive episode of mild (F32.0) or moderate (F32.1) severity.

F34.9   Persistent mood [affective] disorder, unspecified

F38 Other mood [affective] disorders

F38.0   Other single mood [affective] disorders

F38.00 Mixed affective episode
An affective episode lasting for at least 2 weeks, characterized by either a mixture or a rapid alternation (usually within a few hours) of hypomanic, manic, and depressive symptoms.

F38.1   Other recurrent mood [affective] disorders

F38.10 Recurrent brief depressive disorder
Recurrent brief depressive episodes, occurring about once a month over the past year. The individual depressive episodes all last less than 2 weeks (typically 2 – 3 days, with complete recovery) but fulfil the symptomatic criteria for mild, moderate, or severe depressive episode (F32.0, F32.1, F32.2).

Differential diagnosis. In contrast to those with dysthymia (F34.1), patients are not depressed for the majority of the time. If the depressive episodes occur only in relation to the menstrual cycle, F38.8 should be used with a second code for the underlying cause (N94.8, other specified conditions associated with female genital organs and menstrual cycle).

F38.8   Other specified mood [affective] disorders
This is a residual category for affective disorders that do not meet the criteria for any other categories F30 – F38.1 above.

F39 Unspecified mood [affective] disorder

To be used only as a last resort, when no other term can be used.

Includes: affective psychosis NOS

Excludes: mental disorder NOS (F99)

F40 – F48
Neurotic, stress-related and somatoform disorders

Overview of this block

F40 Phobic anxiety disorders
F40.0 Agoraphobia
.00 Without panic disorder
.01 With panic disorder
F40.1 Social phobias
F40.2 Specific (isolated) phobias
F40.8 Other phobic anxiety disorders
F40.9 Phobic anxiety disorder, unspecified

F41 Other anxiety disorders
F41.0 Panic disorder [episodic paroxysmal anxiety]
F41.1 Generalized anxiety disorder
F41.2 Mixed anxiety and depressive disorder
F41.3 Other mixed anxiety disorders
F41.8 Other specified anxiety disorders
F41.9 Anxiety disorder, unspecified

F42 Obsessive – compulsive disorder
F42.0 Predominantly obsessional thoughts or ruminations
F42.1 Predominantly compulsive acts [obsessional rituals]
F42.2 Mixed obsessional thoughts and acts
F42.8 Other obsessive – compulsive disorders
F42.9 Obsessive – compulsive disorder, unspecified

F43 Reaction to severe stress, and adjustment disorders
F43.0 Acute stress reaction
F43.1 Post-traumatic stress disorder
F43.2 Adjustment disorders
.20 Brief depressive reaction
.21 Prolonged depressive reaction
.22 Mixed anxiety and depressive reaction
.23 With predominant disturbance of other emotions
.24 With predominant disturbance of conduct
.25 With mixed disturbance of emotions and conduct
.28 With other specified predominant symptoms

F43.8 Other reactions to severe stress

F43.9 Reaction to severe stress, unspecified

F44 Dissociative [conversion] disorders

F44.0 Dissociative amnesia

F44.1 Dissociative fugue

F44.2 Dissociative stupor

F44.3 Trance and possession disorders

F44.4 Dissociative motor disorders

F44.5 Dissociative convulsions

F44.6 Dissociative anaesthesia and sensory loss

F44.7 Mixed dissociative [conversion] disorders

F44.8 Other dissociative [conversion] disorders

    .80 Ganser's syndrome

    .81 Multiple personality disorder

    .82 Transient dissociative [conversion] disorders occurring in childhood and adolescence

    .88 Other specified dissociative [conversion] disorders

F44.9 Dissociative [conversion] disorder, unspecified

F45 Somatoform disorders

F45.0 Somatization disorder

F45.1 Undifferentiated somatoform disorder

F45.2 Hypochondriacal disorder

F45.3 Somatoform autonomic dysfunction

    .30 Heart and cardiovascular system

    .31 Upper gastrointestinal tract

    .32 Lower gastrointestinal tract

    .33 Respiratory system

    .34 Genitourinary system

    .38 Other organ or system

F45.4 Persistent somatoform pain disorder

F45.8 Other somatoform disorders

F45.9 Somatoform disorder, unspecified

F48 Other neurotic disorders

F48.0 Neurasthenia

F48.1 Depersonalization – derealization syndrome

F48.8 Other specified neurotic disorders

F48.9 Neurotic disorder, unspecified

Introduction

Neurotic, stress-related, and somatoform disorders have been brought together in one large overall group because of their historical association with the concept of neurosis and the association of a substantial (though uncertain) proportion of these disorders with psychological causation. As noted in the general introduction to this classification, the concept of neurosis has not been retained as a major organizing principle, but care has been taken to allow the easy identification of disorders that some users still might wish to regard as neurotic in their own usage of the term (see note on neurosis in the general introduction (page 3).

Mixtures of symptoms are common (coexistent depression and anxiety being by far the most frequent), particularly in the less severe varieties of these disorders often seen in primary care. Although efforts should be made to decide which is the predominant syndrome, a category is provided for those cases of mixed depression and anxiety in which it would be artificial to force a decision (F41.2).

F40 Phobic anxiety disorders

In this group of disorders, anxiety is evoked only, or predominantly, by certain well-defined situations or objects (external to the individual) which are not currently dangerous. As a result, these situations or objects are characteristically avoided or endured with dread. Phobic anxiety is indistinguishable subjectively, physiologically, and behaviourally from other types of anxiety and may vary in severity from mild unease to terror. The individual's concern may focus on individual symptoms such as palpitations or feeling faint and is often associated with secondary fears of dying, losing control, or going mad. The anxiety is not relieved by the knowledge that other people do not regard the situation in question as dangerous or threatening. Mere contemplation of entry to the phobic situation usually generates anticipatory anxiety.

The adoption of the criterion that the phobic object or situation is external to the subject implies that many of the fears relating to the presence of disease (nosophobia) and disfigurement (dysmorphobia) are now classified under F45.2 (hypochondriacal disorder). However, if the fear of disease arises predominantly and repeatedly from possible exposure to infection or contamination, or is simply a fear of medical procedures (injections, operations, etc.) or medical establishments (dentists' surgeries, hospitals, etc.), a category from F40. – will be appropriate (usually F 40.2, specific phobia).

Phobic anxiety often coexists with depression. Pre-existing phobic anxiety almost invariably gets worse during an intercurrent depressive episode. Some depressive episodes are accompanied by temporary phobic anxiety and a depressive mood often accompanies some phobias, particularly agoraphobia. Whether two diagnoses, phobic anxiety and depressive episode, are needed or only one is determined by whether one disorder developed clearly before the other and by whether one is clearly predominant at the time of diagnosis. If the criteria for depressive disorder were met before the phobic symptoms first appeared, the former should be given diagnostic precedence (see note in Introduction, pages 6 and 7).

Most phobic disorders other than social phobias are more common in women than in men.

In this classification, a panic attack (F41.0) occurring in an established phobic situation is regarded as an expression of the severity of the phobia, which should be given diagnostic precedence. Panic disorder as a main diagnosis should be diagnosed only in the absence of any of the phobias listed in F40. – .

F40.0   Agoraphobia

The term "agoraphobia" is used here with a wider meaning than it had when originally introduced and as it is still used in some countries. It is now taken to include fears not only of open spaces but also of related aspects such as the presence of crowds and the difficulty of immediate easy escape to a safe place (usually home). The term therefore refers to an interrelated and often overlapping cluster of phobias embracing fears of leaving home: fear of entering shops, crowds, and public places, or of travelling alone in trains, buses, or planes. Although the severity of the anxiety and the extent of avoidance behaviour are variable, this is the most incapacitating of the phobic disorders and some sufferers become completely housebound; many are terrified by the thought of collapsing and being left helpless in public. The lack of an immediately available exit is one of the key features of many of these agoraphobic situations. Most sufferers are women and the onset is usually early in adult life. Depressive and obsessional symptoms and social phobias may also be present but do not dominate the clinical picture. In the absence of effective treatment, agoraphobia often becomes chronic, though usually fluctuating.

Diagnostic guidelines

All of the following criteria should be fulfilled for a definite diagnosis:

(a) the psychological or autonomic symptoms must be primarily manifestations of anxiety and not secondary to other symptoms, such as delusions or obsessional thoughts;

(b) the anxiety must be restricted to (or occur mainly in) at least two of the following situations: crowds, public places, travelling away from home, and travelling alone; and

(c) avoidance of the phobic situation must be, or have been, a prominent feature.

Differential diagnosis. It must be remembered that some agoraphobics experience little anxiety because they are consistently able to avoid their phobic situations. The presence of other symptoms such as depression, depersonalization, obsessional symptoms, and social phobias does not invalidate the diagnosis, provided that these symptoms do not dominate the clinical picture. However, if the patient was already significantly depressed when the phobic symptoms first appeared, depressive episode may be a more appropriate main diagnosis; this is more common in late-onset cases.

The presence or absence of panic disorder (F41.0) in the agoraphobic situation on a majority of occasions may be recorded by means of a fifth character:

F40.00 Without panic disorder

F40.01 With panic disorder

Includes: panic disorder with agoraphobia

F40.1 Social phobias

Social phobias often start in adolescence and are centred around a fear of scrutiny by other people in comparatively small groups (as opposed to crowds), usually leading to avoidance of social situations. Unlike most other phobias, social phobias are equally common in men and women. They may be discrete (i.e. restricted to eating in public, to public speaking, or to encounters with the opposite sex) or diffuse, involving almost all social situations outside the family circle. A fear of vomiting in public may be important. Direct eye-to-eye confrontation may be particularly stressful in some cultures. Social phobias are usually associated with low self-esteem and fear of criticism. They may present as a complaint of blushing, hand tremor, nausea, or urgency of micturition, the individual sometimes being convinced that one of these secondary manifestations of anxiety is the primary problem; symptoms may progress to panic attacks. Avoidance is often marked, and in extreme cases may result in almost complete social isolation.

Diagnostic guidelines

All of the following criteria should be fulfilled for a definite diagnosis:

(a) the psychological, behavioural, or autonomic symptoms must be primarily manifestations of anxiety and not secondary to other symptoms such as delusions or obsessional thoughts;

(b) the anxiety must be restricted to or predominate in particular social situations; and

(c) the phobic situation is avoided whenever possible.

Includes: anthropophobia
social neurosis

Differential diagnosis. Agoraphobia and depressive disorders are often prominent, and may both contribute to sufferers becoming "housebound". If the distinction between social phobia and agoraphobia is very difficult, precedence should be given to agoraphobia; a depressive diagnosis should not be made unless a full depressive syndrome can be identified clearly.

F40.2 Specific (isolated) phobias

These are phobias restricted to highly specific situations such as proximity to particular animals, heights, thunder, darkness, flying, closed spaces, urinating or defecating in public toilets, eating certain foods, dentistry, the sight of blood or injury, and the fear of exposure to specific diseases. Although the triggering situation is discrete, contact with it can evoke panic as in agoraphobia or social phobias. Specific phobias usually arise in childhood or early adult life and can persist for decades if they remain untreated. The seriousness of the resulting handicap depends on how easy it is for the sufferer to avoid the phobic situation. Fear of the phobic situation tends not to fluctuate, in contrast to agoraphobia. Radiation sickness and venereal infections and, more recently, AIDS are common subjects of disease phobias.

Diagnostic guidelines

All of the following should be fulfilled for a definite diagnosis:

(a) the psychological or autonomic symptoms must be primary manifestations of anxiety, and not secondary to other symptoms such as delusion or obsessional thought;
(b) the anxiety must be restricted to the presence of the particular phobic object or situation; and
(c) the phobic situation is avoided whenever possible.

Includes: acrophobia
animal phobias
claustrophobia
examination phobia
simple phobia

Differential diagnosis. It is usual for there to be no other psychiatric symptoms, in contrast to agoraphobia and social phobias. Blood-injury phobias differ from others in leading to bradycardia and sometimes syncope, rather than tachycardia. Fears of specific diseases such as cancer, heart disease, or venereal infection should be classified under hypochondriacal disorder (F45.2), unless they relate to specific situations where the disease might be acquired. If the conviction of disease reaches delusional intensity, the diagnosis should be delusional disorder (F22.0). Individuals who are convinced that they have an abnormality or disfigurement of a specific bodily (often facial) part, which is not objectively noticed by others (sometimes termed dysmorphophobia), should be classified under hypochondriacal disorder (F45.2) or delusional disorder (F22.0), depending upon the strength and persistence of their conviction.

F40.8   Other phobic anxiety disorders

F40.9 Phobic anxiety disorder, unspecified

Includes: phobia NOS
phobic states NOS

F41 Other anxiety disorders

Manifestations of anxiety are the major symptoms of these disorders and are not restricted to any particular environmental situation. Depressive and obsessional symptoms, and even some elements of phobic anxiety, may also be present, provided that they are clearly secondary or less severe.

F41.0 Panic disorder [episodic paroxysmal anxiety]

The essential features are recurrent attacks of severe anxiety (panic) which are not restricted to any particular situation or set of circumstances, and which are therefore unpredictable. As in other anxiety disorders, the dominant symptoms vary from person to person, but sudden onset of palpitations, chest pain, choking sensations, dizziness, and feelings of unreality (depersonalization or derealization) are common. There is also, almost invariably, a secondary fear of dying, losing control, or going mad. Individual attacks usually last for minutes only, though sometimes longer; their frequency and the course of the disorder are both rather variable. An individual in a panic attack often experiences a crescendo of fear and autonomic symptoms which results in an exit, usually hurried, from wherever he or she may be. If this occurs in a specific situation, such as on a bus or in a crowd, the patient may subsequently avoid that situation. Similarly, frequent and unpredictable panic attacks produce fear of being alone or going into public places. A panic attack is often followed by a persistent fear of having another attack.

Diagnostic guidelines

In this classification, a panic attack that occurs in an established phobic situation is regarded as an expression of the severity of the phobia, which should be given diagnostic precedence. Panic disorder should be the main diagnosis only in the absence of any of the phobias in F40. – .

For a definite diagnosis, several severe attacks of autonomic anxiety should have occurred within a period of about 1 month:

(a) in circumstances where there is no objective danger;

(b) without being confined to known or predictable situations; and

(c) with comparative freedom from anxiety symptoms between attacks (although anticipatory anxiety is common).

Includes: panic attack
          panic state

Differential diagnosis. Panic disorder must be distinguished from panic attacks occurring as part of established phobic disorders as already noted. Panic attacks may be secondary to depressive disorders, particularly in men, and if the criteria for a depressive disorder are fulfilled at the same time, the panic disorder should not be given as the main diagnosis.

F41.1   Generalized anxiety disorder

The essential feature is anxiety, which is generalized and persistent but not restricted to, or even strongly predominating in, any particular environmental circumstances (i.e. it is "free-floating"). As in other anxiety disorders the dominant symptoms are highly variable, but complaints of continuous feelings of nervousness, trembling, muscular tension, sweating, lightheadedness, palpitations, dizziness, and epigastric discomfort are common. Fears that the sufferer or a relative will shortly become ill or have an accident are often expressed, together with a variety of other worries and forebodings. This disorder is more common in women, and often related to chronic environmental stress. Its course is variable but tends to be fluctuating and chronic.

Diagnostic guidelines

The sufferer must have primary symptoms of anxiety most days for at least several weeks at a time, and usually for several months. These symptoms should usually involve elements of:

(a) apprehension (worries about future misfortunes, feeling "on edge", difficulty in concentrating, etc.);

(b) motor tension (restless fidgeting, tension headaches, trembling, inability to relax); and

(c) autonomic overactivity (lightheadedness, sweating, tachycardia or tachypnoea, epigastric discomfort, dizziness, dry mouth, etc.).

In children, frequent need for reassurance and recurrent somatic complaints may be prominent.

The transient appearance (for a few days at a time) of other symptoms, particularly depression, does not rule out generalized anxiety disorder as a main diagnosis, but the sufferer must not meet the full criteria for depressive episode (F32. –), phobic anxiety disorder (F40. –), panic disorder (F41.0), or obsessive – compulsive disorder (F42. –)

Includes: anxiety neurosis
anxiety reaction
anxiety state

Excludes: neurasthenia (F48.0)

F41.2 Mixed anxiety and depressive disorder

This mixed category should be used when symptoms of both anxiety and depression are present, but neither set of symptoms, considered separately, is sufficiently severe to justify a diagnosis. If severe anxiety is present with a lesser degree of depression, one of the other categories for anxiety or phobic disorders should be used. When both depressive and anxiety syndromes are present and severe enough to justify individual diagnoses, both disorders should be recorded and this category should not be used; if, for practical reasons of recording, only one diagnosis can be made, depression should be given precedence. Some autonomic symptoms (tremor, palpitations, dry mouth, stomach churning, etc.) must be present, even if only intermittently; if only worry or over-concern is present, without autonomic symptoms, this category should not be used. If symptoms that fulfil the criteria for this disorder occur in close association with significant life changes or stressful life events, category F43.2, adjustment disorders, should be used.

Individuals with this mixture of comparatively mild symptoms are frequently seen in primary care, but many more cases exist among the population at large which never come to medical or psychiatric attention.

Includes: anxiety depression (mild or not persistent)

Excludes: persistent anxiety depression (dysthymia) (F34.1)

F41.3   Other mixed anxiety disorders

This category should be used for disorders that meet the criteria for
generalized anxiety disorder (F41.1) and that also have prominent
(although often short-lasting) features of other disorders in F40 – F49,
although the full criteria for these additional disorders are not met.
The commonest examples are obsessive – compulsive disorder
(F42. –), dissociative disorders (F44. –), somatization disorder
(F45.0), undifferentiated somatoform disorder (F45.1), and hypochondriacal disorder (F45.2). If symptoms that fulfil the criteria for this
disorder occur in close association with significant life changes or
stressful life events, category F43.2, adjustment disorders, should
be used.

F41.8   Other specified anxiety disorders

Includes: anxiety hysteria

F41.9   Anxiety disorder, unspecified

Includes: anxiety NOS

F42 Obsessive – compulsive disorder

The essential feature of this disorder is recurrent obsessional thoughts
or compulsive acts. (For brevity, ''obsessional'' will be used
subsequently in place of ''obsessive – compulsive'' when referring
to symptoms.) Obsessional thoughts are ideas, images or impulses
that enter the individual's mind again and again in a stereotyped
form. They are almost invariably distressing (because they are violent
or obscene, or simply because they are perceived as senseless) and
the sufferer often tries, unsuccessfully, to resist them. They are,
however, recognized as the individual's own thoughts, even though
they are involuntary and often repugnant. Compulsive acts or rituals
are stereotyped behaviours that are repeated again and again. They
are not inherently enjoyable, nor do they result in the completion
of inherently useful tasks. The individual often views them as
preventing some objectively unlikely event, often involving harm to
or caused by himself or herself. Usually, though not invariably, this
behaviour is recognized by the individual as pointless or ineffectual
and repeated attempts are made to resist it; in very long-standing
cases, resistance may be minimal. Autonomic anxiety symptoms are
often present, but distressing feelings of internal or psychic tension

without obvious autonomic arousal are also common. There is a close relationship between obsessional symptoms, particularly obsessional thoughts, and depression. Individuals with obsessive – compulsive disorder often have depressive symptoms, and patients suffering from recurrent depressive disorder (F33. –) may develop obsessional thoughts during their episodes of depression. In either situation, increases or decreases in the severity of the depressive symptoms are generally accompanied by parallel changes in the severity of the obsessional symptoms.

Obsessive – compulsive disorder is equally common in men and women, and there are often prominent anankastic features in the underlying personality. Onset is usually in childhood or early adult life. The course is variable and more likely to be chronic in the absence of significant depressive symptoms.

Diagnostic guidelines

For a definite diagnosis, obsessional symptoms or compulsive acts, or both, must be present on most days for at least 2 successive weeks and be a source of distress or interference with activities. The obsessional symptoms should have the following characteristics:

(a) they must be recognized as the individual's own thoughts or impulses;
(b) there must be at least one thought or act that is still resisted unsuccessfully, even though others may be present which the sufferer no longer resists;
(c) the thought of carrying out the act must not in itself be pleasurable (simple relief of tension or anxiety is not regarded as pleasure in this sense);
(d) the thoughts, images, or impulses must be unpleasantly repetitive.

Includes: anankastic neurosis
         obsessional neurosis
         obsessive – compulsive neurosis

Differential diagnosis. Differentiating between obsessive – compulsive disorder and a depressive disorder may be difficult because these two types of symptoms so frequently occur together. In an acute episode of disorder, precedence should be given to the symptoms that developed first; when both types are present but neither predominates, it is usually best to regard the depression as primary.

143

In chronic disorders the symptoms that most frequently persist in the absence of the other should be given priority.

Occasional panic attacks or mild phobic symptoms are no bar to the diagnosis. However, obsessional symptoms developing in the presence of schizophrenia, Tourette's syndrome, or organic mental disorder should be regarded as part of these conditions.

Although obsessional thoughts and compulsive acts commonly coexist, it is useful to be able to specify one set of symptoms as predominant in some individuals, since they may respond to different treatments.

F42.0 Predominantly obsessional thoughts or ruminations

These may take the form of ideas, mental images, or impulses to act. They are very variable in content but nearly always distressing to the individual. A woman may be tormented, for example, by a fear that she might eventually be unable to resist an impulse to kill the child she loves, or by the obscene or blasphemous and ego-alien quality of a recurrent mental image. Sometimes the ideas are merely futile, involving an endless and quasi-philosophical consideration of imponderable alternatives. This indecisive consideration of alternatives is an important element in many other obsessional ruminations and is often associated with an inability to make trivial but necessary decisions in day-to-day living.

The relationship between obsessional ruminations and depression is particularly close: a diagnosis of obsessive–compulsive disorder should be preferred only if ruminations arise or persist in the absence of a depressive disorder.

F42.1 Predominantly compulsive acts [obsessional rituals]

The majority of compulsive acts are concerned with cleaning (particularly hand-washing), repeated checking to ensure that a potentially dangerous situation has not been allowed to develop, or orderliness and tidiness. Underlying the overt behaviour is a fear, usually of danger either to or caused by the patient, and the ritual act is an ineffectual or symbolic attempt to avert that danger. Compulsive ritual acts may occupy many hours every day and are sometimes associated with marked indecisiveness and slowness. Overall, they are equally common in the two sexes but hand-washing rituals are more common in women and slowness without repetition is more common in men.

Compulsive ritual acts are less closely associated with depression than obsessional thoughts and are more readily amenable to behavioural therapies.

F42.2 Mixed obsessional thoughts and acts

Most obsessive – compulsive individuals have elements of both obsessional thinking and compulsive behaviour. This subcategory should be used if the two are equally prominent, as is often the case, but it is useful to specify only one if it is clearly predominant, since thoughts and acts may respond to different treatments.

F42.8 Other obsessive – compulsive disorders

F42.9 Obsessive – compulsive disorder, unspecified

F43 Reaction to severe stress, and adjustment disorders

This category differs from others in that it includes disorders identifiable not only on grounds of symptomatology and course but also on the basis of one or other of two causative influences — an exceptionally stressful life event producing an acute stress reaction, or a significant life change leading to continued unpleasant circumstances that result in an adjustment disorder. Less severe psychosocial stress ("life events") may precipitate the onset or contribute to the presentation of a very wide range of disorders classified elsewhere in this work, but the etiological importance of such stress is not always clear and in each case will be found to depend on individual, often idiosyncratic, vulnerability. In other words, the stress is neither necessary nor sufficient to explain the occurrence and form of the disorder. In contrast, the disorders brought together in this category are thought to arise always as a direct consequence of the acute severe stress or continued trauma. The stressful event or the continuing unpleasantness of circumstances is the primary and overriding causal factor, and the disorder would not have occurred without its impact. Reactions to severe stress and adjustment disorders in all age groups, including children and adolescents, are included in this category.

Although each individual symptom of which both the acute stress reaction and the adjustment disorder are composed may occur in other disorders, there are some special features in the way the symptoms are manifest that justify the inclusion of these states as a clinical entity. The third condition in this section — post-traumatic stress disorder — has relatively specific and characteristic clinical features.

These disorders can thus be regarded as maladaptive responses to severe or continued stress, in that they interfere with successful coping mechanisms and thus lead to problems in social functioning.

Acts of self-harm, most commonly self-poisoning by prescribed medication, that are associated closely in time with the onset of either a stress reaction or an adjustment disorder should be recorded by means of an additional X code from ICD-10, Chapter XX. These codes do not allow differentiation between attempted suicide and "parasuicide", both being included in the general category of self-harm.

F43.0   Acute stress reaction

A transient disorder of significant severity which develops in an individual without any other apparent mental disorder in response to exceptional physical and/or mental stress and which usually subsides within hours or days. The stressor may be an overwhelming traumatic experience involving serious threat to the security or physical integrity of the individual or of a loved person(s) (e.g. natural catastrophe, accident, battle, criminal assault, rape), or an unusually sudden and threatening change in the social position and/or network of the individual, such as multiple bereavement or domestic fire. The risk of this disorder developing is increased if physical exhaustion or organic factors (e.g. in the elderly) are also present.

Individual vulnerability and coping capacity play a role in the occurrence and severity of acute stress reactions, as evidenced by the fact that not all people exposed to exceptional stress develop the disorder. The symptoms show great variation but typically they include an initial state of "daze", with some constriction of the field of consciousness and narrowing of attention, inability to comprehend stimuli, and disorientation. This state may be followed either by further withdrawal from the surrounding situation (to the extent of a dissociative stupor — see F44.2), or by agitation and over-activity (flight reaction or fugue). Autonomic signs of panic anxiety (tachycardia, sweating, flushing) are commonly present. The symptoms usually appear within minutes of the impact of the stressful stimulus or event, and disappear within 2 – 3 days (often within hours). Partial or complete amnesia (see F44.0) for the episode may be present.

Diagnostic guidelines

There must be an immediate and clear temporal connection between the impact of an exceptional stressor and the onset of symptoms; onset is usually within a few minutes, if not immediate. In addition, the symptoms:

(a) show a mixed and usually changing picture; in addition to the initial state of "daze", depression, anxiety, anger, despair, overactivity, and withdrawal may all be seen, but no one type of symptom predominates for long;

(b) resolve rapidly (within a few hours at the most) in those cases where removal from the stressful environment is possible; in cases where the stress continues or cannot by its nature be reversed, the symptoms usually begin to diminish after 24 – 48 hours and are usually minimal after about 3 days.

This diagnosis should not be used to cover sudden exacerbations of symptoms in individuals already showing symptoms that fulfil the criteria of any other psychiatric disorder, except for those in F60. – (personality disorders). However, a history of previous psychiatric disorder does not invalidate the use of this diagnosis.

Includes: acute crisis reaction
combat fatigue
crisis state
psychic shock

F43.1 Post-traumatic stress disorder

This arises as a delayed and/or protracted response to a stressful event or situation (either short- or long-lasting) of an exceptionally threatening or catastrophic nature, which is likely to cause pervasive distress in almost anyone (e.g. natural or man-made disaster, combat, serious accident, witnessing the violent death of others, or being the victim of torture, terrorism, rape, or other crime).

Predisposing factors such as personality traits (e.g. compulsive, asthenic) or previous history of neurotic illness may lower the threshold for the development of the syndrome or aggravate its course, but they are neither necessary nor sufficient to explain its occurrence.

Typical symptoms include episodes of repeated reliving of the trauma in intrusive memories ("flashbacks") or dreams, occurring against the persisting background of a sense of "numbness" and emotional blunting, detachment from other people, unresponsiveness to surroundings, anhedonia, and avoidance of activities and situations reminiscent of the trauma. Commonly there is fear and avoidance of cues that remind the sufferer of the original trauma. Rarely, there may be dramatic, acute bursts of fear, panic or aggression, triggered by stimuli arousing a sudden recollection and/or re-enactment of the trauma or of the original reaction to it.

There is usually a state of autonomic hyperarousal with hypervigilance, an enhanced startle reaction, and insomnia. Anxiety and depression are commonly associated with the above symptoms and signs, and suicidal ideation is not infrequent. Excessive use of alcohol or drugs may be a complicating factor.

The onset follows the trauma with a latency period which may range from a few weeks to months (but rarely exceeds 6 months). The course is fluctuating but recovery can be expected in the majority of cases. In a small proportion of patients the condition may show a chronic course over many years and a transition to an enduring personality change (see F62.0).

Diagnostic guidelines

This disorder should not generally be diagnosed unless there is evidence that it arose within 6 months of a traumatic event of exceptional severity. A "probable" diagnosis might still be possible if the delay between the event and the onset was longer than 6 months, provided that the clinical manifestations are typical and no alternative iden-tification of the disorder (e.g. as an anxiety or obsessive – compulsive disorder or depressive episode) is plausible. In addition to evidence of trauma, there must be a repetitive, intrusive recollection or re-enactment of the event in memories, daytime imagery, or dreams. Conspicuous emotional detachment, numbing of feeling, and avoidance of stimuli that might arouse recollection of the trauma are often present but are not essential for the diagnosis. The autonomic disturbances, mood disorder, and behavioural abnormalities all contribute to the diagnosis but are not of prime importance.

The late chronic sequelae of devastating stress, i.e. those manifest decades after the stressful experience, should be classified under F62.0.

Includes: traumatic neurosis

F43.2   Adjustment disorders

States of subjective distress and emotional disturbance, usually interfering with social functioning and performance, and arising in the period of adaptation to a significant life change or to the consequences of a stressful life event (including the presence or possibility of serious physical illness). The stressor may have affected the integrity of an individual's social network (through bereavement or separation experiences) or the wider system of social supports and values (migration or refugee status). The stressor may involve only the individual or also his or her group or community.

Individual predisposition or vulnerability plays a greater role in the risk of occurrence and the shaping of the manifestations of adjustment disorders than it does in the other conditions in F43. – , but it is nevertheless assumed that the condition would not have arisen without the stressor. The manifestations vary, and include depressed mood, anxiety, worry (or a mixture of these), a feeling of inability to cope, plan ahead, or continue in the present situation, and some degree of disability in the performance of daily routine. The individual may feel liable to dramatic behaviour or outbursts of violence, but these rarely occur. However, conduct disorders (e.g. aggressive or dissocial behaviour) may be an associated feature, particularly in adolescents. None of the symptoms is of sufficient severity or prominence in its own right to justify a more specific diagnosis. In children, regressive phenomena such as return to bed-wetting, babyish speech, or thumb-sucking are frequently part of the symptom pattern. If these features predominate, F43.23 should be used.

The onset is usually within 1 month of the occurrence of the stressful event or life change, and the duration of symptoms does not usually exceed 6 months, except in the case of prolonged depressive reaction (F43.21). If the symptoms persist beyond this period, the diagnosis should be changed according to the clinical picture present, and any continuing stress can be coded by means of one of the Z codes in Chapter XXI of ICD-10.

Contacts with medical and psychiatric services because of normal bereavement reactions, appropriate to the culture of the individual concerned and not usually exceeding 6 months in duration, should not be recorded by means of the codes in this book but by a code from Chapter XXI of ICD-10 such as Z63.4 (disappearance or death of family member) plus for example Z71.9 (counselling) or Z73.3 (stress not elsewhere classified). Grief reactions of any duration, considered to be abnormal because of their form or content, should be coded as F43.22, F43.23, F43.24 or F43.25, and those that are still intense and last longer than 6 months as F43.21 (prolonged depressive reaction).

Diagnostic guidelines

Diagnosis depends on a careful evaluation of the relationship between:

(a) form, content, and severity of symptoms;
(b) previous history and personality; and
(c) stressful event, situation, or life crisis.

The presence of this third factor should be clearly established and there should be strong, though perhaps presumptive, evidence that the disorder would not have arisen without it. If the stressor is relatively minor, or if a temporal connection (less than 3 months) cannot be demonstrated, the disorder should be classified elsewhere, according to its presenting features.

Includes: culture shock
grief reaction
hospitalism in children

Excludes: separation anxiety disorder of childhood (F93.0)

If the criteria for adjustment disorder are satisfied, the clinical form or predominant features can be specified by a fifth character:

F43.20 Brief depressive reaction
A transient, mild depressive state of duration not exceeding 1 month.

F43.21 Prolonged depressive reaction

A mild depressive state occurring in response to a prolonged exposure to a stressful situation but of duration not exceeding 2 years.

F43.22 Mixed anxiety and depressive reaction

Both anxiety and depressive symptoms are prominent, but at levels no greater than specified in mixed anxiety and depressive disorder (F41.2) or other mixed anxiety disorder (F41.3).

F43.23 With predominant disturbance of other emotions

The symptoms are usually of several types of emotion, such as anxiety, depression, worry, tensions, and anger. Symptoms of anxiety and depression may fulfil the criteria for mixed anxiety and depressive disorder (F41.2) or other mixed anxiety disorder (F41.3), but they are not so predominant that other more specific depressive or anxiety disorders can be diagnosed. This category should also be used for reactions in children in which regressive behaviour such as bed-wetting or thumb-sucking are also present.

F43.24 With predominant disturbance of conduct

The main disturbance is one involving conduct, e.g. an adolescent grief reaction resulting in aggressive or dissocial behaviour.

F43.25 With mixed disturbance of emotions and conduct

Both emotional symptoms and disturbance of conduct are prominent features.

F43.28 With other specified predominant symptoms

F43.8   Other reactions to severe stress

F43.9   Reaction to severe stress, unspecified

F44   Dissociative [conversion] disorders

The common theme shared by dissociative (or conversion) disorders is a partial or complete loss of the normal integration between memories of the past, awareness of identity and immediate sensations, and control of bodily movements. There is normally a considerable degree of conscious control over the memories and sensations that can be selected for immediate attention, and the movements that are to be carried out. In the dissociative disorders it is presumed that this ability to exercise a conscious and selective control is impaired, to a degree that can vary from day to day or even from hour to hour. It is usually very difficult to assess the extent to which some of the loss of functions might be under voluntary control.

These disorders have previously been classified as various types of "conversion hysteria", but it now seems best to avoid the term "hysteria" as far as possible, in view of its many and varied meanings. Dissociative disorders as described here are presumed to be "psychogenic" in origin, being associated closely in time with traumatic events, insoluble and intolerable problems, or disturbed relationships. It is therefore often possible to make interpretations and presumptions about the individual's means of dealing with intolerable stress, but concepts derived from any one particular theory, such as "unconscious motivation" and "secondary gain", are not included among the guidelines or criteria for diagnosis.

The term "conversion" is widely applied to some of these disorders, and implies that the unpleasant affect, engendered by the problems and conflicts that the individual cannot solve, is somehow transformed into the symptoms.

The onset and termination of dissociative states are often reported as being sudden, but they are rarely observed except during contrived interactions or procedures such as hypnosis or abreaction. Change in or disappearance of a dissociative state may be limited to the duration of such procedures. All types of dissociative state tend to remit after a few weeks or months, particularly if their onset was associated with a traumatic life event. More chronic states, particularly paralyses and anaesthesias, may develop (sometimes more slowly) if they are associated with insoluble problems or interpersonal difficulties. Dissociative states that have endured for more than 1 – 2 years before coming to psychiatric attention are often resistant to therapy.

Individuals with dissociative disorders often show a striking denial of problems or difficulties that may be obvious to others. Any problems that they themselves recognize may be attributed by patients to the dissociative symptoms.

Depersonalization and derealization are *not* included here, since in these syndromes only limited aspects of personal identity are usually affected, and there is no associated loss of performance in terms of sensations, memories, or movements.

Diagnostic guidelines

For a definite diagnosis the following should be present:

(a) the clinical features as specified for the individual disorders in F44. – ;
(b) no evidence of a physical disorder that might explain the symptoms;
(c) evidence for psychological causation, in the form of clear association in time with stressful events and problems or disturbed relationships (even if denied by the individual).

Convincing evidence of psychological causation may be difficult to find, even though strongly suspected. In the presence of known disorders of the central or peripheral nervous system, the diagnosis of dissociative disorder should be made with great caution. In the absence of evidence for psychological causation, the diagnosis should remain provisional, and enquiry into both physical and psychological aspects should continue.

Includes: conversion hysteria
conversion reaction
hysteria
hysterical psychosis

Excludes: malingering [conscious simulation] (Z76.5)

F44.0 Dissociative amnesia

The main feature is loss of memory, usually of important recent events, which is not due to organic mental disorder and is too extensive to be explained by ordinary forgetfulness or fatigue. The amnesia is usually centred on traumatic events, such as accidents or unexpected bereavements, and is usually partial and selective. The extent and completeness of the amnesia often vary from day to day and between investigators, but there is a persistent common core that cannot be recalled in the waking state. Complete and generalized amnesia is rare; it is usually part of a fugue (F44.1) and, if so, should be classified as such.

The affective states that accompany amnesia are very varied, but severe depression is rare. Perplexity, distress, and varying degrees of attention-seeking behaviour may be evident, but calm acceptance is also sometimes striking. Young adults are most commonly affected, the most extreme instances usually occurring in men subject to battle stress. Nonorganic dissociative states are rare in the elderly. Purposeless local wandering may occur; it is usually accompanied by self-neglect and rarely lasts more than a day or two.

Diagnostic guidelines

A definite diagnosis requires:

(a) amnesia, either partial or complete, for recent events that are of a traumatic or stressful nature (these aspects may emerge only when other informants are available);
(b) absence of organic brain disorders, intoxication, or excessive fatigue.

Differential diagnosis. In organic mental disorders, there are usually other signs of disturbance in the nervous system, plus obvious and consistent signs of clouding of consciousness, disorientation, and fluctuating awareness. Loss of very recent memory is more typical of organic states, irrespective of any possibly traumatic events or problems. "Blackouts" due to abuse of alcohol or drugs are closely associated with the time of abuse, and the lost memories can never be regained. The short-term memory loss of the amnesic state (Korsakov's syndrome), in which immediate recall is normal but recall after only 2 – 3 minutes is lost, is not found in dissociative amnesia.

Amnesia following concussion or serious head injury is usually retrograde, although in severe cases it may be anterograde also; dissociative amnesia is usually predominantly retrograde. Only dissociative amnesia can be modified by hypnosis or abreaction. Postictal amnesia in epileptics, and other states of stupor or mutism occasionally found in schizophrenic or depressive illnesses can usually be differentiated by other characteristics of the underlying illness.

The most difficult differentiation is from conscious simulation of amnesia (malingering), and repeated and detailed assessment of premorbid personality and motivation may be required. Conscious simulation of amnesia is usually associated with obvious problems concerning money, danger of death in wartime, or possible prison or death sentences.

Excludes: alcohol- or other psychoactive substance-induced amnesic disorder (F10 – F19 with common fourth character .6)
amnesia NOS (R41.3)
anterograde amnesia (R41.1)
nonalcoholic organic amnesic syndrome (F04)
postictal amnesia in epilepsy (G40. –)
retrograde amnesia (R41.2)

F44.1 Dissociative fugue

Dissociative fugue has all the features of dissociative amnesia, plus an apparently purposeful journey away from home or place of work during which self-care is maintained. In some cases, a new identity may be assumed, usually only for a few days but occasionally for long periods of time and to a surprising degree of completeness. Organized travel may be to places previously known and of emotional significance. Although there is amnesia for the period of the fugue, the individual's behaviour during this time may appear completely normal to independent observers.

Diagnostic guidelines

For a definite diagnosis there should be:

(a) the features of dissociative amnesia (F44.0);
(b) purposeful travel beyond the usual everyday range (the differentiation between travel and wandering must be made by those with local knowledge); and
(c) maintenance of basic self-care (eating, washing, etc.) and simple social interaction with strangers (such as buying tickets or petrol, asking directions, ordering meals).

Differential diagnosis. Differentiation from postictal fugue, seen particularly after temporal lobe epilepsy, is usually clear because of the history of epilepsy, the lack of stressful events or problems, and the less purposeful and more fragmented activities and travel of the epileptic.

As with dissociative amnesia, differentiation from conscious simulation of a fugue may be very difficult.

F44.2 Dissociative stupor

The individual's behaviour fulfils the criteria for stupor, but examination and investigation reveal no evidence of a physical cause. In addition, as in other dissociative disorders, there is positive evidence of psychogenic causation in the form of either recent stressful events or prominent interpersonal or social problems.

Stupor is diagnosed on the basis of a profound diminution or absence of voluntary movement and normal responsiveness to external stimuli such as light, noise, and touch. The individual lies or sits largely motionless for long periods of time. Speech and spontaneous and purposeful movement are completely or almost completely absent. Although some degree of disturbance of consciousness may be present, muscle tone, posture, breathing, and sometimes eye-opening and coordinated eye movements are such that it is clear that the individual is neither asleep nor unconscious.

Diagnostic guidelines

For a definite diagnosis there should be:

(a) stupor, as described above;
(b) absence of a physical or other psychiatric disorder that might explain the stupor; and
(c) evidence of recent stressful events or current problems.

Differential diagnosis. Dissociative stupor must be differentiated from catatonic stupor and depressive or manic stupor. The stupor of catatonic schizophrenia is often preceded by symptoms or behaviour suggestive of schizophrenia. Depressive and manic stupor usually develop comparatively slowly, so a history from another informant should be decisive. Both depressive and manic stupor are increasingly rare in many countries as early treatment of affective illness becomes more widespread.

F44.3 Trance and possession disorders

Disorders in which there is a temporary loss of both the sense of personal identity and full awareness of the surroundings; in some instances the individual acts as if taken over by another personality, spirit, deity, or "force". Attention and awareness may be limited to or concentrated upon only one or two aspects of the immediate environment, and there is often a limited but repeated set of movements, postures, and utterances. Only trance disorders that are involuntary or unwanted, and that intrude into ordinary activities by occurring outside (or being a prolongation of) religious or other culturally accepted situations should be included here.

Trance disorders occurring during the course of schizophrenic or acute psychoses with hallucinations or delusions, or multiple personality should not be included here, nor should this category be used if the trance disorder is judged to be closely associated with any physical disorder (such as temporal lobe epilepsy or head injury) or with psychoactive substance intoxication.

F44.4 – F44.7 Dissociative disorders of movement and sensation

In these disorders there is a loss of or interference with movements or loss of sensations (usually cutaneous). The patient therefore presents as having a physical disorder, although none can be found that would explain the symptoms. The symptoms can often be seen to represent the patient's concept of physical disorder, which may be at variance with physiological or anatomical principles. In addition, assessment of the patient's mental state and social situation usually suggests that the disability resulting from the loss of functions is helping the patient to escape from an unpleasant conflict, or to express dependency or resentment indirectly. Although problems or conflicts may be evident to others, the patient often denies their presence and attributes any distress to the symptoms or the resulting disability.

The degree of disability resulting from all these types of symptom may vary from occasion to occasion, depending upon the number and type of other people present, and upon the emotional state of the patient. In other words, a variable amount of attention-seeking behaviour may be present in addition to a central and unvarying core of loss of movement or sensation which is not under voluntary control.

In some patients, the symptoms usually develop in close relationship to psychological stress, but in others this link does not emerge. Calm acceptance ("belle indifférence") of serious disability may be striking, but is not universal; it is also found in well-adjusted individuals facing obvious and serious physical illness.

Premorbid abnormalities of personal relationships and personality are usually found, and close relatives and friends may have suffered from physical illness with symptoms resembling those of the patient. Mild and transient varieties of these disorders are often seen in adolescence, particularly in girls, but the chronic varieties are usually found in young adults. A few individuals establish a repetitive pattern of reaction to stress by the production of these disorders, and may still manifest this in middle and old age.

Disorders involving only *loss* of sensations are included here; disorders involving additional sensations such as pain, and other complex sensations mediated by the autonomic nervous system are included in somatoform disorders (F45. –).

Diagnostic guidelines

The diagnosis should be made with great caution in the presence of physical disorders of the nervous system, or in a previously well-adjusted individual with normal family and social relationships.

For a definite diagnosis:

(a) there should be no evidence of physical disorder; and
(b) sufficient must be known about the psychological and social setting and personal relationships of the patient to allow a convincing formulation to be made of the reasons for the appearance of the disorder.

The diagnosis should remain probable or provisional if there is any doubt about the contribution of actual or possible physical disorders, or if it is impossible to achieve an understanding of why the disorder has developed. In cases that are puzzling or not clear-cut, the possibility of the later appearance of serious physical or psychiatric disorders should always be kept in mind.

Differential diagnosis. The early stages of progressive neurological disorders, particularly multiple sclerosis and systemic lupus erythematosus, may be confused with dissociative disorders of movement and sensation. Patients reacting to early multiple sclerosis with distress and attention-seeking behaviour pose especially difficult problems; comparatively long periods of assessment and observation may be needed before the diagnostic probabilities become clear.

Multiple and ill-defined somatic complaints should be classified elsewhere, under somatoform disorders (F45. –) or neurasthenia (F48.0).

Isolated dissociative symptoms may occur during major mental disorders such as schizophrenia or severe depression, but these disorders are usually obvious and should take precedence over the dissociative symptoms for diagnostic and coding purposes.

Conscious simulation of loss of movement and sensation is often very difficult to distinguish from dissociation; the decision will rest upon detailed observation, and upon obtaining an understanding of the personality of the patient, the circumstances surrounding the onset of the disorder, and the consequences of recovery versus continued disability.

F44.4   Dissociative motor disorders

The commonest varieties of dissociative motor disorder are loss of ability to move the whole or a part of a limb or limbs. Paralysis may be partial, with movements being weak or slow, or complete. Various forms and variable degrees of incoordination (ataxia) may be evident, particularly in the legs, resulting in bizarre gait or inability to stand unaided (astasia-abasia). There may also be exaggerated trembling or shaking of one or more extremities or the whole body. There may be close resemblance to almost any variety of ataxia, apraxia, akinesia, aphonia, dysarthria, dyskinesia, or paralysis.

Includes: psychogenic aphonia
psychogenic dysphonia

F44.5   Dissociative convulsions

Dissociative convulsions (pseudoseizures) may mimic epileptic seizures very closely in terms of movements, but tongue-biting, serious bruising due to falling, and incontinence of urine are rare in dissociative convulsion, and loss of consciousness is absent or replaced by a state of stupor or trance.

F44.6   Dissociative anaesthesia and sensory loss

Anaesthetic areas of skin often have boundaries which make it clear that they are associated more with the patient's ideas about bodily functions than with medical knowledge. There may also be differential loss between the sensory modalities which cannot be due to a neurological lesion. Sensory loss may be accompanied by complaints of paraesthesia.

Loss of vision is rarely total in dissociative disorders, and visual disturbances are more often a loss of acuity, general blurring of vision, or "tunnel vision". In spite of complaints of visual loss, the patient's general mobility and motor performance are often surprisingly well preserved.

Dissociative deafness and anosmia are far less common than loss of sensation or vision.

Includes: psychogenic deafness

F44.7 Mixed dissociative [conversion] disorders
Mixtures of the disorders specified above (F44.0 – F44.6) should be coded here.

F44.8 Other dissociative [conversion] disorders

F44.80 Ganser's syndrome
The complex disorder described by Ganser, which is characterized by "approximate answers", usually accompanied by several other dissociative symptoms, often in circumstances that suggest a psychogenic etiology, should be coded here.

F44.81 Multiple personality disorder
This disorder is rare, and controversy exists about the extent to which it is iatrogenic or culture-specific. The essential feature is the apparent existence of two or more distinct personalities within an individual, with only one of them being evident at a time. Each personality is complete, with its own memories, behaviour, and preferences; these may be in marked contrast to the single premorbid personality.

In the common form with two personalities, one personality is usually dominant but neither has access to the memories of the other and the two are almost always unaware of each other's existence. Change from one personality to another in the first instance is usually sudden and closely associated with traumatic events. Subsequent changes are often limited to dramatic or stressful events, or occur during sessions with a therapist that involve relaxation, hypnosis, or abreaction.

F44.82 Transient dissociative [conversion] disorders occurring in childhood and adolescence

F44.88 Other specified dissociative [conversion] disorders

Includes: psychogenic confusion
twilight state

F44.9 Dissociative [conversion] disorder, unspecified

F45 Somatoform disorders

The main feature of somatoform disorders is repeated presentation of physical symptoms, together with persistent requests for medical investigations, in spite of repeated negative findings and reassurances by doctors that the symptoms have no physical basis. If any physical disorders are present, they do not explain the nature and extent of the symptoms or the distress and preoccupation of the patient. Even when the onset and continuation of the symptoms bear a close relationship with unpleasant life events or with difficulties or conflicts, the patient usually resists attempts to discuss the possibility of psychological causation; this may even be the case in the presence of obvious depressive and anxiety symptoms. The degree of understanding, either physical or psychological, that can be achieved about the cause of the symptoms is often disappointing and frustrating for both patient and doctor.

In these disorders there is often a degree of attention-seeking (histrionic) behaviour, particularly in patients who are resentful of their failure to persuade doctors of the essentially physical nature of their illness and of the need for further investigations or examinations.

Differential diagnosis. Differentiation from hypochondriacal delusions usually depends upon close acquaintance with the patient. Although the beliefs are long-standing and appear to be held against reason, the degree of conviction is usually susceptible, to some degree and in the short term, to argument, reassurance, and the performance of yet another examination or investigation. In addition, the presence of unpleasant and frightening physical sensations can be regarded as a culturally acceptable explanation for the development and persistence of a conviction of physical illness.

161

Excludes: dissociative disorders (F44. –)
  hair-plucking (F98.4)
  lalling (F80.0)
  lisping (F80.8)
  nail-biting (F98.8)
  psychological or behavioural factors associated with
    disorders or diseases classified elsewhere (F54)
  sexual dysfunction, not caused by organic disorder or
    disease (F52. –)
  thumb-sucking (F98.8)
  tic disorders (in childhood and adolescence) (F95. –)
  Tourette's syndrome (F95.2)
  trichotillomania (F63.3)

F45.0 Somatization disorder

The main features are multiple, recurrent, and frequently changing physical symptoms, which have usually been present for several years before the patient is referred to a psychiatrist. Most patients have a long and complicated history of contact with both primary and specialist medical services, during which many negative investigations or fruitless operations may have been carried out. Symptoms may be referred to any part or system of the body, but gastrointestinal sensations (pain, belching, regurgitation, vomiting, nausea, etc.), and abnormal skin sensations (itching, burning, tingling, numbness, soreness, etc.) and blotchiness are among the commonest. Sexual and menstrual complaints are also common.

Marked depression and anxiety are frequently present and may justify specific treatment.

The course of the disorder is chronic and fluctuating, and is often associated with long-standing disruption of social, interpersonal, and family behaviour. The disorder is far more common in women than in men, and usually starts in early adult life.

Dependence upon or abuse of medication (usually sedatives and analgesics) often results from the frequent courses of medication.

Diagnostic guidelines

A definite diagnosis requires the presence of all of the following:

(a) at least 2 years of multiple and variable physical symptoms for which no adequate physical explanation has been found;

(b) persistent refusal to accept the advice or reassurance of several doctors that there is no physical explanation for the symptoms;

(c) some degree of impairment of social and family functioning attributable to the nature of the symptoms and resulting behaviour.

Includes: Briquet's disorder
multiple complaint syndrome
multiple psychosomatic disorder

Differential diagnosis. In diagnosis, differentiation from the following disorders is essential:

Physical disorders. Patients with long-standing somatization disorder have the same chance of developing independent physical disorders as any other person of their age, and further investigations or consultations should be considered if there is a shift in the emphasis or stability of the physical complaints which suggests possible physical disease.

Affective (depressive) and anxiety disorders. Varying degrees of depression and anxiety commonly accompany somatization disorders, but need not be specified separately unless they are sufficiently marked and persistent as to justify a diagnosis in their own right. The onset of multiple somatic symptoms after the age of 40 years may be an early manifestation of a primarily depressive disorder.

Hypochondriacal disorder. In somatization disorders, the emphasis is on the symptoms themselves and their individual effects, whereas in hypochondriacal disorder, attention is directed more to the presence of an underlying progressive and serious disease process and its disabling consequences. In hypochondriacal disorder, the patient tends to ask for investigations to determine or confirm the nature of the underlying disease, whereas the patient with somatization disorder asks for treatment to remove the symptoms. In somatization disorder there is usually excessive drug use, together with noncompliance over long periods, whereas patients with hypochondriacal disorder fear drugs and their side-effects, and seek for reassurance by frequent visits to different physicians.

Delusional disorders (such as schizophrenia with somatic delusions, and depressive disorders with hypochondriacal delusions). The bizarre qualities of the beliefs, together with fewer physical symptoms of more constant nature, are most typical of the delusional disorders.

Short-lived (e.g. less than 2 years) and less striking symptom patterns are better classified as undifferentiated somatoform disorder (F45.1).

F45.1 Undifferentiated somatoform disorder

When physical complaints are multiple, varying and persistent, but the complete and typical clinical picture of somatization disorder is not fulfilled, this category should be considered. For instance, the forceful and dramatic manner of complaint may be lacking, the complaints may be comparatively few in number, or the associated impairment of social and family functioning may be totally absent. There may or may not be grounds for presuming a psychological causation, but there must be no physical basis for the symptoms upon which the psychiatric diagnosis is based.

If a distinct possibility of underlying physical disorder still exists, or if the psychiatric assessment is not completed at the time of diagnostic coding, other categories from the relevant chapters of ICD-10 should be used.

Includes: undifferentiated psychosomatic disorder

Differential diagnosis. As for the full syndrome of somatization disorder (F45.0).

F45.2 Hypochondriacal disorder

The essential feature is a persistent preoccupation with the possibility of having one or more serious and progressive physical disorders. Patients manifest persistent somatic complaints or persistent preoccupation with their physical appearance. Normal or commonplace sensations and appearances are often interpreted by a patient as abnormal and distressing, and attention is usually focused on only one or two organs or systems of the body. The feared physical disorder or disfigurement may be named by the patient, but even so the degree of conviction about its presence and the emphasis upon one disorder rather than another usually varies between consultations; the patient will usually entertain the possibility that other or additional physical disorders may exist in addition to the one given pre-eminence.

Marked depression and anxiety are often present, and may justify additional diagnosis. The disorders rarely present for the first time after the age of 50 years, and the course of both symptoms and disability is usually chronic and fluctuating. There must be no fixed delusions about bodily functions or shape. Fears of the presence of one or more diseases (nosophobia) should be classified here.

This syndrome occurs in both men and women, and there are no special familial characteristics (in contrast to somatization disorder).

Many individuals, especially those with milder forms of the disorder, remain within primary care or nonpsychiatric medical specialties. Psychiatric referral is often resented, unless accomplished early in the development of the disorder and with tactful collaboration between physician and psychiatrist. The degree of associated disability is very variable; some individuals dominate or manipulate family and social networks as a result of their symptoms, in contrast to a minority who function almost normally.

Diagnostic guidelines

For a definite diagnosis, both of the following should be present:

(a) persistent belief in the presence of at least one serious physical illness underlying the presenting symptom or symptoms, even though repeated investigations and examinations have identified no adequate physical explanation, or a persistent preoccupation with a presumed deformity or disfigurement;

(b) persistent refusal to accept the advice and reassurance of several different doctors that there is no physical illness or abnormality underlying the symptoms.

Includes: body dysmorphic disorder
dysmorphophobia (nondelusional)
hypochondriacal neurosis
hypochondriasis
nosophobia

Differential diagnosis. Differentiation from the following disorders is essential:

Somatization disorder. Emphasis is on the presence of the disorder itself and its future consequences, rather than on the individual symptoms as in somatization disorder. In hypochondriacal disorder, there is also likely to be preoccupation with only one or two possible physical disorders, which will be named consistently, rather than with the more numerous and often changing possibilities in somatization disorder. In hypochondriacal disorder there is no marked sex differential rate, nor are there any special familial connotations.

Depressive disorders. If depressive symptoms are particularly prominent and precede the development of hypochondriacal ideas, the depressive disorder may be primary.

Delusional disorders. The beliefs in hypochondriacal disorder do not have the same fixity as those in depressive and schizophrenic disorders accompanied by somatic delusions. A disorder in which the patient is convinced that he or she has an unpleasant appearance or is physically misshapen should be classified under delusional disorder (F22. –).

Anxiety and panic disorders. The somatic symptoms of anxiety are sometimes interpreted as signs of serious physical illness, but in these disorders the patients are usually reassured by physiological explanations, and convictions about the presence of physical illness do not develop.

F45.3 Somatoform autonomic dysfunction

The symptoms are presented by the patient as if they were due to a physical disorder of a system or organ that is largely or completely under autonomic innervation and control, i.e. the cardiovascular, gastrointestinal, or respiratory system. (Some aspects of the genitourinary system are also included here.) The most common and striking examples affect the cardiovascular system ("cardiac neurosis"), the respiratory system (psychogenic hyperventilation and hiccough) and the gastrointestinal system ("gastric neurosis" and "nervous diarrhoea"). The symptoms are usually of two types, neither of which indicates a physical disorder of the organ or system concerned. The first type, upon which this diagnosis largely depends, is characterized by complaints based upon objective signs of autonomic arousal, such as palpitations, sweating, flushing, and tremor. The second type is characterized by more idiosyncratic, subjective, and nonspecific symptoms, such as sensations of fleeting aches and pains, burning, heaviness, tightness, and sensations of being bloated or distended; these are referred by the patient to a specific organ or system (as the autonomic symptoms may also be). It is the combination of clear autonomic involvement, additional nonspecific subjective complaints, and persistent referral to a particular organ or system as the cause of the disorder that gives the characteristic clinical picture.

In many patients with this disorder there will also be evidence of psychological stress, or current difficulties and problems that appear to be related to the disorder; however, this is not the case in a substantial proportion of patients who nevertheless clearly fulfil the criteria for this condition.

In some of these disorders, some minor disturbance of physiological function may also be present, such as hiccough, flatulence, and hyperventilation, but these do not of themselves disturb the essential physiological function of the relevant organ or system.

Diagnostic guidelines

Definite diagnosis requires all of the following:

(a) symptoms of autonomic arousal, such as palpitations, sweating, tremor, flushing, which are persistent and troublesome;

(b) additional subjective symptoms referred to a specific organ or system;

(c) preoccupation with and distress about the possibility of a serious (but often unspecified) disorder of the stated organ or system, which does not respond to repeated explanation and reassurance by doctors;

(d) no evidence of a significant disturbance of structure or function of the stated system or organ.

Differential diagnosis. Differentiation from generalized anxiety disorder is based on the predominance of the psychological components of autonomic arousal, such as fear and anxious foreboding in generalized anxiety disorder, and the lack of a consistent physical focus for the other symptoms. In somatization disorders, autonomic symptoms may occur but they are neither prominent nor persistent in comparison with the many other sensations and feelings, and the symptoms are not so persistently attributed to one stated organ or system.

Excludes: psychological and behavioural factors associated with disorders or diseases classified elsewhere (F54)

A fifth character may be used to classify the individual disorders in this group, indicating the organ or system regarded by the patient as the origin of the symptoms:

F45.30 Heart and cardiovascular system

Includes: cardiac neurosis
Da Costa's syndrome
neurocirculatory asthenia

F45.31 Upper gastrointestinal tract

Includes: gastric neurosis
psychogenic aerophagy, hiccough, dyspepsia, and pylorospasm

F45.32 Lower gastrointestinal tract

Includes: psychogenic flatulence, irritable bowel syndrome, and diarrhoea gas syndrome

F45.33 Respiratory system

Includes: psychogenic forms of cough and hyperventilation

F45.34 Genitourinary system

Includes: psychogenic increase of frequency of micturition and dysuria

F45.38 Other organ or system

F45.4   Persistent somatoform pain disorder
The predominant complaint is of persistent, severe, and distressing pain, which cannot be explained fully by a physiological process or a physical disorder. Pain occurs in association with emotional conflict or psychosocial problems that are sufficient to allow the conclusion that they are the main causative influences. The result is usually a marked increase in support and attention, either personal or medical.

Pain presumed to be of psychogenic origin occurring during the course of depressive disorder or schizophrenia should not be included here. Pain due to known or inferred psychophysiological mechanisms such as muscle tension pain or migraine, but still believed to have a psychogenic cause, should be coded by the use of F54 (psychological or behavioural factors associated with disorders or diseases classified elsewhere) plus an additional code from elsewhere in ICD-10 (e.g. migraine, G43. –).

Includes: psychalgia
psychogenic backache or headache
somatoform pain disorder

Differential diagnosis. The commonest problem is to differentiate this disorder from the histrionic elaboration of organically caused pain. Patients with organic pain for whom a definite physical diagnosis has not yet been reached may easily become frightened or resentful, with resulting attention-seeking behaviour. A variety of aches and pains are common in somatization disorders but are not so persistent or so dominant over the other complaints.

Excludes: backache NOS (M54.9)
pain NOS (acute/chronic) (R52. –)
tension-type headache (G44.2)

F45.8 Other somatoform disorders
In these disorders the presenting complaints are not mediated through the autonomic nervous system, and are limited to specific systems or parts of the body. This is in contrast to the multiple and often changing complaints of the origin of symptoms and distress found in somatization disorder (F45.0) and undifferentiated somatoform disorder (F45.1). Tissue damage is not involved.

Any other disorders of sensation not due to physical disorders, which are closely associated in time with stressful events or problems, or which result in significantly increased attention for the patient, either personal or medical, should also be classified here. Sensations of swelling, movements on the skin, and paraesthesias (tingling and/or numbness) are common examples. Disorders such as the following should also be included here:

(a) "globus hystericus" (a feeling of a lump in the throat causing dysphagia) and other forms of dysphagia;

(b) psychogenic torticollis, and other disorders of spasmodic movements (but excluding Tourette's syndrome);

(c) psychogenic pruritus (but excluding specific skin lesions such as alopecia, dermatitis, eczema, or urticaria of psychogenic origin (F54));

(d) psychogenic dysmenorrhoea (but excluding dyspareunia (F52.6) and frigidity (F52.0));

(e) teeth-grinding

F45.9   Somatoform disorder, unspecified

Includes: unspecified psychophysiological or psychosomatic disorder

F48   Other neurotic disorders

F48.0   Neurasthenia

Considerable cultural variations occur in the presentation of this disorder; two main types occur, with substantial overlap. In one type, the main feature is a complaint of increased fatigue after mental effort, often associated with some decrease in occupational performance or coping efficiency in daily tasks. The mental fatiguability is typically described as an unpleasant intrusion of distracting associations or recollections, difficulty in concentrating, and generally inefficient thinking. In the other type, the emphasis is on feelings of bodily or physical weakness and exhaustion after only minimal effort, accompanied by a feeling of muscular aches and pains and inability to relax. In both types, a variety of other unpleasant physical feelings, such as dizziness, tension headaches, and a sense of general instability, is common. Worry about decreasing mental and bodily well-being, irritability, anhedonia, and varying minor degrees of both depression and anxiety are all common. Sleep is often disturbed in its initial and middle phases but hypersomnia may also be prominent.

Diagnostic guidelines

Definite diagnosis requires the following:

(a) either persistent and distressing complaints of increased fatigue after mental effort, or persistent and distressing complaints of bodily weakness and exhaustion after minimal effort;

(b) at least two of the following:
- feelings of muscular aches and pains
- dizziness
- tension headaches
- sleep disturbance
- inability to relax
- irritability
- dyspepsia;

(c) any autonomic or depressive symptoms present are not sufficiently persistent and severe to fulfil the criteria for any of the more specific disorders in this classification.

Includes: fatigue syndrome

Differential diagnosis. In many countries neurasthenia is not generally used as a diagnostic category. Many of the cases so diagnosed in the past would meet the current criteria for depressive disorder or anxiety disorder. There are, however, cases that fit the description of neurasthenia better than that of any other neurotic syndrome, and such cases seem to be more frequent in some cultures than in others. If the diagnostic category of neurasthenia is used, an attempt should be made first to rule out a depressive illness or an anxiety disorder. Hallmarks of the syndrome are the patient's emphasis on fatiguability and weakness and concern about lowered mental and physical efficiency (in contrast to the somatoform disorders, where bodily complaints and preoccupation with physical disease dominate the picture). If the neurasthenic syndrome develops in the aftermath of a physical illness (particularly influenza, viral hepatitis, or infectious mononucleosis), the diagnosis of the latter should also be recorded.

Excludes: asthenia NOS (R53)
burn-out (Z73.0)
malaise and fatigue (R53)
postviral fatigue syndrome (G93.3)
psychasthenia (F48.8)

F48.1 Depersonalization – derealization syndrome

A disorder in which the sufferer complains that his or her mental activity, body, and/or surroundings are changed in their quality, so as to be unreal, remote, or automatized. Individuals may feel

171

that they are no longer doing their own thinking, imaging, or remembering; that their movements and behaviour are somehow not their own; that their body seems lifeless, detached, or otherwise anomalous; and that their surroundings seem to lack colour and life and appear as artificial, or as a stage on which people are acting contrived roles. In some cases, they may feel as if they were viewing themselves from a distance or as if they were dead. The complaint of loss of emotions is the most frequent among these varied phenomena.

The number of individuals who experience this disorder in a pure or isolated form is small. More commonly, depersonalization – derealization phenomena occur in the context of depressive illnesses, phobic disorder, and obsessive – compulsive disorder. Elements of the syndrome may also occur in mentally healthy individuals in states of fatigue, sensory deprivation, hallucinogen intoxication, or as a hypnogogic/hypnopompic phenomenon. The depersonalization – derealization phenomena are similar to the so-called "near-death experiences" associated with moments of extreme danger to life.

Diagnostic guidelines

For a definite diagnosis, there must be either or both of (a) and (b), plus (c) and (d):

(a) depersonalization symptoms, i.e. the individual feels that his or her own feelings and/or experiences are detached, distant, not his or her own, lost, etc;

(b) derealization symptoms, i.e. objects, people, and/or surroundings seem unreal, distant, artificial, colourless, lifeless, etc;

(c) an acceptance that this is a subjective and spontaneous change, not imposed by outside forces or other people (i.e. insight);

(d) a clear sensorium and absence of toxic confusional state or epilepsy.

Differential diagnosis. The disorder must be differentiated from other disorders in which "change of personality" is experienced or presented, such as schizophrenia (delusions of transformation or passivity and control experiences), dissociative disorders (where awareness of change is lacking), and some instances of early dementia. The preictal aura of temporal lobe epilepsy and some postictal states may include depersonalization and derealization syndromes as secondary phenomena.

If the depersonalization – derealization syndrome occurs as part of a diagnosable depressive, phobic, obsessive – compulsive, or schizophrenic disorder, the latter should be given precedence as the main diagnosis.

F48.8 Other specified neurotic disorders

This category includes mixed disorders of behaviour, beliefs, and emotions which are of uncertain etiology and nosological status and which occur with particular frequency in certain cultures; examples include Dhat syndrome (undue concern about the debilitating effects of the passage of semen), koro (anxiety and fear that the penis will retract into the abdomen and cause death), and latah (imitative and automatic response behaviour). The strong association of these syndromes with locally accepted cultural beliefs and patterns of behaviour indicates that they are probably best regarded as not delusional.

> *Includes:* Dhat syndrome
> koro
> latah
> occupational neurosis, including writer's cramp
> psychasthenia
> psychasthenic neurosis
> psychogenic syncope

F48.9 Neurotic disorder, unspecified

> *Includes:* neurosis NOS

F50 – F59
Behavioural syndromes associated with physiological disturbances and physical factors

Overview of this block

F50 Eating disorders
F50.0 Anorexia nervosa
F50.1 Atypical anorexia nervosa
F50.2 Bulimia nervosa
F50.3 Atypical bulimia nervosa
F50.4 Overeating associated with other psychological disturbances
F50.5 Vomiting associated with other psychological disturbances
F50.8 Other eating disorders
F50.9 Eating disorder, unspecified

F51 Nonorganic sleep disorders
F51.0 Nonorganic insomnia
F51.1 Nonorganic hypersomnia
F51.2 Nonorganic disorder of the sleep – wake schedule
F51.3 Sleepwalking [somnambulism]
F51.4 Sleep terrors [night terrors]
F51.5 Nightmares
F51.8 Other nonorganic sleep disorders
F51.9 Nonorganic sleep disorder, unspecified

F52 Sexual dysfunction, not caused by organic disorder or disease
F52.0 Lack or loss of sexual desire
F52.1 Sexual aversion and lack of sexual enjoyment
    .10 Sexual aversion
    .11 Lack of sexual enjoyment
F52.2 Failure of genital response
F52.3 Orgasmic dysfunction
F52.4 Premature ejaculation
F52.5 Nonorganic vaginismus
F52.6 Nonorganic dyspareunia
F52.7 Excessive sexual drive
F52.8 Other sexual dysfunction, not caused by organic disorder or disease

F52.9 Unspecified sexual dysfunction, not caused by organic disorder or disease

F53 Mental and behavioural disorders associated with the puerperium, not elsewhere classified

F53.0 Mild mental and behavioural disorders associated with the puerperium, not elsewhere classified

F53.1 Severe mental and behavioural disorders associated with the puerperium, not elsewhere classified

F53.8 Other mental and behavioural disorders associated with the puerperium, not elsewhere classified

F53.9 Puerperal mental disorder, unspecified

F54 Psychological and behavioural factors associated with disorders or diseases classified elsewhere

F55 Abuse of non-dependence-producing substances

F55.0 Antidepressants

F55.1 Laxatives

F55.2 Analgesics

F55.3 Antacids

F55.4 Vitamins

F55.5 Steroids or hormones

F55.6 Specific herbal or folk remedies

F55.8 Other substances that do not produce dependence

F55.9 Unspecified

F59 Unspecified behavioural syndromes associated with physiological disturbances and physical factors

F50 Eating disorders

Under the heading of eating disorders, two important and clear-cut syndromes are described: anorexia nervosa and bulimia nervosa. Less specific bulimic disorders also deserve place, as does overeating when it is associated with psychological disturbances. A brief note is provided on vomiting associated with psychological disturbances.

Excludes: anorexia or loss of appetite NOS (R63.0)
feeding difficulties and mismanagement (R63.3)
feeding disorder in infancy and childhood (F98.2)
pica in children (F98.3)

F50.0 Anorexia nervosa

Anorexia nervosa is a disorder characterized by deliberate weight loss, induced and/or sustained by the patient. The disorder occurs most commonly in adolescent girls and young women, but adolescent boys and young men may be affected more rarely, as may children approaching puberty and older women up to the menopause. Anorexia nervosa constitutes an independent syndrome in the following sense:

(a) the clinical features of the syndrome are easily recognized, so that diagnosis is reliable with a high level of agreement between clinicians;

(b) follow-up studies have shown that, among patients who do not recover, a considerable number continue to show the same main features of anorexia nervosa, in a chronic form.

Although the fundamental causes of anorexia nervosa remain elusive, there is growing evidence that interacting sociocultural and biological factors contribute to its causation, as do less specific psychological mechanisms and a vulnerability of personality. The disorder is associated with undernutrition of varying severity, with resulting secondary endocrine and metabolic changes and disturbances of bodily function. There remains some doubt as to whether the characteristic endocrine disorder is entirely due to the undernutrition and the direct effect of various behaviours that have brought it about (e.g. restricted dietary choice, excessive exercise and alterations in body composition, induced vomiting and purgation and the consequent electrolyte disturbances), or whether uncertain factors are also involved.

Diagnostic guidelines

For a definite diagnosis, all the following are required:

(a) Body weight is maintained at least 15% below that expected (either lost or never achieved), or Quetelet's body-mass index[1] is 17.5 or less. Prepubertal patients may show failure to make the expected weight gain during the period of growth.

(b) The weight loss is self-induced by avoidance of "fattening foods". One or more of the following may also be present: self-induced vomiting; self-induced purging; excessive exercise; use of appetite suppressants and/or diuretics.

(c) There is body-image distortion in the form of a specific psychopathology whereby a dread of fatness persists as an intrusive, overvalued idea and the patient imposes a low weight threshold on himself or herself.

(d) A widespread endocrine disorder involving the hypothalamic – pituitary – gonadal axis is manifest in women as amenorrhoea and in men as a loss of sexual interest and potency. (An apparent exception is the persistence of vaginal bleeds in anorexic women who are receiving replacement hormonal therapy, most commonly taken as a contraceptive pill.) There may also be elevated levels of growth hormone, raised levels of cortisol, changes in the peripheral metabolism of the thyroid hormone, and abnormalities of insulin secretion.

(e) If onset is prepubertal, the sequence of pubertal events is delayed or even arrested (growth ceases; in girls the breasts do not develop and there is a primary amenorrhoea; in boys the genitals remain juvenile). With recovery, puberty is often completed normally, but the menarche is late.

Differential diagnosis. There may be associated depressive or obsessional symptoms, as well as features of a personality disorder, which may make differentiation difficult and/or require the use of more than one diagnostic code. Somatic causes of weight loss in young patients that must be distinguished include chronic debilitating diseases, brain tumors, and intestinal disorders such as Crohn's disease or a malabsorption syndrome.

---

[1] Quetelet's body-mass index $= \dfrac{\text{weight (kg)}}{[\text{height (m)}]^2}$ to be used for age 16 or above.

Excludes: loss of appetite (R63.0)
psychogenic loss of appetite (F50.8)

F50.1 Atypical anorexia nervosa

This term should be used for those individuals in whom one or more of the key features of anorexia nervosa (F50.0), such as amenorrhoea or significant weight loss, is absent, but who otherwise present a fairly typical clinical picture. Such people are usually encountered in psychiatric liaison services in general hospitals or in primary care. Patients who have all the key symptoms but to only a mild degree may also be best described by this term. This term should not be used for eating disorders that resemble anorexia nervosa but that are due to known physical illness.

F50.2 Bulimia nervosa

Bulimia nervosa is a syndrome characterized by repeated bouts of overeating and an excessive preoccupation with the control of body weight, leading the patient to adopt extreme measures so as to mitigate the "fattening" effects of ingested food. The term should be restricted to the form of the disorder that is related to anorexia nervosa by virtue of sharing the same psychopathology. The age and sex distribution is similar to that of anorexia nervosa, but the age of presentation tends to be slightly later. The disorder may be viewed as a sequel to persistent anorexia nervosa (although the reverse sequence may also occur). A previously anorexic patient may first appear to improve as a result of weight gain and possibly a return of menstruation, but a pernicious pattern of overeating and vomiting then becomes established. Repeated vomiting is likely to give rise to disturbances of body electrolytes, physical complications (tetany, epileptic seizures, cardiac arrhythmias, muscular weakness), and further severe loss of weight.

Diagnostic guidelines

For a definite diagnosis, all the following are required:

(a) There is a persistent preoccupation with eating, and an irresistible craving for food; the patient succumbs to episodes of overeating in which large amounts of food are consumed in short periods of time.

(b) The patient attempts to counteract the "fattening" effects of food by one or more of the following: self-induced vomiting; purgative abuse, alternating periods of starvation; use of drugs such as appetite suppressants, thyroid preparations or diuretics. When bulimia occurs in diabetic patients they may choose to neglect their insulin treatment.

(c) The psychopathology consists of a morbid dread of fatness and the patient sets herself or himself a sharply defined weight threshold, well below the premorbid weight that constitutes the optimum or healthy weight in the opinion of the physician. There is often, but not always, a history of an earlier episode of anorexia nervosa, the interval between the two disorders ranging from a few months to several years. This earlier episode may have been fully expressed, or may have assumed a minor cryptic form with a moderate loss of weight and/or a transient phase of amenorrhoea.

Includes: bulimia NOS
hyperorexia nervosa

Differential diagnosis. Bulimia nervosa must be differentiated from:

(a) upper gastrointestinal disorders leading to repeated vomiting (the characteristic psychopathology is absent);

(b) a more general abnormality of personality (the eating disorder may coexist with alcohol dependence and petty offences such as shoplifting);

(c) depressive disorder (bulimic patients often experience depressive symptoms).

F50.3 Atypical bulimia nervosa

This term should be used for those individuals in whom one or more of the key features listed for bulimia nervosa (F50.2) is absent, but who otherwise present a fairly typical clinical picture. Most commonly this applies to people with normal or even excessive weight but with typical periods of overeating followed by vomiting or purging. Partial syndromes together with depressive symptoms are also not uncommon, but if the depressive symptoms justify a separate diagnosis of a depressive disorder two separate diagnoses should be made.

Includes: normal weight bulimia

F50.4 Overeating associated with other psychological disturbances

Overeating that has led to obesity as a reaction to distressing events should be coded here. Bereavements, accidents, surgical operations, and emotionally distressing events may be followed by a "reactive obesity", especially in individuals predisposed to weight gain.

Obesity as a cause of psychological disturbance should not be coded here. Obesity may cause the individual to feel sensitive about his or her appearance and give rise to a lack of confidence in personal relationships; the subjective appraisal of body size may be exaggerated. Obesity as a cause of psychological disturbance should be coded in a category such as F38. – (other mood [affective] disorders), F41.2 (mixed anxiety and depressive disorder), or F48.9 (neurotic disorder, unspecified), plus a code from E66. – of ICD-10 to indicate the type of obesity.

Obesity as an undesirable effect of long-term treatment with neuroleptic antidepressants or other type of medication should not be coded here, but under E66.1 (drug-induced obesity) plus an additional code from Chapter XX (External causes) of ICD-10, to identify the drug.

Obesity may be the motivation for dieting, which in turn results in minor affective symptoms (anxiety, restlessness, weakness, and irritability) or, more rarely, severe depressive symptoms ("dieting depression"). The appropriate code from F30 – F39 or F40 – F49 should be used to cover the symptoms as above, plus F50.8 (other eating disorder) to indicate the dieting, plus a code from E66. – to indicate the type of obesity.

Includes: psychogenic overeating

Excludes: obesity (E66. –)
polyphagia NOS (R63.2)

F50.5   Vomiting associated with other psychological disturbances
Apart from the self-induced vomiting of bulimia nervosa, repeated vomiting may occur in dissociative disorders (F44. –), in hypochondriacal disorder (F45.2) when vomiting may be one of several bodily symptoms, and in pregnancy when emotional factors may contribute to recurrent nausea and vomiting.

Includes: psychogenic hyperemesis gravidarum
psychogenic vomiting

Excludes: nausea and vomiting NOS (R11)

F50.8 Other eating disorders

Includes: pica of nonorganic origin in adults
psychogenic loss of appetite

F50.9 Eating disorder, unspecified

F51 Nonorganic sleep disorders

This group of disorders includes:

(a) dyssomnias: primarily psychogenic conditions in which the predominant disturbance is in the amount, quality, or timing of sleep due to emotional causes, i.e. insomnia, hypersomnia, and disorder of sleep – wake schedule; and

(b) parasomnias: abnormal episodic events occurring during sleep; in childhood these are related mainly to the child's development, while in adulthood they are predominantly psychogenic, i.e. sleepwalking, sleep terrors, and nightmares.

This section includes only those sleep disorders in which emotional causes are considered to be a primary factor. Sleep disorders of organic origin such as Kleine – Levin syndrome (G47.8) are coded in Chapter VI (G47. –) of ICD-10. Nonpsychogenic disorders including narcolepsy and cataplexy (G47.4) and disorders of the sleep – wake schedule (G47.2) are also listed in Chapter VI, as are sleep apnoea (G47.3) and episodic movement disorders which include nocturnal myoclonus (G25.3). Finally, enuresis (F98.0) is listed with other emotional and behavioural disorders with onset specific to childhood and adolescence, while primary nocturnal enuresis (R33.8), which is considered to be due to a maturational delay of bladder control during sleep, is listed in Chapter XVIII of ICD-10 among the symptoms involving the urinary system.

In many cases, a disturbance of sleep is one of the symptoms of another disorder, either mental or physical. Even when a specific sleep disorder appears to be clinically independent, a number of associated psychiatric and/or physical factors may contribute to its occurrence. Whether a sleep disorder in a given individual is an independent condition or simply one of the features of another disorder (classified elsewhere in Chapter V or in other chapters of ICD-10) should be determined on the basis of its clinical presentation and course, as well as of therapeutic considerations and priorities at the time of the consultation. In any event, whenever the disturbance of sleep is among the predominant complaints, a sleep disorder should be diagnosed. Generally, however, it is preferable to list the diagnosis of the specific sleep disorder along with as many other pertinent diagnoses as are necessary to describe adequately the psychopathology and/or pathophysiology involved in a given case.

Excludes: sleep disorders (organic) (G47. –)

F51.0   Nonorganic insomnia

Insomnia is a condition of unsatisfactory quantity and/or quality of sleep, which persists for a considerable period of time. The actual degree of deviation from what is generally considered as a normal amount of sleep should not be the primary consideration in the diagnosis of insomnia, because some individuals (the so-called short sleepers) obtain a minimal amount of sleep and yet do not consider themselves as insomniacs. Conversely, there are people who suffer immensely from the poor quality of their sleep, while sleep quantity is judged subjectively and/or objectively as within normal limits.

Among insomniacs, difficulty falling asleep is the most prevalent complaint, followed by difficulty staying asleep and early final wakening. Usually, however, patients report a combination of these complaints. Typically, insomnia develops at a time of increased life-stress and tends to be more prevalent among women, older individuals and psychologically disturbed and socioeconomically disadvantaged people. When insomnia is repeatedly experienced, it can lead to an increased fear of sleeplessness and a preoccupation with its conse-quences. This creates a vicious circle which tends to perpetuate the individual's problem.

Individuals with insomnia describe themselves as feeling tense, anxious, worried, or depressed at bedtime, and as though their thoughts are racing. They frequently ruminate over getting enough sleep, personal problems, health status, and even death. Often they attempt to cope with their tension by taking medication or alcohol. In the morning, they frequently report feeling physically and mentally tired; during the day, they characteristically feel depressed, worried, tense, irritable, and preoccupied with themselves.

Children are often said to have difficulty sleeping when in reality the problem is a difficulty in the management of bedtime routines (rather than of sleep *per se*); bedtime difficulties should not be coded here, but in Chapter XXI of ICD-10 (Z62.0, inadequate parental supervision and control).

Diagnostic guidelines

The following are essential clinical features for a definite diagnosis:

(a) the complaint is either of difficulty falling asleep or maintaining sleep, or of poor quality of sleep;
(b) the sleep disturbance has occurred at least three times per week for at least 1 month;
(c) there is preoccupation with the sleeplessness and excessive concern over its consequences at night and during the day;
(d) the unsatisfactory quantity and/or quality of sleep either causes marked distress or interferes with ordinary activities in daily living.

Whenever unsatisfactory quantity and/or quality of sleep is the patient's only complaint, the disorder should be coded here. The presence of other psychiatric symptoms such as depression, anxiety or obsessions does not invalidate the diagnosis of insomnia, provided that insomnia is the primary complaint or the chronicity and severity of insomnia cause the patient to perceive it as the primary disorder. Other coexisting disorders should be coded if they are sufficiently marked and persistent to justify treatment in their own right. It should be noted that most chronic insomniacs are usually preoccupied with their sleep disturbance and deny the existence of any emotional problems. Thus, careful clinical assessment is necessary before ruling out a psychological basis for the complaint.

Insomnia is a common symptom of other mental disorders, such as affective, neurotic, organic, and eating disorders, substance use, and schizophrenia, and of other sleep disorders such as nightmares. Insomnia may also be associated with physical disorders in which there is pain and discomfort or with taking certain medications. If insomnia occurs only as one of the multiple symptoms of a mental disorder or a physical condition, i.e. does not dominate the clinical picture, the diagnosis should be limited to that of the underlying mental or physical disorder. Moreover, the diagnosis of another sleep disorder, such as nightmare, disorder of the sleep – wake schedule, sleep apnoea and nocturnal myoclonus, should be made only when these disorders lead to a reduction in the quantity or quality of sleep. However, in all of the above instances, if insomnia is one of the major complaints and is perceived as a condition in itself, the present code should be added after that of the principal diagnosis.

The present code does not apply to so-called "transient insomnia". Transient disturbances of sleep are a normal part of everyday life. Thus, a few nights of sleeplessness related to a psychosocial stressor would not be coded here, but could be considered as part of an acute stress reaction (F43.0) or adjustment disorder (F43.2) if accompanied by other clinically significant features.

F51.1   Nonorganic hypersomnia

Hypersomnia is defined as a condition of either excessive daytime sleepiness and sleep attacks (not accounted for by an inadequate amount of sleep) or prolonged transition to the fully aroused state upon awakening. When no definite evidence of organic etiology can be found, this condition is usually associated with mental disorders. It is often found to be a symptom of a bipolar affective disorder currently depressed (F31.3, F31.4 or F31.5), a recurrent depressive disorder (F33. –) or a depressive episode (F32. –). At times, however, the criteria for the diagnosis of another mental disorder cannot be met, although there is often some evidence of a psychopathological basis for the complaint.

Some patients will themselves make the connection between their tendency to fall asleep at inappropriate times and certain unpleasant daytime experiences. Others will deny such a connection even when a skilled clinician identifies the presence of these experiences. In other cases, no emotional or other psychological factors can be readily identified, but the presumed absence of organic factors suggests that the hypersomnia is most likely of psychogenic origin.

Diagnostic guidelines

The following clinical features are essential for a definite diagnosis:

(a) excessive daytime sleepiness or sleep attacks, not accounted for by an inadequate amount of sleep, and/or prolonged transition to the fully aroused state upon awakening (sleep drunkenness);

(b) sleep disturbance occurring daily for more than 1 month or for recurrent periods of shorter duration, causing either marked distress or interference with ordinary activities in daily living;

(c) absence of auxiliary symptoms of narcolepsy (cataplexy, sleep paralysis, hypnagogic hallucinations) or of clinical evidence for sleep apnoea (nocturnal breath cessation, typical intermittent snorting sounds, etc.);

(d) absence of any neurological or medical condition of which daytime somnolence may be symptomatic.

If hypersomnia occurs only as one of the symptoms of a mental disorder, such as an affective disorder, the diagnosis should be that of the underlying disorder. The diagnosis of psychogenic hypersomnia should be added, however, if hypersomnia is the predominant complaint in patients with other mental disorders. When another diagnosis cannot be made, the present code should be used alone.

Differential diagnosis. Differentiating hypersomnia from narcolepsy is essential. In narcolepsy (G47.4), one or more auxiliary symptoms such as cataplexy, sleep paralysis, and hypnagogic hallucinations are usually present; the sleep attacks are irresistible and more refreshing; and nocturnal sleep is fragmented and curtailed. By contrast, daytime sleep attacks in hypersomnia are usually fewer per day, although each of longer duration; the patient is often able to prevent their occurrence; nocturnal sleep is usually prolonged, and there is a marked difficulty in achieving the fully aroused state upon awakening (sleep drunkenness).

It is important to differentiate nonorganic hypersomnia from hypersomnia related to sleep apnoea and other organic hypersomnias. In addition to the symptom of excessive daytime sleepiness, most patients with sleep apnoea have a history of nocturnal cessation of breathing, typical intermittent snorting sounds, obesity, hypertension, impotence, cognitive impairment, nocturnal hypermotility and profuse sweating, morning headaches and incoordination. When there is a strong suspicion of sleep apnoea, confirmation of the diagnosis and quantification of the apnoeic events by means of sleep laboratory recordings should be considered.

Hypersomnia due to a definable organic cause (encephalitis, meningitis, concussion and other brain damage, brain tumours, cerebrovascular lesions, degenerative and other neurologic diseases, metabolic disorders, toxic conditions, endocrine abnormalities, post-radiation syndrome) can be differentiated from nonorganic hypersomnia by the presence of the insulting organic factor, as evidenced by the patient's clinical presentation and the results of appropriate laboratory tests.

F51.2   Nonorganic disorder of the sleep – wake schedule

A disorder of the sleep – wake schedule is defined as a lack of synchrony between the individual's sleep – wake schedule and the desired sleep – wake schedule for the environment, resulting in a complaint of either insomnia or hypersomnia. This disorder may be either psychogenic or of presumed organic origin, depending on the relative contribution of psychological or organic factors. Individuals with disorganized and variable sleeping and waking times most often present with significant psychological disturbance, usually in association with various psychiatric conditions such as personality disorders and affective disorders. In individuals who frequently change work shifts or travel across time zones, the circadian dysregulation is basically biological, although a strong emotional component may also be operating since many such individuals are distressed. Finally, in some individuals there is a phase advance to the desired sleep – wake schedule, which may be due to either an intrinsic malfunction of the circadian oscillator (biological clock) or an abnormal processing of the time-cues that drive the biological clock (the latter may in fact be related to an emotional and/or cognitive disturbance).

The present code is reserved for those disorders of the sleep – wake schedule in which psychological factors play the most important role, whereas cases of presumed organic origin should be classified under G47.2, i.e. as non-psychogenic disorders of the sleep – wake schedule. Whether or not psychological factors are of primary importance and, therefore, whether the present code or G47.2 should be used is a matter for clinical judgement in each case.

Diagnostic guidelines

The following clinical features are essential for a definite diagnosis:

(a) the individual's sleep – wake pattern is out of synchrony with the sleep – wake schedule that is normal for a particular society and shared by most people in the same cultural environment;

(b) insomnia during the major sleep period and hypersomnia during the waking period are experienced nearly every day for at least 1 month or recurrently for shorter periods of time;

(c) the unsatisfactory quantity, quality, and timing of sleep cause marked distress or interfere with ordinary activities in daily living.

Whenever there is no identifiable psychiatric or physical cause of the disorder, the present code should be used alone. None the less, the presence of psychiatric symptoms such as anxiety, depression, or hypomania does not invalidate the diagnosis of a nonorganic disorder of the sleep – wake schedule, provided that this disorder is predominant in the patient's clinical picture. When other psychiatric symptoms are sufficiently marked and persistent, the specific mental disorder(s) should be diagnosed separately.

Includes: psychogenic inversion of circadian, nyctohemeral, or sleep rhythm

F51.3 Sleepwalking [somnambulism]

Sleepwalking or somnambulism is a state of altered consciousness in which phenomena of sleep and wakefulness are combined. During a sleepwalking episode the individual arises from bed, usually during the first third of nocturnal sleep, and walks about, exhibiting low levels of awareness, reactivity, and motor skill. A sleepwalker will sometimes leave the bedroom and at times may actually walk out of the house, and is thus exposed to considerable risks of injury during the episode. Most often, however, he or she will return quietly to bed, either unaided or when gently led by another person. Upon awakening either from the sleepwalking episode or the next morning, there is usually no recall of the event.

Sleepwalking and sleep terrors (F51.4) are very closely related. Both are considered as disorders of arousal, particularly arousal from the deepest stages of sleep (stages 3 and 4). Many individuals have a positive family history for either condition as well as a personal history of having experienced both. Moreover, both conditions are much more common in childhood, which indicates the role of developmental factors in their etiology. In addition, in some cases, the onset of these conditions coincides with a febrile illness. When they continue beyond childhood or are first observed in adulthood, both conditions tend to be associated with significant psychological disturbance; the conditions may also occur for the first time in old age or in the early stages of dementia. Based upon the clinical and pathogenetic similarities between sleepwalking and sleep terrors, and the fact that the differential diagnosis of these disorders is usually a matter of which of the two is predominant, they have both been considered recently to be part of the same nosologic continuum. For consistency with tradition, however, as well as to emphasize the differences in the intensity of clinical manifestations, separate codes are provided in this classification.

Diagnostic guidelines

The following clinical features are essential for a definite diagnosis:

(a) the predominant symptom is one or more episodes of rising from bed, usually during the first third of nocturnal sleep, and walking about;

(b) during an episode, the individual has a blank, staring face, is relatively unresponsive to the efforts of others to influence the event or to communicate with him or her, and can be awakened only with considerable difficulty;

(c) upon awakening (either from an episode or the next morning), the individual has no recollection of the episode;

(d) within several minutes of awakening from the episode, there is no impairment of mental activity or behaviour, although there may initially be a short period of some confusion and disorientation;

(e) there is no evidence of an organic mental disorder such as dementia, or a physical disorder such as epilepsy.

Differential diagnosis. Sleepwalking should be differentiated from psychomotor epileptic seizures. Psychomotor epilepsy very seldom occurs only at night. During the epileptic attack the individual is completely unresponsive to environmental stimuli, and perseverative movements such as swallowing and rubbing the hands are common.

The presence of epileptic discharges in the EEG confirms the diagnosis, although a seizure disorder does not preclude coexisting sleepwalking.

Dissociative fugue (see F44.1) must also be differentiated from sleepwalking. In dissociative disorders the episodes are much longer in duration and patients are more alert and capable of complex and purposeful behaviours. Further, these disorders are rare in children and typically begin during the hours of wakefulness.

F51.4 Sleep terrors [night terrors]

Sleep terrors or night terrors are nocturnal episodes of extreme terror and panic associated with intense vocalization, motility, and high levels of autonomic discharge. The individual sits up or gets up with a panicky scream, usually during the first third of nocturnal sleep, often rushing to the door as if trying to escape, although he or she very seldom leaves the room. Efforts of others to influence the sleep terror event may actually lead to more intense fear, since the individual not only is relatively unresponsive to such efforts but may become disoriented for a few minutes. Upon awaking there is usually no recollection of the episode. Because of these clinical characteristics, individuals are at great risk of injury during the episodes of sleep terrors.

Sleep terrors and sleepwalking (F51.3) are closely related: genetic, developmental, organic, and psychological factors all play a role in their development, and the two conditions share the same clinical and pathophysiological characteristics. On the basis of their many similarities, these two conditions have been considered recently to be part of the same nosologic continuum.

Diagnostic guidelines

The following clinical features are essential for a definite diagnosis:

(a) the predominant symptom is that one or more episodes of awakening from sleep begin with a panicky scream, and are characterized by intense anxiety, body motility, and autonomic hyperactivity, such as tachycardia, rapid breathing, dilated pupils, and sweating;

(b) these repeated episodes typically last 1 – 10 minutes and usually occur during the first third of nocturnal sleep;

(c) there is relative unresponsiveness to efforts of others to influence the sleep terror event and such efforts are almost invariably followed by at least several minutes of disorientation and perseverative movements;

(d) recall of the event, if any, is minimal (usually limited to one or two fragmentary mental images);

(e) there is no evidence of a physical disorder, such as brain tumour or epilepsy.

Differential diagnosis. Sleep terrors should be differentiated from nightmares. The latter are the common "bad dreams" with limited, if any, vocalization and body motility. In contrast to sleep terrors, nightmares occur at any time of the night, and the individual is quite easy to arouse and has a very detailed and vivid recall of the event.

In differentiating sleep terrors from epileptic seizures, the physician should keep in mind that seizures very seldom occur only during the night; an abnormal clinical EEG, however, favours the diagnosis of epilepsy.

F51.5   Nightmares

Nightmares are dream experiences loaded with anxiety or fear, of which the individual has very detailed recall. The dream experiences are extremely vivid and usually include themes involving threats to survival, security, or self-esteem. Quite often there is a recurrence of the same or similar frightening nightmare themes. During a typical episode there is a degree of autonomic discharge but no appreciable vocalization or body motility. Upon awakening, the individual rapidly becomes alert and oriented. He or she can fully communicate with others, usually giving a detailed account of the dream experience both immediately and the next morning.

In children, there is no consistently associated psychological disturbance, as childhood nightmares are usually related to a specific phase of emotional development. In contrast, adults with nightmares are often found to have significant psychological disturbance, usually in the form of a personality disorder. The use of certain psychotropic drugs such as reserpine, thioridazine, tricyclic antidepressants, and benzodiazepines has also been found to contribute to the occurrence of nightmares. Moreover, abrupt withdrawal of drugs such as non-benzodiazepine hypnotics, which suppress REM sleep (the stage of sleep related to dreaming), may lead to enhanced dreaming and nightmare through REM rebound.

Diagnostic guidelines

The following clinical features are essential for a definite diagnosis:

(a) awakening from nocturnal sleep or naps with detailed and vivid recall of intensely frightening dreams, usually involving threats to survival, security, or self-esteem; the awakening may occur at any time during the sleep period, but typically during the second half;

(b) upon awakening from the frightening dreams, the individual rapidly becomes oriented and alert;

(c) the dream experience itself, and the resulting disturbance of sleep, cause marked distress to the individual.

Includes: dream anxiety disorder

Differential diagnosis. It is important to differentiate nightmares from sleep terrors. In the latter, the episodes occur during the first third of the sleep period and are marked by intense anxiety, panicky screams, excessive body motility, and extreme autonomic discharge. Further, in sleep terrors there is no detailed recollection of the dream, either immediately following the episode or upon awakening in the morning.

F51.8 Other nonorganic sleep disorders

F51.9 Nonorganic sleep disorder, unspecified

Includes: emotional sleep disorder NOS

F52 Sexual dysfunction, not caused by organic disorder or disease

Sexual dysfunction covers the various ways in which an individual is unable to participate in a sexual relationship as he or she would wish. There may be lack of interest, lack of enjoyment, failure of the physiological responses necessary for effective sexual interaction (e.g. erection), or inability to control or experience orgasm.

Sexual response is a psychosomatic process, and both psychological and somatic processes are usually involved in the causation of sexual dysfunction. It may be possible to identify an unequivocal psychogenic or organic etiology, but more commonly, particularly with such problems as erectile failure or dyspareunia, it is difficult to ascertain the relative importance of psychological and/or organic factors. In such cases, it is appropriate to categorize the condition as being of either mixed or uncertain etiology.

Some types of dysfunction (e.g. lack of sexual desire) occur in both men and women. Women, however, tend to present more commonly with complaints about the subjective quality of the sexual experience (e.g. lack of enjoyment or interest) rather than failure of a specific response. The complaint of orgasmic dysfunction is not unusual, but when one aspect of a woman's sexual response is affected, others are also likely to be impaired. For example, if a woman is unable to experience orgasm, she will often find herself unable to enjoy other aspects of lovemaking and will thus lose much of her sexual appetite. Men, on the other hand, though complaining of failure of a specific response such as erection or ejaculation, often report a continuing sexual appetite. It is therefore necessary to look beyond the presenting complaint to find the most appropriate diagnostic category.

Excludes: Dhat syndrome (F48.8)
koro (F48.8)

F52.0 Lack or loss of sexual desire

Loss of sexual desire is the principal problem and is not secondary to other sexual difficulties, such as erectile failure or dyspareunia. Lack of sexual desire does not preclude sexual enjoyment or arousal, but makes the initiation of sexual activity less likely.

Includes: frigidity
hypoactive sexual desire disorder

F52.1 Sexual aversion and lack of sexual enjoyment

F52.10 Sexual aversion
The prospect of sexual interaction with a partner is associated with strong negative feelings and produces sufficient fear or anxiety that sexual activity is avoided.

F52.11 Lack of sexual enjoyment

Sexual responses occur normally and orgasm is experienced but there is a lack of appropriate pleasure. This complaint is much more common in women than in men.

Includes: anhedonia (sexual)

F52.2 Failure of genital response

In men, the principal problem is erectile dysfunction, i.e. difficulty in developing or maintaining an erection suitable for satisfactory intercourse. If erection occurs normally in certain situations, e.g. during masturbation or sleep or with a different partner, the causation is likely to be psychogenic. Otherwise, the correct diagnosis of nonorganic erectile dysfunction may depend on special investigations (e.g. measurement of nocturnal penile tumescence) or the response to psychological treatment.

In women, the principal problem is vaginal dryness or failure of lubrication. The cause can be psychogenic or pathological (e.g. infection) or estrogen deficiency (e.g. postmenopausal). It is unusual for women to complain primarily of vaginal dryness except as a symptom of postmenopausal estrogen deficiency.

Includes: female sexual arousal disorder
male erectile disorder
psychogenic impotence

F52.3 Orgasmic dysfunction

Orgasm either does not occur or is markedly delayed. This may be situational (i.e. occur only in certain situations), in which case etiology is likely to be psychogenic, or invariable, when physical or constitutional factors cannot be easily excluded except by a positive response to psychological treatment. Orgasmic dysfunction is more common in women than in men.

Includes: inhibited orgasm (male) (female)
psychogenic anorgasmy

F52.4 Premature ejaculation

The inability to control ejaculation sufficiently for both partners to enjoy sexual interaction. In severe cases, ejaculation may occur before vaginal entry or in the absence of an erection. Premature ejaculation is unlikely to be of organic origin but can occur as a psychological reaction to organic impairment, e.g. erectile failure or pain. Ejaculation may also appear to be premature if erection requires prolonged stimulation, causing the time interval between satisfactory erection and ejaculation to be shortened; the primary problem in such a case is delayed erection.

F52.5 Nonorganic vaginismus

Spasm of the muscles that surround the vagina, causing occlusion of the vaginal opening. Penile entry is either impossible or painful. Vaginismus may be a secondary reaction to some local cause of pain, in which case this category should not be used.

Includes: psychogenic vaginismus

F52.6 Nonorganic dyspareunia

Dyspareunia (pain during sexual intercourse) occurs in both women and men. It can often be attributed to a local pathological condition and should then be appropriately categorized. In some cases, however, no obvious cause is apparent and emotional factors may be important. This category is to be used only if there is no other more primary sexual dysfunction (e.g. vaginismus or vaginal dryness).

Includes: psychogenic dyspareunia

F52.7 Excessive sexual drive

Both men and women may occasionally complain of excessive sexual drive as a problem in its own right, usually during late teenage or early adulthood. When the excessive sexual drive is secondary to an affective disorder (F30 – F39) or when it occurs during the early stages of dementia (F00 – F03), the underlying disorder should be coded.

Includes: nymphomania
satyriasis

F52.8 Other sexual dysfunction, not caused by organic disorder or disease

F52.9 Unspecified sexual dysfunction, not caused by organic disorder or disease

F53 Mental and behavioural disorders associated with the puerperium, not elsewhere classified

This classification should be used only for mental disorders associated with the puerperium (commencing within 6 weeks of delivery) that do not meet the criteria for disorders classified elsewhere in this book, either because insufficient information is available, or because it is considered that special additional clinical features are present which make classification elsewhere inappropriate. It will usually be possible to classify mental disorders associated with the puerperium by using two other codes: the first is from elsewhere in Chapter V(F) and indicates the specific type of mental disorder (usually affective (F30 – F39), and the second is O99.3 (mental diseases and diseases of the nervous system complicating the puerperium) of ICD-10.

F53.0 Mild mental and behavioural disorders associated with the puerperium, not elsewhere classified

Includes: postnatal depression NOS
postpartum depression NOS

F53.1 Severe mental and behavioural disorders associated with the puerperium, not elsewhere classified

Includes: puerperal psychosis NOS

F53.8 Other mental and behavioural disorders associated with the puerperium, not elsewhere classified

F53.9 Puerperal mental disorder, unspecified

F54 Psychological and behavioural factors associated with disorders or diseases classified elsewhere

This category should be used to record the presence of psychological or behavioural influences thought to have played a major part in the manifestation of physical disorders that can be classified by using other chapters of ICD-10. Any resulting mental disturbances are usually mild and often prolonged (such as worry, emotional conflict, apprehension), and do not of themselves justify the use of any of the categories described in the rest of this book. An additional code should be used to identify the physical disorder. (In the rare instances in which an overt psychiatric disorder is thought to have caused a physical disorder, a second additional code should be used to record the psychiatric disorder.)

Examples of the use of this category are: asthma (F54 plus J45. −); dermatitis and eczema (F54 plus L23 − L25); gastric ulcer (F54 plus K25. −); mucous colitis (F54 plus K58. −); ulcerative colitis (F54 plus K51. −); and urticaria (F54 plus L50. −).

Includes: psychological factors affecting physical conditions

Excludes: tension-type headache (G44.2)

F55 Abuse of non-dependence-producing substances

A wide variety of medicaments, proprietary drugs, and folk remedies may be involved, but three particularly important groups are: psychotropic drugs that do not produce dependence, such as antidepressants; laxatives; and analgesics that can be purchased without medical prescription, such as aspirin and paracetamol. Although the medication may have been medically prescribed or recommended in the first instance, prolonged, unnecessary, and often excessive dosage develops, which is facilitated by the availability of the substances without medical prescription.

Persistent and unjustified use of these substances is usually associated with unnecessary expense, often involves unnecessary contacts with medical professionals or supporting staff, and is sometimes marked by the harmful physical effects of the substances. Attempts to discourage or forbid the use of the substances are often met with resistance; for laxatives and analgesics this may be in spite of warnings about (or even the development of) physical problems such as renal dysfunction or electrolyte disturbances. Although it is usually clear that the patient has a strong motivation to take the substance, there is no development of dependence (F1x.2) or withdrawal symptoms (F1*x*.3) as in the case of the psychoactive substances specified in F10 – F19.

A fourth character may be used to identify the type of substance involved.

F55.0 Antidepressants

(such as tricyclic and tetracyclic antidepressants and monamine oxidase inhibitors)

F55.1 Laxatives

F55.2 Analgesics

(such as aspirin, paracetamol, phenacetin, not specified as psycho-active in F10 – F19)

F55.3 Antacids

F55.4 Vitamins

F55.5 Steroids or hormones

F55.6 Specific herbal or folk remedies

F55.8 Other substances that do not produce dependence

(such as diuretics)

F55.9 Unspecified

Excludes: abuse of (dependence-producing) psychoactive substances (F10 – F19)

F59 Unspecified behavioural syndromes associated with physiological disturbances and physical factors

Includes: psychogenic physiological dysfunction NOS

F60 – F69
Disorders of adult personality and behaviour

Overview of this block

F60 Specific personality disorders
    F60.0 Paranoid personality disorder
    F60.1 Schizoid personality disorder
    F60.2 Dissocial personality disorder
    F60.3 Emotionally unstable personality disorder
        .30 Impulsive type
        .31 Borderline type
    F60.4 Histrionic personality disorder
    F60.5 Anankastic personality disorder
    F60.6 Anxious [avoidant] personality disorder
    F60.7 Dependent personality disorder
    F60.8 Other specific personality disorders
    F60.9 Personality disorder, unspecified

F61 Mixed and other personality disorders
    F61.0[1] Mixed personality disorders
    F61.1[1] Troublesome personality changes

F62 Enduring personality changes, not attributable to brain damage and disease
    F62.0 Enduring personality change after catastrophic experience
    F62.1 Enduring personality change after psychiatric illness
    F62.8 Other enduring personality changes
    F62.9 Enduring personality change, unspecified

F63 Habit and impulse disorders
    F63.0 Pathological gambling
    F63.1 Pathological fire-setting [pyromania]
    F63.2 Pathological stealing [kleptomania]
    F63.3 Trichotillomania
    F63.8 Other habit and impulse disorders
    F63.9 Habit and impulse disorder, unspecified

---

[1] This four-character code is not included in Chapter V(F) of ICD-10.

F64 Gender identity disorders
F64.0 Transsexualism
F64.1 Dual-role transvestism
F64.2 Gender identity disorder of childhood
F64.8 Other gender identity disorders
F64.9 Gender identity disorder, unspecified

F65 Disorders of sexual preference
F65.0 Fetishism
F65.1 Fetishistic transvestism
F65.2 Exhibitionism
F65.3 Voyeurism
F65.4 Paedophilia
F65.5 Sadomasochism
F65.6 Multiple disorders of sexual preference
F65.8 Other disorders of sexual preference
F65.9 Disorder of sexual preference, unspecified

F66 Psychological and behavioural disorders associated with sexual development and orientation
F66.0 Sexual maturation disorder
F66.1 Egodystonic sexual orientation
F66.2 Sexual relationship disorder
F66.8 Other psychosexual development disorders
F66.9 Psychosexual development disorder, unspecified

A fifth character may be used to indicate association with:
.x0 Heterosexuality
.x1 Homosexuality
.x2 Bisexuality
.x8 Other, including prepubertal

F68 Other disorders of adult personality and behaviour
F68.0 Elaboration of physical symptoms for psychological reasons
F68.1 Intentional production or feigning of symptoms or disabilities either physical or psychological [factitious disorder]
F68.8 Other specified disorders of adult personality and behaviour

F69 Unspecified disorder of adult personality and behaviour

Introduction

This block includes a variety of clinically significant conditions and behaviour patterns which tend to be persistent and are the expression of an individual's characteristic lifestyle and mode of relating to self and others. Some of these conditions and patterns of behaviour emerge early in the course of individual development, as a result of both constitutional factors and social experience, while others are acquired later in life.

F60 – F62 Specific personality disorders, mixed and other personality disorders, and enduring personality changes

These types of condition comprise deeply ingrained and enduring behaviour patterns, manifesting themselves as inflexible responses to a broad range of personal and social situations. They represent either extreme or significant deviations from the way the average individual in a given culture perceives, thinks, feels, and particularly relates to others. Such behaviour patterns tend to be stable and to encompass multiple domains of behaviour and psychological functioning. They are frequently, but not always, associated wtih various degrees of subjective distress and problems in social functioning and performance.

Personality disorders differ from personality change in their timing and the mode of their emergence: they are developmental conditions, which appear in childhood or adolescence and continue into adulthood. They are not secondary to another mental disorder or brain disease, although they may precede and coexist with other disorders. In contrast, personality change is acquired, usually during adult life, following severe or prolonged stress, extreme environmental deprivation, serious psychiatric disorder, or brain disease or injury (see F07. –).

Each of the conditions in this group can be classified according to its predominant behavioural manifestations. However, classification in this area is currently limited to the description of a series of types and subtypes, which are not mutually exclusive and which overlap in some of their characteristics.

Personality disorders are therefore subdivided according to clusters of traits that correspond to the most frequent or conspicuous behavioural manifestations. The subtypes so described are widely recognized as major forms of personality deviation. In making a diagnosis of personality disorder, the clinician should consider all aspects of personal functioning, although the diagnostic formulation, to be simple and efficient, will refer to only those dimensions or traits for which the suggested thresholds for severity are reached.

The assessment should be based on as many sources of information as possible. Although it is sometimes possible to evaluate a personality condition in a single interview with the patient, it is often necessary to have more than one interview and to collect history data from informants.

Cyclothymia and schizotypal disorders were formerly classified with the personality disorders but are now listed elsewhere (cyclothymia in F30 – F39 and schizotypal disorder in F20 – F29), since they seem to have many aspects in common with the other disorders in those blocks (e.g. phenomena, family history).

The subdivision of personality change is based on the cause or antecedent of such change, i.e. catastrophic experience, prolonged stress or strain, and psychiatric illness (excluding residual schizophrenia, which is classified under F20.5).

It is important to separate personality conditions from the disorders included in other categories of this book. If a personality condition precedes or follows a time-limited or chronic psychiatric disorder, both should be diagnosed. Use of the multiaxial format accompanying the core classification of mental disorders and psychosocial factors will facilitate the recording of such conditions and disorders.

Cultural or regional variations in the manifestations of personality conditions are important, but specific knowledge in this area is still scarce. Personality conditions that appear to be frequently recognized in a given part of the world but do not correspond to any one of the specified subtypes below may be classified as "other" personality disorders and identified through a five-character code provided in an adaptation of this classification for that particular country or region. Local variations in the manifestations of a personality disorder may also be reflected in the wording of the diagnostic guidelines set for such conditions.

F60 Specific personality disorders

A specific personality disorder is a severe disturbance in the characterological constitution and behavioural tendencies of the individual, usually involving several areas of the personality, and nearly always associated with considerable personal and social disruption. Personality disorder tends to appear in late childhood or adolescence and continues to be manifest into adulthood. It is therefore unlikely that the diagnosis of personality disorder will be appropriate before the age of 16 or 17 years. General diagnostic guidelines applying to all personality disorders are presented below; supplementary descriptions are provided with each of the subtypes.

Diagnostic guidelines

Conditions not directly attributable to gross brain damage or disease, or to another psychiatric disorder, meeting the following criteria:

(a) markedly disharmonious attitudes and behaviour, involving usually several areas of functioning, e.g. affectivity, arousal, impulse control, ways of perceiving and thinking, and style of relating to others;

(b) the abnormal behaviour pattern is enduring, of long standing, and not limited to episodes of mental illness;

(c) the abnormal behaviour pattern is pervasive and clearly maladaptive to a broad range of personal and social situations;

(d) the above manifestations always appear during childhood or adolescence and continue into adulthood;

(e) the disorder leads to considerable personal distress but this may only become apparent late in its course;

(f) the disorder is usually, but not invariably, associated with significant problems in occupational and social performance.

For different cultures it may be necessary to develop specific sets of criteria with regard to social norms, rules and obligations. For diagnosing most of the subtypes listed below, clear evidence is usually required of the presence of *at least three* of the traits or behaviours given in the clinical description.

F60.0 Paranoid personality disorder

Personality disorder characterized by:

(a) excessive sensitiveness to setbacks and rebuffs;

(b) tendency to bear grudges pesistently, e.g. refusal to forgive insults and injuries or slights;

(c) suspiciousness and a pervasive tendency to distort experience by misconstruing the neutral or friendly actions of others as hostile or contemptuous;

(d) a combative and tenacious sense of personal rights out of keeping with the actual situation;

(e) recurrent suspicions, without justification, regarding sexual fidelity of spouse or sexual partner;

(f) tendency to experience excessive self-importance, manifest in a persistent self-referential attitude;

(g) preoccupation with unsubstantiated "conspiratorial" explanations of events both immediate to the patient and in the world at large.

Includes: expansive paranoid, fanatic, querulant and sensitive paranoid personality (disorder)

Excludes: delusional disorder (F22. –)
schizophrenia (F20. –)

F60.1 Schizoid personality disorder

Personality disorder meeting the following description:

(a) few, if any, activities, provide pleasure;

(b) emotional coldness, detachment or flattened affectivity;

(c) limited capacity to express either warm, tender feelings or anger towards others;

(d) apparent indifference to either praise or criticism;

(e) little interest in having sexual experiences with another person (taking into account age);

(f) almost invariable preference for solitary activities;

(g) excessive preoccupation with fantasy and introspection;

(h) lack of close friends or confiding relationships (or having only one) and of desire for such relationships;

(i) marked insensitivity to prevailing social norms and conventions.

Excludes: Asperger's syndrome (F84.5)
delusional disorder (F22.0)
schizoid disorder of childhood (F84.5)
schizophrenia (F20. –)
schizotypal disorder (F21)

F60.2 Dissocial personality disorder

Personality disorder, usually coming to attention because of a gross disparity between behaviour and the prevailing social norms, and characterized by:

(a) callous unconcern for the feelings of others;
(b) gross and persistent attitude of irresponsibility and disregard for social norms, rules and obligations;
(c) incapacity to maintain enduring relationships, though having no difficulty in establishing them;
(d) very low tolerance to frustration and a low threshold for discharge of aggression, including violence;
(e) incapacity to experience guilt or to profit from experience, particularly punishment;
(f) marked proneness to blame others, or to offer plausible rationalizations, for the behaviour that has brought the patient into conflict with society.

There may also be persistent irritability as an associated feature. Conduct disorder during childhood and adolescence, though not invariably present, may further support the diagnosis.

Includes: amoral, antisocial, asocial, psychopathic, and sociopathic personality (disorder)

Excludes: conduct disorders (F91. –)
emotionally unstable personality disorder (F60.3)

F60.3 Emotionally unstable personality disorder

A personality disorder in which there is a marked tendency to act impulsively without consideration of the consequences, together with affective instability. The ability to plan ahead may be minimal, and outbursts of intense anger may often lead to violence or "behavioural explosions"; these are easily precipitated when impulsive acts are criticized or thwarted by others. Two variants of this personality disorder are specified, and both share this general theme of impulsiveness and lack of self-control.

F60.30 Impulsive type

The predominant characteristics are emotional instability and lack of impulse control. Outbursts of violence or threatening behaviour are common, particularly in response to criticism by others.

Includes: explosive and aggressive personality (disorder)

Excludes: dissocial personality disorder (F60.2)

F60.31 Borderline type
Several of the characteristics of emotional instability are present; in addition, the patient's own self-image, aims, and internal preferences (including sexual) are often unclear or disturbed. There are usually chronic feelings of emptiness. A liability to become involved in intense and unstable relationships may cause repeated emotional crises and may be associated with excessive efforts to avoid abandonment and a series of suicidal threats or acts of self-harm (although these may occur without obvious precipitants).

Includes: borderline personality (disorder)

F60.4 Histrionic personality disorder
Personality disorder characterized by:

(a) self-dramatization, theatricality, exaggerated expression of emotions;
(b) suggestibility, easily influenced by others or by circumstances;
(c) shallow and labile affectivity;
(d) continual seeking for excitement and activities in which the patient is the centre of attention;
(e) inappropriate seductiveness in appearance or behaviour;
(f) over-concern with physical attractiveness.

Associated features may include egocentricity, self-indulgence, continuous longing for appreciation, feelings that are easily hurt, and persistent manipulative behaviour to achieve own needs.

Includes: hysterical and psychoinfantile personality (disorder)

F60.5 Anankastic personality disorder
Personality disorder characterized by:

(a) feelings of excessive doubt and caution;
(b) preoccupation with details, rules, lists, order, organization or schedule;
(c) perfectionism that interferes with task completion;

(d) excessive conscientiousness, scrupulousness, and undue preoccupation with productivity to the exclusion of pleasure and interpersonal relationships;

(e) excessive pedantry and adherence to social conventions;

(f) rigidity and stubbornness;

(g) unreasonable insistence by the patient that others submit to exactly his or her way of doing things, or unreasonable reluctance to allow others to do things;

(h) intrusion of insistent and unwelcome thoughts or impulses.

Includes: compulsive and obsessional personality (disorder)
    obsessive – compulsive personality disorder

Excludes: obsessive – compulsive disorder (F42. –)

F60.6 Anxious [avoidant] personality disorder

Personality disorder characterized by:

(a) persistent and pervasive feelings of tension and apprehension;

(b) belief that one is socially inept, personally unappealing, or inferior to others;

(c) excessive preoccupation with being criticized or rejected in social situations;

(d) unwillingness to become involved with people unless certain of being liked;

(e) restrictions in lifestyle because of need to have physical security;

(f) avoidance of social or occupational activities that involve significant interpersonal contact because of fear of criticism, disapproval, or rejection.

Associated features may include hypersensitivity to rejection and criticism.

F60.7 Dependent personality disorder

Personality disorder characterized by:

(a) encouraging or allowing others to make most of one's important life decisions;

(b) subordination of one's own needs to those of others on whom one is dependent, and undue compliance with their wishes;

(c) unwillingness to make even reasonable demands on the people one depends on;

(d) feeling uncomfortable or helpless when alone, because of exaggerated fears of inability to care for oneself;

(e) preoccupation with fears of being abandoned by a person with whom one has a close relationship, and of being left to care for oneself;

(f) limited capacity to make everyday decisions without an excessive amount of advice and reassurance from others.

Associated features may include perceiving oneself as helpless, incompetent, and lacking stamina.

Includes: asthenic, inadequate, passive, and self-defeating personality (disorder)

F60.8 Other specific personality disorders

A personality disorder that fits none of the specific rubrics F60.0 – F60.7.

Includes: eccentric, "haltlose" type, immature, narcissistic, passive – aggressive, and psychoneurotic personality (disorder)

F60.9 Personality disorder, unspecified

Includes: character neurosis NOS
pathological personality NOS

F61 Mixed and other personality disorders

This category is intended for personality disorders and abnormalities that are often troublesome but do not demonstrate the specific patterns of symptoms that characterize the disorders described in F60. – . As a result they are often more difficult to diagnose than the disorders in that category. Two types are specified here by the fourth character; any other different types should be coded as F60.8.

F61.0¹ Mixed personality disorders

With features of several of the disorders in F60. – but without a predominant set of symptoms that would allow a more specific diagnosis.

F61.1¹ Troublesome personality changes

Not classifiable in F60. – or F62. – and regarded as secondary to a main diagnosis of a coexisting affective or anxiety disorder.

Excludes: accentuation of personality traits (Z73.1)

F62 Enduring personality changes, not attributable to brain damage and disease

This group includes disorders of adult personality and behaviour which develop following catastrophic or excessive prolonged stress, or following a severe psychiatric illness, in people with no previous personality disorder. These diagnoses should be made only when there is evidence of a definite and enduring change in a person's pattern of perceiving, relating to, or thinking about the environment and the self. The personality change should be significant and associated with inflexible and maladaptive behaviour which was not present before the pathogenic experience. The change should not be a manifestation of another mental disorder, or a residual symptom of any antecedent mental disorder. Such enduring personality change is most often seen following devastating traumatic experience but may also develop in the aftermath of a severe, recurrent, or prolonged mental disorder. It may be difficult to differentiate between an acquired personality change and the unmasking or exacerbation of an existing personality disorder following stress, strain, or psychotic experience. Enduring personality change should be diagnosed only when the change represents a permanent and different way of being, which can be etiologically traced back to a profound, existentially extreme experience. The diagnosis should not be made if the personality disorder is secondary to brain damage or disease (category F07.0 should be used instead).

Excludes: personality and behavioural disorder due to brain disease, damage and dysfunction (F07. –)

---

¹ This four-character code is not included in Chapter V(F) of ICD-10.

F62.0 Enduring personality change after catastrophic experience

Enduring personality change may follow the experience of catastrophic stress. The stress must be so extreme that it is unnecessary to consider personal vulnerability in order to explain its profound effect on the personality. Examples include concentration camp experiences, torture, disasters, prolonged exposure to life-threatening circumstances (e.g. hostage situations — prolonged captivity with an imminent possibility of being killed). Post-traumatic stress disorder (F43.1) may precede this type of personality change, which may then be seen as a chronic, irreversible sequel of stress disorder. In other instances, however, enduring personality change meeting the description given below may develop without an interim phase of a manifest post-traumatic stress disorder. However, long-term change in personality following short-term exposure to a life-threatening experience such as a car accident should *not* be included in this category, since recent research indicates that such a development depends on a pre-existing psychological vulnerability.

Diagnostic guidelines

The personality change should be enduring and manifest as inflexible and maladaptive features leading to an impairment in interpersonal, social, and occupational functioning. Usually the personality change has to be confirmed by a key informant. In order to make the diagnosis, it is essential to establish the presence of features not previously seen, such as:

(a) a hostile or mistrustful attitude towards the world;
(b) social withdrawal;
(c) feelings of emptiness or hopelessness;
(d) a chronic feeling of being "on edge", as if constantly threatened;
(e) estrangement.

This personality change must have been present for at least 2 years, and should not be attributable to a pre-existing personality disorder or to a mental disorder other than post-traumatic stress disorder (F43.1). The presence of brain damage or disease which may cause similar clinical features should be ruled out.

Includes: personality change after concentration camp experiences, disasters, prolonged captivity with imminent possibility of being killed, prolonged exposure to life-threatening situations such as being a victim of terrorism or torture

Excludes: post-traumatic stress disorder (F43.1)

F62.1   Enduring personality change after psychiatric illness
Personality change attributable to the traumatic experience of suffering from a severe psychiatric illness. The change cannot be explained by pre-existing personality disorder and should be differentiated from residual schizophrenia and other states of incomplete recovery from an antecedent mental disorder.

Diagnostic guidelines

The personality change should be enduring and manifest as an inflexible and maladaptive pattern of experiencing and functioning, leading to long-standing problems in interpersonal, social, or occupational functioning and subjective distress. There should be no evidence of a pre-existing personality disorder that can explain the personality change, and the diagnosis should not be based on any residual symptoms of the antecedent mental disorder. The change in personality develops following clinical recovery from a mental disorder that must have been experienced as emotionally extremely stressful and shattering to the patient's self-image. Other people's attitudes or reactions to the patient following the illness are important in determining and reinforcing his or her perceived level of stress. This type of personality change cannot be fully understood without taking into consideration the subjective emotional experience and the previous personality, its adjustment, and its specific vulnerabilities.

Diagnostic evidence for this type of personality change should include such clinical features as the following:

(a) excessive dependence on and a demanding attitude towards others;
(b) conviction of being changed or stigmatized by the preceding illness, leading to an inability to form and maintain close and confiding personal relationships and to social isolation;
(c) passivity, reduced interests, and diminished involvement in leisure activities;
(d) persistent complaints of being ill, which may be associated with hypochondriacal claims and illness behaviour;

(e) dysphoric or labile mood, not due to the presence of a current mental disorder or antecedent mental disorder with residual affective symptoms;

(f) significant impairment in social and occupational functioning compared with the premorbid situation.

The above manifestations must have been present over a period of 2 or more years. The change is not attributable to gross brain damage or disease. A previous diagnosis of schizophrenia does not preclude the diagnosis.

F62.8 Other enduring personality changes

Includes: enduring personality disorder after experiences not mentioned in F62.0 and F62.1, such as chronic pain personality syndrome and enduring personality change after bereavement

F62.9 Enduring personality change, unspecified

F63 Habit and impulse disorders

This category includes certain behavioural disorders that are not classifiable under other rubrics. They are characterized by repeated acts that have no clear rational motivation and that generally harm the patient's own interests and those of other people. The patient reports that the behaviour is associated with impulses to action that cannot be controlled. The causes of these conditions are not understood; the disorders are grouped together because of broad descriptive similarities, not because they are known to share any other important features. By convention, the habitual excessive use of alcohol or drugs (F10 – F19) and impulse and habit disorders involving sexual (F65. –) or eating (F52. –) behaviour are excluded.

F63.0 Pathological gambling

The disorder consists of frequent, repeated episodes of gambling which dominate the individual's life to the detriment of social, occupational, material, and family values and commitments.

Those who suffer from this disorder may put their jobs at risk, acquire large debts, and lie or break the law to obtain money or evade payment of debts. They describe an intense urge to gamble, which is difficult to control, together with preoccupation with ideas and images of the act of gambling and the circumstances that surround the act. These preoccupations and urges often increase at times when life is stressful.

This disorder is also called "compulsive gambling" but this term is less appropriate because the behaviour is not compulsive in the technical sense, nor is the disorder related to obsessive – compulsive neurosis.

Diagnostic guidelines

The essential feature of the disorder is persistently repeated gambling, which continues and often increases despite adverse social consequences such as impoverishment, impaired family relationships, and disruption of personal life.

Includes: compulsive gambling

Differential diagnosis. Pathological gambling should be distinguished from:

(a) gambling and betting (Z72.6) (frequent gambling for excitement, or in an attempt to make money; people in this category are likely to curb their habit when confronted with heavy losses, or other adverse effects);

(b) excessive gambling by manic patients (F30. –);

(c) gambling by sociopathic personalities (F60.2) (in which there is a wider persistent disturbance of social behaviour, shown in acts that are aggressive or in other ways demonstrate a marked lack of concern for the well-being and feelings of other people).

F63.1   Pathological fire-setting [pyromania]

The disorder is characterized by multiple acts of, or attempts at, setting fire to property or other objects, without apparent motive, and by a persistent preoccupation with subjects related to fire and burning. There may also be an abnormal interest in fire-engines and other fire-fighting equipment, in other associations of fires, and in calling out the fire service.

Diagnostic guidelines

The essential features are:

(a) repeated fire-setting without any obvious motive such as monetary gain, revenge, or political extremism;
(b) an intense interest in watching fires burn; and
(c) reported feelings of increasing tension before the act, and intense excitement immediately after it has been carried out.

Differential diagnosis. Pathological fire-setting should be distinguished from:

(a) deliberate fire-setting without a manifest psychiatric disorder (in these cases there is an obvious motive) (Z03.2, observation for suspected mental disorder);
(b) fire-setting by a young person with conduct disorder (F91.1), where there is evidence of other disordered behaviour such as stealing, aggression, or truancy;
(c) fire-setting by an adult with sociopathic personality disorder (F60.2), where there is evidence of other persistent disturbance of social behaviour such as aggression, or other indications of lack of concern with the interests and feelings of other people;
(d) fire-setting in schizophrenia (F20. –), when fires are typically started in response to delusional ideas or commands from hallucinated voices;
(e) fire-setting in organic psychiatric disorders (F00 – F09), when fires are started accidentally as a result of confusion, poor memory, or lack of awareness of the consequences of the act, or a combination of these factors.

Dementia or acute organic states may also lead to inadvertent fire-setting; acute drunkenness, chronic alcoholism or other drug intoxication (F10 – F19) are other causes.

F63.2 Pathological stealing [kleptomania]

The disorder is characterized by repeated failure to resist impulses to steal objects that are not acquired for personal use or monetary gain. The objects may instead be discarded, given away, or hoarded.

Diagnostic guidelines

There is an increasing sense of tension before, and a sense of gratification during and immediately after, the act. Although some

213

effort at concealment is usually made, not all the opportunities for this are taken. The theft is a solitary act, not carried out with an accomplice. The individual may express anxiety, despondency, and guilt between episodes of stealing from shops (or other premises) but this does not prevent repetition. Cases meeting this description alone, and not secondary to one of the disorders listed below, are uncommon.

Differential diagnosis. Pathological stealing should be distinguished from:

(a) recurrent shoplifting without a manifest psychiatric disorder, when the acts are more carefully planned, and there is an obvious motive of personal gain (Z03.2, observation for suspected mental disorder);

(b) organic mental disorder (F00 – F09), when there is recurrent failure to pay for goods as a consequence of poor memory and other kinds of intellectual deterioration;

(c) depressive disorder with stealing (F30 – F33); some depressed individuals steal, and may do so repeatedly as long as the depressive disorder persists.

F63.3   Trichotillomania

A disorder characterized by noticeable hair loss due to a recurrent failure to resist impulses to pull out hairs. The hair-pulling is usually preceded by mounting tension and is followed by a sense of relief or gratification. This diagnosis should not be made if there is a pre-existing inflammation of the skin, or if the hair-pulling is in response to a delusion or a hallucination.

Excludes: stereotyped movement disorder with hair-plucking (F98.4)

F63.8   Other habit and impulse disorders

This category should be used for other kinds of persistently repeated maladaptive behaviour that are not secondary to a recognized psychiatric syndrome, and in which it appears that there is repeated failure to resist impulses to carry out the behaviour. There is a prodromal period of tension with a feeling of release at the time of the act.

Includes: intermittent explosive (behaviour) disorder

F63.9   Habit and impulse disorder, unspecified

F64   Gender identity disorders

F64.0   Transsexualism

A desire to live and be accepted as a member of the opposite sex, usually accompanied by a sense of discomfort with, or inappropriateness of, one's anatomic sex and a wish to have hormonal treatment and surgery to make one's body as congruent as possible with the preferred sex.

Diagnostic guidelines

For this diagnosis to be made, the transsexual identity should have been present persistently for at least 2 years, and must not be a symptom of another mental disorder, such as schizophrenia, or associated with any intersex, genetic, or sex chromosome abnormality.

F64.1   Dual-role transvestism

The wearing of clothes of the opposite sex for part of the individual's existence in order to enjoy the temporary experience of membership of the opposite sex, but without any desire for a more permanent sex change or associated surgical reassignment. No sexual excitement accompanies the cross-dressing, which distinguishes the disorder from fetishistic transvestism (F65.1).

Includes: gender identity disorder of adolescence or adulthood, nontranssexual type

Excludes: fetishistic transvestism (F65.1)

F64.2   Gender identity disorder of childhood

Disorders, usually first manifest during early childhood (and always well before puberty), characterized by a persistent and intense distress about assigned sex, together with a desire to be (or insistence that one is) of the other sex. There is a persistent preoccupation with the dress and/or activities of the opposite sex and/or repudiation of the patient's own sex. These disorders are thought to be relatively uncommon and should not be confused with the much more frequent nonconformity with stereotypic sex-role behaviour. The diagnosis of gender identity disorder in childhood requires a

215

profound disturbance of the normal sense of maleness or femaleness; mere "tomboyishness" in girls or "girlish" behaviour in boys is not sufficient. The diagnosis cannot be made when the individual has reached puberty.

Because gender identity disorder of childhood has many features in common with the other identity disorders in this section, it has been classified in F64. – rather than in F90 – F98.

Diagnostic guidelines

The essential diagnostic feature is the child's pervasive and persistent desire to be (or insistence that he or she is of) the opposite sex to that assigned, together with an intense rejection of the behaviour, attributes, and/or attire of the assigned sex. Typically, this is first manifest during the preschool years; for the diagnosis to be made, the disorder must have been apparent before puberty. In both sexes, there may be repudiation of the anatomical structures of their own sex, but this is an uncommon, probably rare, manifestation. Characteristically, children with a gender identity disorder deny being disturbed by it, although they may be distressed by the conflict with the expectations of their family or peers and by the teasing and/or rejection to which they may be subjected.

More is known about these disorders in boys than in girls. Typically, from the preschool years onwards, boys are preoccupied with types of play and other activities stereotypically associated with females, and there may often be a preference for dressing in girls' or women's clothes. However, such cross-dressing does not cause sexual excitement (unlike fetishistic transvestism in adults (F65.1)). They may have a very strong desire to participate in the games and pastimes of girls, female dolls are often their favourite toys, and girls are regularly their preferred playmates. Social ostracism tends to arise during the early years of schooling and is often at a peak in middle childhood, with humiliating teasing by other boys. Grossly feminine behaviour may lessen during early adolescence but follow-up studies indicate that between one-third and two-thirds of boys with gender identity disorder of childhood show a homosexual orientation during and after adolescence. However, very few exhibit transsexualism in adult life (although most adults with transsexualism report having had a gender identity problem in childhood).

In clinic samples, gender identity disorders are less frequent in girls than in boys, but it is not known whether this sex ratio applies in the general population. In girls, as in boys, there is usually an early manifestation of a preoccupation with behaviour stereotypically associated with the opposite sex. Typically, girls with these disorders have male companions and show an avid interest in sports and rough-and-tumble play; they lack interest in dolls and in taking female roles in make-believe games such as "mothers and fathers" or playing "house". Girls with a gender identity disorder tend not to experience the same degree of social ostracism as boys, although they may suffer from teasing in later childhood or adolescence. Most give up an exaggerated insistence on male activities and attire as they approach adolescence, but some retain a male identification and go on to show a homosexual orientation.

Rarely, a gender identity disorder may be associated with a persistent repudiation of the anatomic structures of the assigned sex. In girls, this may be manifest by repeated assertions that they have, or will grow, a penis, by rejection of urination in the sitting position, or by the assertion that they do not want to grow breasts or to menstruate. In boys, it may be shown by repeated assertions that they will grow up physically to become a woman, that penis and testes are disgusting or will disappear, and/or that it would be better not to have a penis or testes.

Excludes: egodystonic sexual orientation (F66.1)
    sexual maturation disorder (F66.0)

F64.8   Other gender identity disorders

F64.9   Gender identity disorder, unspecified

Includes: gender-role disorder NOS

F65   Disorders of sexual preference

Includes: paraphilias

Excludes: problems associated with sexual orientation (F66. –)

F65.0   Fetishism

Reliance on some non-living object as a stimulus for sexual arousal and sexual gratification. Many fetishes are extensions of the human body, such as articles of clothing or footware. Other common examples are characterized by some particular texture such as rubber, plastic, or leather. Fetish objects vary in their importance to the individual: in some cases they serve simply to enhance sexual excitement achieved in ordinary ways (e.g. having the partner wear a particular garment).

Diagnostic guidelines

Fetishism should be diagnosed only if the fetish is the most important source of sexual stimulation or essential for satisfactory sexual response.

Fetishistic fantasies are common, but they do not amount to a disorder unless they lead to rituals that are so compelling and unacceptable as to interfere with sexual intercourse and cause the individual distress.

Fetishism is limited almost exclusively to males.

F65.1   Fetishistic transvestism

The wearing of clothes of the opposite sex principally to obtain sexual excitement.

Diagnostic guidelines

This disorder is to be distinguished from simple fetishism in that the fetishistic articles of clothing are not only worn, but worn also to create the appearance of a person of the opposite sex. Usually more than one article is worn and often a complete outfit, plus wig and makeup. Fetishistic transvestism is distinguished from transsexual transvestism by its clear association with sexual arousal and the strong desire to remove the clothing once orgasm occurs and sexual arousal declines. A history of fetishistic transvestism is commonly reported as an earlier phase by transsexuals and probably represents a stage in the development of transsexualism in such cases.

Includes: transvestic fetishism

F65.2   Exhibitionism

A recurrent or persistent tendency to expose the genitalia to strangers (usually of the opposite sex) or to people in public places, without inviting or intending closer contact. There is usually, but not invariably, sexual excitement at the time of the exposure and the act is commonly followed by masturbation. This tendency may be manifest only at times of emotional stress or crises, interspersed with long periods without such overt behaviour.

Diagnostic guidelines

Exhibitionism is almost entirely limited to heterosexual males who expose to females, adult or adolescent, usually confronting them from a safe distance in some public place. For some, exhibitionism is their only sexual outlet, but others continue the habit simultaneously with an active sex life within long-standing relationships, although their urges may become more pressing at times of conflict in those relationships. Most exhibitionists find their urges difficult to control and ego-alien. If the witness appears shocked, frightened, or impressed, the exhibitionist's excitement is often heightened.

F65.3   Voyeurism

A recurrent or persistent tendency to look at people engaging in sexual or intimate behaviour such as undressing. This usually leads to sexual excitement and masturbation and is carried out without the observed people being aware.

F65.4   Paedophilia

A sexual preference for children, usually of prepubertal or early pubertal age. Some paedophiles are attracted only to girls, others only to boys, and others again are interested in both sexes.

Paedophilia is rarely identified in women. Contacts between adults and sexually mature adolescents are socially disapproved, especially if the participants are of the same sex, but are not necessarily associated with paedophilia. An isolated incident, especially if the perpetrator is himself an adolescent, does not establish the presence of the persistent or predominant tendency required for the diagnosis. Included among paedophiles, however, are men who retain a preference for adult sex partners but, because they are chronically frustrated in achieving appropriate contacts, habitually turn to children as substitutes. Men who sexually molest their own prepubertal children occasionally approach other children as well, but in either case their behaviour is indicative of paedophilia.

F65.5 Sadomasochism

A preference for sexual activity that involves bondage or the infliction of pain or humiliation. If the individual prefers to be the recipient of such stimulation this is called masochism; if the provider, sadism. Often an individual obtains sexual excitement from both sadistic and masochistic activities.

Mild degrees of sadomasochistic stimulation are commonly used to enhance otherwise normal sexual activity. This category should be used only if sadomasochistic activity is the most important source of stimulation or necessary for sexual gratification.

Sexual sadism is sometimes difficult to distinguish from cruelty in sexual situations or anger unrelated to eroticism. Where violence is necessary for erotic arousal, the diagnosis can be clearly established.

Includes: masochism
sadism

F65.6 Multiple disorders of sexual preference

Sometimes more than one disorder of sexual preference occurs in one person and none has clear precedence. The most common combination is fetishism, transvestism, and sadomasochism.

F65.8 Other disorders of sexual preference

A variety of other patterns of sexual preference and activity may occur, each being relatively uncommon. These include such activities as making obscene telephone calls, rubbing up against people for sexual stimulation in crowded public places (frotteurism), sexual activity with animals, use of strangulation or anoxia for intensifying sexual excitement, and a preference for partners with some particular anatomical abnormality such as an amputated limb.

Erotic practices are too diverse and many too rare or idiosyncratic to justify a separate term for each. Swallowing urine, smearing faeces, or piercing foreskin or nipples may be part of the behavioural repertoire in sadomasochism. Masturbatory rituals of various kinds are common, but the more extreme practices, such as the insertion of objects into the rectum or penile urethra, or partial self-strangulation, when they take the place of ordinary sexual contacts, amount to abnormalities. Necrophilia should also be coded here.

Includes: frotteurism
  necrophilia

F65.9 Disorder of sexual preference, unspecified

Includes: sexual deviation NOS

F66 Psychological and behavioural disorders associated with sexual development and orientation

Note: Sexual orientation alone is not to be regarded as a disorder.

The following five-character codes may be used to indicate variations of sexual development or orientation that may be problematic for the individual:

F66.*x*0 Heterosexual

F66.*x*1 Homosexual

F66.*x*2 Bisexual
To be used only when there is clear evidence of sexual attraction to members of both sexes.

F66.*x*8 Other, including prepubertal

F66.0 Sexual maturation disorder

The individual suffers from uncertainty about his or her gender identity or sexual orientation, which causes anxiety or depression. Most commonly this occurs in adolescents who are not certain whether they are homosexual, heterosexual, or bisexual in orientation, or in individuals who after a period of apparently stable sexual orientation, often within a long-standing relationship, find that their sexual orientation is changing.

F66.1 Egodystonic sexual orientation
The gender identity or sexual preference is not in doubt but the individual wishes it were different because of associated psychological and behavioural disorders and may seek treatment in order to change it.

F66.2 Sexual relationship disorder
The gender identity or sexual preference abnormality is responsible for difficulties in forming or maintaining a relationship with a sexual partner.

F66.8 Other psychosexual development disorders

F66.9 Psychosexual development disorder, unspecified

F68 Other disorders of adult personality and behaviour

F68.0 Elaboration of physical symptoms for psychological reasons
Physical symptoms compatible with and originally due to a confirmed physical disorder, disease, or disability become exaggerated or prolonged due to the psychological state of the patient. An attention-seeking (histrionic) behavioural syndrome develops, which may also contain additional (and usually nonspecific) complaints that are not of physical origin. The patient is commonly distressed by this pain or disability and is often preoccupied with worries, which may be justified, of the possibility of prolonged or progressive disability or pain. Dissatisfaction with the result of treatment or investigations, or disappointment with the amount of personal attention received in wards and clinics may also be a motivating factor. Some cases appear to be clearly motivated by the possibility of financial compensation following accidents or injuries, but the syndrome does not necessarily resolve rapidly even after successful litigation.

Includes: compensation neurosis

F68.1 Intentional production or feigning of symptoms or disabilities, either physical or psychological [factitious disorder]
In the absence of a confirmed physical or mental disorder, disease, or disability, the individual feigns symptoms repeatedly and consistently. For physical symptoms this may even extend to self-infliction

of cuts or abrasions to produce bleeding, or to self-injection of toxic substances. The imitation of pain and the insistence upon the presence of bleeding may be so convincing and persistent that repeated investigations and operations are performed at several different hospitals or clinics, in spite of repeatedly negative findings.

The motivation for this behaviour is almost always obscure and presumably internal, and the condition is best interpreted as a disorder of illness behaviour and the sick role. Individuals with this pattern of behaviour usually show signs of a number of other marked abnormalities of personality and relationships.

Malingering, defined as the intentional production or feigning of either physical or psychological symptoms or disabilities, motivated by external stresses or incentives, should be coded as Z76.5 of ICD-10, and not by one of the codes in this book. The commonest external motives for malingering include evading criminal prosecution, obtaining illicit drugs, avoiding military conscription or dangerous military duty, and attempts to obtain sickness benefits or improvements in living conditions such as housing. Malingering is comparatively common in legal and military circles, and comparatively uncommon in ordinary civilian life.

Includes: hospital hopper syndrome
Munchhausen's syndrome
peregrinating patient

Excludes: battered baby or child syndrome NOS (T74.1)
factitial dermatitis (unintentionally produced) (L98.1)
malingering (person feigning illness) (Z76.5)
Munchhausen by proxy (child abuse) (T74.8)

F68.8   Other specified disorders of adult personality and behaviour
This category should be used for coding any specified disorder of adult personality and behaviour that cannot be classified under any one of the preceding headings.

Includes: character disorder NOS
relationship disorder NOS

F69 Unspecified disorder of adult personality and behaviour

This code should be used only as a last resort, if the presence of a disorder of adult personality and behaviour can be assumed, but information to allow its diagnosis and allocation to a specific category is lacking.

F70 – F79
Mental retardation

Overview of this block

F70 Mild mental retardation
F71 Moderate mental retardation
F72 Severe mental retardation
F73 Profound mental retardation
F78 Other mental retardation
F79 Unspecified mental retardation

A fourth character may be used to specify the extent of associated behavioural impairment:

F7x.0 No, or minimal, impairment of behaviour
F7x.1 Significant impairment of behaviour requiring attention or treatment
F7x.8 Other impairments of behaviour
F7x.9 Without mention of impairment of behaviour

Introduction

Mental retardation is a condition of arrested or incomplete development of the mind, which is especially characterized by impairment of skills manifested during the developmental period, which contribute to the overall level of intelligence, i.e. cognitive, language, motor, and social abilities. Retardation can occur with or without any other mental or physical disorder. However, mentally retarded individuals can experience the full range of mental disorders, and the prevalence of other mental disorders is at least three to four times greater in this population than in the general population. In addition, mentally retarded individuals are at greater risk of exploitation and physical/sexual abuse. Adaptive behaviour is always impaired, but in protected social environments where support is available this impairment may not be at all obvious in subjects with mild mental retardation.

A fourth character may be used to specify the extent of the behavioural impairment, if this is not due to an associated disorder:

F7x.0 No, or minimal, impairment of behaviour
F7x.1 Significant impairment of behaviour requiring attention or treatment
F7x.8 Other impairments of behaviour
F7x.9 Without mention of impairment of behaviour

If the cause of the mental retardation is known, an additional code from ICD-10 should be used (e.g. F72 severe mental retardation plus E00. − (congenital iodine-deficiency syndrome)).

The presence of mental retardation does not rule out additional diagnoses coded elsewhere in this book. However, communication difficulties are likely to make it necessary to rely more than usual for the diagnosis upon objectively observable symptoms such as, in the case of a depressive episode, psychomotor retardation, loss of appetite and weight, and sleep disturbance.

Diagnostic guidelines

Intelligence is not a unitary characteristic but is assessed on the basis of a large number of different, more-or-less specific skills. Although the general tendency is for all these skills to develop to a similar level in each individual, there can be large discrepancies, especially in persons who are mentally retarded. Such people may show severe impairments in one particular area (e.g. language), or may have a particular area of higher skill (e.g. in simple visuospatial tasks) against a background of severe mental retardation. This presents

226

problems when determining the diagnostic category in which a retarded person should be classified. The assessment of intellectual level should be based on whatever information is available, including clinical findings, adaptive behaviour (judged in relation to the individual's cultural background), and psychometric test performance.

For a definite diagnosis, there should be a reduced level of intellectual functioning resulting in diminished ability to adapt to the daily demands of the normal social environment. Associated mental or physical disorders have a major influence on the clinical picture and the use made of any skills. The diagnostic category chosen should therefore be based on global assessments of ability and not on any single area of specific impairment or skill. The IQ levels given are provided as a guide and should not be applied rigidly in view of the problems of cross-cultural validity. The categories given below are arbitrary divisions of a complex continuum, and cannot be defined with absolute precision. The IQ should be determined from standardized, individually administered intelligence tests for which local cultural norms have been determined, and the test selected should be appropriate to the individual's level of functioning and additional specific handicapping conditions, e.g. expressive language problems, hearing impairment, physical involvement. Scales of social maturity and adaptation, again locally standardized, should be completed if at all possible by interviewing a parent or care-provider who is familiar with the individual's skills in everyday life. Without the use of standardized procedures, the diagnosis must be regarded as a provisional estimate only.

F70 Mild mental retardation

Mildly retarded people acquire language with some delay but most achieve the ability to use speech for everyday purposes, to hold conversations, and to engage in the clinical interview. Most of them also achieve full independence in self-care (eating, washing, dressing, bowel and bladder control) and in practical and domestic skills, even if the rate of development is considerably slower than normal. The main difficulties are usually seen in academic school work, and many have particular problems in reading and writing. However, mildly retarded people can be greatly helped by education designed to develop their skills and compensate for their handicaps. Most of those in the higher ranges of mild mental retardation are potentially capable of work demanding practical rather than academic abilities, including unskilled or semiskilled manual labour. In a sociocultural context requiring little academic achievement, some degree of mild retardation may not itself represent a problem. However, if there is also noticeable emotional and social immaturity, the consequences of the handicap, e.g. inability to cope with the demands of marriage or child-rearing, or difficulty fitting in with cultural traditions and expectations, will be apparent.

In general, the behavioural, emotional, and social difficulties of the mildly mentally retarded, and the needs for treatment and support arising from them, are more closely akin to those found in people of normal intelligence than to the specific problems of the moderately and severely retarded. An organic etiology is being identified in increasing proportions of patients, although not yet in the majority.

Diagnostic guidelines

If the proper standardized IQ tests are used, the range 50 to 69 is indicative of mild retardation. Understanding and use of language tend to be delayed to a varying degree, and executive speech problems that interfere with the development of independence may persist into adult life. An organic etiology is identifiable in only a minority of subjects. Associated conditions such as autism, other developmental disorders, epilepsy, conduct disorders, or physical disability are found in varying proportions. If such disorders are present, they should be coded independently.

Includes: feeble-mindedness
mild mental subnormality
mild oligophrenia
moron

F71 Moderate mental retardation

Individuals in this category are slow in developing comprehension and use of language, and their eventual achievement in this area is limited. Achievement of self-care and motor skills is also retarded, and some need supervision throughout life. Progress in school work is limited, but a proportion of these individuals learn the basic skills needed for reading, writing, and counting. Educational programmes can provide opportunities for them to develop their limited potential and to acquire some basic skills; such programmes are appropriate for slow learners with a low ceiling of achievement. As adults, moderately retarded people are usually able to do simple practical work, if the tasks are carefully structured and skilled supervision is provided. Completely independent living in adult life is rarely achieved. Generally, however, such people are fully mobile and physically active and the majority show evidence of social development in their ability to establish contact, to communicate with others, and to engage in simple social activities.

Diagnostic guidelines

The IQ is usually in the range 35 to 49. Discrepant profiles of abilities are common in this group, with some individuals achieving higher levels in visuo-spatial skills than in tasks dependent on language, while others are markedly clumsy but enjoy social interaction and simple conversation. The level of development of language is variable: some of those affected can take part in simple conversations while others have only enough language to communicate their basic needs. Some never learn to use language, though they may understand simple instructions and may learn to use manual signs to compensate to some extent for their speech disabilities. An organic etiology can be identified in the majority of moderately mentally retarded people. Childhood autism or other pervasive developmental disorders are present in a substantial minority, and have a major effect upon the clinical picture and the type of management needed. Epilepsy, and neurological and physical disabilities are also common, although most moderately retarded people are able to walk without assistance. It is sometimes possible to identify other psychiatric conditions, but the limited level of language development may make diagnosis difficult and dependent upon information obtained from others who are familiar with the individual. Any such associated disorders should be coded independently.

Includes: imbecility
moderate mental subnormality
moderate oligophrenia

F72 Severe mental retardation

This category is broadly similar to that of moderate mental retardation in terms of the clinical picture, the presence of an organic etiology, and the associated conditions. The lower levels of achievement mentioned under F71 are also the most common in this group. Most people in this category suffer from a marked degree of motor impairment or other associated deficits, indicating the presence of clinically significant damage to or maldevelopment of the central nervous system.

Diagnostic guidelines

The IQ is usually in the range of 20 to 34.

Includes: severe mental subnormality
severe oligophrenia

F73 Profound mental retardation

The IQ in this category is estimated to be under 20, which means in practice that affected individuals are severely limited in their ability to understand or comply with requests or instructions. Most such individuals are immobile or severely restricted in mobility, incontinent, and capable at most of only very rudimentary forms of nonverbal communication. They possess little or no ability to care for their own basic needs, and require constant help and supervision.

Diagnostic guidelines

The IQ is under 20. Comprehension and use of language is limited to, at best, understanding basic commands and making simple requests. The most basic and simple visuo-spatial skills of sorting and matching may be acquired, and the affected person may be able with appropriate supervision and guidance to take a small part in domestic and practical tasks. An organic etiology can be identified in most cases. Severe neurological or other physical disabilities affecting mobility are common, as are epilepsy and visual and hearing impairments. Pervasive developmental disorders in their most severe form, especially atypical autism, are particularly frequent, especially in those who are mobile.

Includes: idiocy
profound mental subnormality
profound oligophrenia

F78　Other mental retardation

This category should be used only when assessment of the degree of intellectual retardation by means of the usual procedures is rendered particularly difficult or impossible by associated sensory or physical impairments, as in blind, deaf-mute, and severely behaviourally disturbed or physically disabled people.

F79　Unspecified mental retardation

There is evidence of mental retardation, but insufficient information is available to assign the patient to one of the above categories.

Includes: mental deficiency NOS
mental subnormality NOS
oligophrenia NOS

F80 – F89
Disorders of psychological development

Overview of this block

F80 Specific developmental disorders of speech and language
F80.0 Specific speech articulation disorder
F80.1 Expressive language disorder
F80.2 Receptive language disorder
F80.3 Acquired aphasia with epilepsy [Landau – Kleffner syndrome]
F80.8 Other developmental disorders of speech and language
F80.9 Developmental disorder of speech and language, unspecified

F81 Specific developmental disorders of scholastic skills
F81.0 Specific reading disorder
F81.1 Specific spelling disorder
F81.2 Specific disorder of arithmetical skills
F81.3 Mixed disorder of scholastic skills
F81.8 Other developmental disorders of scholastic skills
F81.9 Developmental disorder of scholastic skills, unspecified

F82 Specific developmental disorder of motor function

F83 Mixed specific developmental disorders

F84 Pervasive developmental disorders
F84.0 Childhood autism
F84.1 Atypical autism
F84.2 Rett's syndrome
F84.3 Other childhood disintegrative disorder
F84.4 Overactive disorder associated with mental retardation and
    stereotyped movements
F84.5 Asperger's syndrome
F84.8 Other pervasive developmental disorders
F84.9 Pervasive developmental disorder, unspecified

F88 Other disorders of psychological development

F89 Unspecified disorder of psychological development

Introduction

The disorders included in F80 – F89 have the following features in common:

(a) an onset that is invariably during infancy or childhood;

(b) an impairment or delay in the development of functions that are strongly related to biological maturation of the central nervous system; and

(c) a steady course that does not involve the remissions and relapses that tend to be characteristic of many mental disorders.

In most cases, the functions affected include language, visuo-spatial skills and/or motor coordination. It is characteristic for the impairments to lessen progressively as children grow older (although milder deficits often remain in adult life). Usually, the history is of a delay or impairment that has been present from as early as it could be reliably detected, with no prior period of normal development. Most of these conditions are several times more common in boys than in girls.

It is characteristic of developmental disorders that a family history of similar or related disorders is common, and there is presumptive evidence that genetic factors play an important role in the etiology of many (but not all) cases. Environmental factors often influence the developmental functions affected but in most cases they are not of paramount influence. However, although there is generally good agreement on the overall conceptualization of disorders in this section, the etiology in most cases is unknown and there is continuing uncertainty regarding both the boundaries and the precise subdivisions of developmental disorders. Moreover, two types of condition are included in this block that do not entirely meet the broad conceptual definition outlined above. First, there are disorders in which there has been an undoubted phase of prior normal development, such as the childhood disintegrative disorder, the Landau – Kleffner syndrome, and some cases of autism. These conditions are included because, although their onset is different, their characteristics and course have many similarities with the group of developmental disorders; moreover it is not known whether or not they are etiologically distinct. Second, there are disorders that are defined primarily in terms of *deviance* rather than delay in developmental functions; this applies especially to autism. Autistic disorders are included in this block because, although defined in terms of deviance, developmental delay of some degree is almost invariable. Furthermore, there is overlap with the other developmental disorders in terms of both the features of individual cases and familiar clustering.

233

F80 Specific developmental disorders of speech and language

These are disorders in which normal patterns of language acquisition are disturbed from the early stages of development. The conditions are not directly attributable to neurological or speech mechanism abnormalities, sensory impairments, mental retardation, or environmental factors. The child may be better able to communicate or understand in certain very familiar situations than in others, but language ability in every setting is impaired.

Differential diagnosis. As with other developmental disorders, the first difficulty in diagnosis concerns the differentiation from normal variations in development. Normal children vary widely in the age at which they first acquire spoken language and in the pace at which language skills become firmly established. Such normal variations are of little or no clinical significance, as the great majority of "slow speakers" go on to develop entirely normally. In sharp contrast, children with specific developmental disorders of speech and language, although most ultimately acquire a normal level of language skills, have multiple associated problems. Language delay is often followed by difficulties in reading and spelling, abnormalities in interpersonal relationships, and emotional and behavioural disorders. Accordingly, early and accurate diagnosis of specific developmental disorders of speech and language is important. There is no clear-cut demarcation from the extremes of normal variation, but four main criteria are useful in suggesting the occurrence of a clinically significant disorder: severity, course, pattern, and associated problems.

As a general rule, a language delay that is sufficiently severe to fall outside the limits of 2 standard deviations may be regarded as abnormal. Most cases of this severity have associated problems. The level of severity in statistical terms is of less diagnostic use in older children, however, because there is a natural tendency towards progressive improvement. In this situation the course provides a useful indicator. If the current level of impairment is mild but there is nevertheless a history of a previously severe degree of impairment, the likelihood is that the current functioning represents the sequelae of a significant disorder rather than just normal variation. Attention should be paid to the pattern of speech and language functioning; if the pattern is abnormal (i.e. deviant and not just of a kind appropriate for an earlier phase of development), or if the child's speech or language includes qualitatively abnormal features, a clinically significant disorder is likely. Moreover, if a delay in some specific aspect of speech or language development is accompanied by scholastic deficits (such as specific retardation in reading or spelling), by abnormalities in interpersonal relationships, and/or by emotional or behavioural disturbance, the delay is unlikely to constitute just a normal variation.

The second difficulty in diagnosis concerns the differentiation from mental retardation or global developmental delay. Because intelligence includes verbal skills, it is likely that a child whose IQ is substantially below average will also show language development that is somewhat below average. The diagnosis of a specific developmental disorder implies that the specific delay is significantly out of keeping with the general level of cognitive functioning. Accordingly, when a language delay is simply part of a more pervasive mental retardation or global developmental delay, a mental retardation coding (F70 – F79) should be used, *not* an F80. – coding. However, it is common for mental retardation to be associated with an uneven pattern of intellectual performance and especially with a degree of language impairment that is more severe than the retardation in nonverbal skills. When this disparity is of such a marked degree that it is evident in everyday functioning, a specific developmental disorder of speech and language should be coded *in addition to* a coding for mental retardation (F70 – F79).

The third difficulty concerns the differentiation from a disorder secondary to severe deafness or to some specific neurological or other structural abnormality. Severe deafness in early childhood will almost always lead to a marked delay and distortion of language development; such conditions should *not* be included here, as they are a direct consequence of the hearing impairment. However, it is not uncommon for the more severe developmental disorders of receptive language to be accompanied by partial selective hearing impairments (especially of high frequencies). The guideline is to *exclude* these disorders from F80 – F89 if the severity of hearing loss constitutes a sufficient explanation for the language delay, but to *include* them if partial hearing loss is a complicating factor but not a sufficient direct cause. However, a hard and fast distinction is impossible to make. A similar principle applies with respect to neurological abnormalities and structural defects. Thus, an articulation abnormality directly due to a cleft palate or to a dysarthria resulting from cerebral palsy would be excluded from this block. On the other hand, the presence of subtle neurological abnormalities that could not have directly caused the speech or language delay would not constitute a reason for exclusion.

F80.0 Specific speech articulation disorder

A specific developmental disorder in which the child's use of speech sounds is below the appropriate level for his or her mental age, but in which there is a normal level of language skills.

Diagnostic guidelines

The age of acquisition of speech sounds, and the order in which these sounds develop, show considerable individual variation.

Normal development. At the age of 4 years, errors in speech sound production are common, but the child is able to be understood easily by strangers. By the age of 6 – 7, most speech sounds will be acquired. Although difficulties may remain with certain sound combinations, these should not result in any problems of communication. By the age of 11 – 12 years, mastery of almost all speech sounds should be acquired.

Abnormal development occurs when the child's acquisition of speech sounds is delayed and/or deviant, leading to: misarticulations in the child's speech with consequent difficulties for others in understanding him or her; omissions, distortions, or substitutions of speech sounds; and inconsistencies in the co-occurrence of sounds (i.e. the child may produce phonemes correctly in some word positions but not in others).

The diagnosis should be made only when the severity of the articulation disorder is outside the limits of normal variation for the child's mental age; nonverbal intelligence is within the normal range; expressive and receptive language skills are within the normal range; the articulation abnormalities are not directly attributable to a sensory, structural or neurological abnormality; and the mispronunciations are clearly abnormal in the context of colloquial usage in the child's subculture.

Includes: developmental articulation disorder
developmental phonological disorder
dyslalia
functional articulation disorder
lalling

Excludes: articulation disorder due to:
aphasia NOS (R47.0)
apraxia (R48.2)
articulation impairments associated with a developmental
disorder of expressive or receptive language (F80.1,
F80.2)
cleft palate or other structural abnormalities of the oral
structures involved in speech (Q35 – Q38)
hearing loss (H90 – H91)
mental retardation (F70 – F79)

F80.1 Expressive language disorder

A specific developmental disorder in which the child's ability to use expressive spoken language is markedly below the appropriate level for his or her mental age, but in which language comprehension is within normal limits. There may or may not be abnormalities in articulation.

Diagnostic guidelines

Although considerable individual variation occurs in normal language development, the absence of single words (or word approximations) by the age of 2 years, and the failure to generate simple two-word phrases by 3 years, should be taken as significant signs of delay. Later difficulties include: restricted vocabulary development; overuse of a small set of general words, difficulties in selecting appropriate words, and word substitutions; short utterance length; immature sentence structure; syntactical errors, especially *omissions* of word endings or prefixes; and misuse of or failure to use grammatical features such as prepositions, pronouns, articles, and verb and noun inflexions. Incorrect overgeneralizations of rules may also occur, as may a lack of sentence fluency and difficulties in sequencing when recounting past events.

It is frequent for impairments in spoken language to be accompanied by delays or abnormalities in word-sound production.

The diagnosis should be made only when the severity of the delay in the development of expressive language is outside the limits of normal variation for the child's mental age, but receptive language skills are within normal limits (although may often be somewhat below average). The use of nonverbal cues (such as smiles and gesture) and "internal" language as reflected in imaginative or make-believe play should be relatively intact, and the ability to communicate socially without words should be relatively unimpaired. The child will seek to communicate in spite of the language impairment and will tend to compensate for lack of speech by use of demonstration, gesture, mime, or non-speech vocalizations. However, associated difficulties in peer relationships, emotional disturbance, behavioural disruption, and/or overactivity and inattention are not uncommon, particularly in school-age children. In a minority of cases there may be some associated partial (often selective) hearing loss, but this should not be of a severity sufficient to account for the language delay. Inadequate involvement in conversational interchanges, or more general environmental privation, may play a major or contributory role in the impaired development of expressive language. Where this is the case, the environmental causal factor should be noted by means of the appropriate Z code from Chapter XXI of ICD-10. The impairment in spoken language should have been evident from infancy without any clear prolonged phase of normal language usage. However, a history of apparently normal first use of a *few* single words, followed by a setback or failure to progress, is not uncommon.

Includes: developmental dysphasia or aphasia, expressive type

Excludes: acquired aphasia with epilepsy [Landau – Kleffner syndrome] (F80.3)
developmental aphasia or dysphasia, receptive type (F80.2)
dysphasia and aphasia NOS (R47.0)
elective mutism (F94.0)
mental retardation (F70 – F79)
pervasive developmental disorders (F84. –)

F80.2 Receptive language disorder

A specific developmental disorder in which the child's understanding of language is below the appropriate level for his or her mental age. In almost all cases, expressive language is markedly disturbed and abnormalities in word-sound production are common.

Diagnostic guidelines

Failure to respond to familiar names (in the absence of nonverbal clues) by the first birthday, inability to identify at least a few common objects by 18 months, or failure to follow simple, routine instructions by the age of 2 years should be taken as significant signs of delay. Later difficulties include inability to understand grammatical structures (negatives, questions, comparatives, etc.), and lack of understanding of more subtle aspects of language (tone of voice, gesture, etc.).

The diagnosis should be made only when the severity of the delay in receptive language is outside the normal limits of variation for the child's mental age, and when the criteria for a pervasive developmental disorder are *not* met. In almost all cases, the development of expressive language is also severely delayed and abnormalities in word-sound production are common. Of all the varieties of specific developmental disorders of speech and language, this has the highest rate of associated socio-emotional-behavioural disturbance. Such disturbances do not take any specific form, but hyperactivity and inattention, social ineptness and isolation from peers, and anxiety, sensitivity, or undue shyness are all relatively frequent. Children with the most severe forms of receptive language impairment may be somewhat delayed in their social development, may echo language that they do not understand, and may show somewhat restricted interest patterns. However, they differ from autistic children in usually showing normal social reciprocity, normal make-believe play, normal use of parents for comfort, near-normal use of gesture, and only mild impairments in nonverbal communication. Some degree of high-frequency hearing loss is not infrequent, but the degree of deafness is not sufficient to account for the language impairment.

Includes: congenital auditory imperception
developmental aphasia or dysphasia, receptive type
developmental Wernicke's aphasia
word deafness

Excludes: acquired aphasia with epilepsy [Landau – Kleffner syndrome] (F80.3)
autism (F84.0, F84.1)

dysphasia and aphasia, NOS (R47.0) or expressive type (F80.1)

elective mutism (F94.0)

language delay due to deafness (H90 – H91)

mental retardation (F70 – F79)

F80.3 Acquired aphasia with epilepsy [Landau – Kleffner syndrome]

A disorder in which the child, having previously made normal progress in language development, loses both receptive and expressive language skills but retains general intelligence. Onset of the disorder is accompanied by paroxysmal abnormalities on the EEG (almost always from the temporal lobes, usually bilateral, but often with more widespread disturbance), and in the majority of cases also by epileptic seizures. Typically the onset is between the ages of 3 and 7 years but the disorder can arise earlier or later in childhood. In a quarter of cases the loss of language occurs gradually over a period of some months, but more often the loss is abrupt, with skills being lost over days or weeks. The temporal association between onset of seizures and loss of language is rather variable, with either one preceding the other by a few months to 2 years. It is highly characteristic that the impairment of receptive language is profound, with difficulties in auditory comprehension often being the first manifestation of the condition. Some children become mute, some are restricted to jargon-like sounds, and some show milder deficits in word fluency and output often accompanied by misarticulations. In a few cases voice quality is affected, with a loss of normal inflexions. Sometimes language functions appear fluctuating in the early phases of the disorder. Behavioural and emotional disturbances are quite common in the months after the initial language loss, but they tend to improve as the child acquires some means of communication.

The etiology of the condition is not known but the clinical characteristics suggest the possibility of an inflammatory encephalitic process. The course of the disorder is quite variable: about two-thirds of the children are left with a more or less severe receptive language deficit and about a third make a complete recovery.

Excludes: acquired aphasia due to cerebral trauma, tumour or other known disease process
autism (F84.0, F84.1)
other disintegrative disorder of childhood (F84.3)

F80.8   Other developmental disorders of speech and language

Includes: lisping

F80.9   Developmental disorder of speech and language, unspecified

This category should be avoided as far as possible and should be used only for unspecified disorders in which there is significant impairment in the development of speech or language that cannot be accounted for by mental retardation, or by neurological, sensory or physical impairments that directly affect speech or language.

Includes: language disorder NOS

F81 Specific developmental disorders of scholastic skills

The concept of specific developmental disorders of scholastic skills is directly comparable to that of specific developmental disorders of speech and language (see F80. –) and essentially the same issues of definition and measurement apply. These are disorders in which the normal patterns of skill acquisition are disturbed from the early stages of development. They are not simply a consequence of a lack of opportunity to learn, nor are they due to any form of acquired brain trauma or disease. Rather, the disorders are thought to stem from abnormalities in cognitive processing that derive largely from some type of biological dysfunction. As with most other developmental disorders, the conditions are substantially more common in boys than in girls.

Five kinds of difficulty arise in diagnosis. First, there is the need to differentiate the disorders from normal variations in scholastic achievement. The considerations are similar to those in language disorders, and the same criteria are proposed for the assessment of abnormality (with the necessary modifications that arise from evaluation of scholastic achievement rather than language). Second, there is the need to take developmental course into account. This is important for two different reasons:

(a) Severity: the significance of one year's retardation in reading at age 7 years is quite different from that of one year's retardation at 14 years.

(b) Change in pattern: it is common for a language delay in the preschool years to resolve so far as spoken language is concerned but to be followed by a specific reading retardation which, in turn, diminishes in adolescence; the principal problem remaining in early adulthood is a severe spelling disorder. The condition is the same throughout but the pattern alters with increasing age; the diagnostic criteria need to take into account this developmental change.

Third, there is the difficulty that scholastic skills have to be taught and learned: they are *not* simply a function of biological maturation. Inevitably a child's level of skills will depend on family circumstances and schooling, as well as on his or her own individual characteristics. Unfortunately, there is no straightforward and unambiguous way of differentiating scholastic difficulties due to lack of adequate experiences from those due to some individual disorder. There are good reasons for supposing that the distinction is real and clinically valid but the diagnosis in individual cases is difficult. Fourth, although research findings provide support for the hypothesis of underlying abnormalities in cognitive processing, there is no easy way in the individual child to differentiate those that *cause* reading difficulties from those that derive from or are associated with poor reading skills. The difficulty is compounded by the finding that reading disorders may stem from more than one type of cognitive abnormality. Fifth, there are continuing uncertainties over the best way of subdividing the specific developmental disorders of scholastic skills.

Children learn to read, write, spell, and perform arithmetical computations when they are introduced to these activities at home and at school. Countries vary widely in the age at which formal schooling is started, in the syllabus followed within schools, and hence in the skills that children are expected to have acquired by different ages. This disparity of expectations is greater during elementary or primary school years (i.e. up to age about 11 years) and complicates the issue of devising operational definitions of disorders of scholastic skills that have cross-national validity.

Nevertheless, within all education settings, it is clear that each chronological age group of schoolchildren contains a wide spread of scholastic attainments and that some children are underachieving in specific aspects of attainment relative to their general level of intellectual functioning.

Specific developmental disorders of scholastic skills (SDDSS) comprise groups of disorders manifested by specific and significant impairments in learning of scholastic skills. These impairments in learning are not the direct result of other disorders (such as mental retardation, gross neurological deficits, uncorrected visual or auditory problems, or emotional disturbances), although they may occur concurrently with such conditions. SDDSS frequently occur in conjunction with other clinical syndromes (such as attention deficit disorder or conduct disorder) or other developmental disorders (such as specific developmental disorder of motor function or specific developmental disorders of speech and language).

The etiology of SDDSS is not known, but there is an assumption of the primacy of biological factors which interact with nonbiological factors (such as opportunity for learning and quality of teaching) to produce the manifestations. Although these disorders are related to biological maturation, there is no implication that children with these disorders are simply at the lower end of a normal continuum and will therefore "catch up" with time. In many instances, traces of these disorders may continue through adolescence into adulthood. Nevertheless, it is a necessary diagnostic feature that the disorders were manifest in some form during the early years of schooling. Children can fall behind in their scholastic performance at a later stage in their educational careers (because of lack of interest, poor teaching, emotional disturbance, an increase or change in pattern of task demands, etc.), but such problems do not form part of the concept of SDDSS.

Diagnostic guidelines

There are several basic requirements for the diagnosis of any of the specific developmental disorders of scholastic skills. First, there must be a clinically significant degree of impairment in the specified scholastic skill. This may be judged on the basis of severity as defined in scholastic terms (i.e. a degree that may be expected to occur in less than 3% of schoolchildren); on developmental precursors (i.e. the scholastic difficulties were preceded by developmental delays or deviance — most often in speech or language — in the preschool years); on associated problems (such as inattention, overactivity, emotional disturbance, or conduct difficulties); on pattern (i.e. the presence of qualitative abnormalities that are not usually part of normal development); and on response (i.e. the scholastic difficulties do not rapidly and readily remit with increased help at home and/or at school).

Second, the impairment must be specific in the sense that it is not solely explained by mental retardation or by lesser impairments in general intelligence. Because IQ and scholastic achievement do not run exactly in parallel, this distinction can be made only on the basis of individually administered standardized tests of achievement and IQ that are appropriate for the relevant culture and educational system. Such tests should be used in connection with statistical tables that provide data on the average expected level of achievement for any given IQ level at any given chronological age. This last requirement is necessary because of the importance of statistical regression effects: diagnoses based on subtractions of achievement age from mental age are bound to be seriously misleading. In routine clinical practice, however, it is unlikely that these requirements will be met in most instances. Accordingly, the clinical guideline is simply that the child's level of attainment must be very substantially below that expected for a child of the same mental age.

Third, the impairment must be developmental, in the sense that it must have been present during the early years of schooling and not acquired later in the educational process. The history of the child's school progress should provide evidence on this point.

Fourth, there must be no external factors that could provide a sufficient reason for the scholastic difficulties. As indicated above, a diagnosis of SDDSS should generally rest on positive evidence of clinically significant disorder of scholastic achievement associated with factors intrinsic to the child's development. To learn effectively, however, children must have adequate learning opportunities. Accordingly, if it is clear that the poor scholastic achievement is directly due to very prolonged school absence without teaching at home or to grossly inadequate education, the disorders should not be coded here. Frequent absences from school or educational discontinuities resulting from changes in school are usually *not* sufficient to give rise to scholastic retardation of the degree necessary for diagnosis of SDDSS. However, poor schooling may complicate or add to the problem, in which case the school factors should be coded by means of a Z code from Chapter XXI of ICD-10.

Fifth, the SDDSS must not be *directly* due to uncorrected visual or hearing impairments.

Differential diagnosis. It is clinically important to differentiate between SDDSS that arise in the absence of any diagnosable neurological disorder and those that are secondary to some neurological condition such as cerebral palsy. In practice this differentiation is often difficult to make (because of the uncertain significance of multiple "soft" neurological signs), and research findings do not show any clear-cut differentiation in either the pattern or course of SDDSS according to the presence or absence of overt neurological dysfunction. Accordingly, although this does *not* form part of the diagnostic criteria, it *is* necessary that the presence of any associated disorder be separately coded in the appropriate neurological section of the classification.

F81.0 Specific reading disorder

The main feature of this disorder is a specific and significant impairment in the development of reading skills, which is not solely accounted for by mental age, visual acuity problems, or inadequate schooling. Reading comprehension skill, reading word recognition, oral reading skill, and performance of tasks requiring reading may all be affected. Spelling difficulties are frequently associated with specific reading disorder and often remain into adolescence even after some progress in reading has been made. Children with specific reading disorder frequently have a history of specific developmental disorders of speech and language, and comprehensive assessment of current language functioning often reveals subtle contemporaneous difficulties. In addition to academic failure, poor school attendance and problems with social adjustment are frequent complications, particularly in the later elementary and secondary school years. The condition is found in all known languages, but there is uncertainty as to whether or not its frequency is affected by the nature of the language and of the written script.

Diagnostic guidelines

The child's reading performance should be significantly below the level expected on the basis of age, general intelligence, and school placement. Performance is best assessed by means of an individually administered, standardized test of reading accuracy and comprehension. The precise nature of the reading problem depends

245

on the expected level of reading, and on the language and script. However, in the early stages of learning an alphabetic script, there may be difficulties in reciting the alphabet, in giving the correct names of letters, in giving simple rhymes for words, and in analysing or categorizing sounds (in spite of normal auditory acuity). Later, there may be errors in oral reading skills such as shown by:

(a) omissions, substitutions, distortions, or additions of words or parts of words;
(b) slow reading rate;
(c) false starts, long hesitations or "loss of place" in text, and inaccurate phrasing; and
(d) reversals of words in sentences or of letters within words.

There may also be deficits in reading comprehension, as shown by, for example:

(e) an inability to recall facts read;
(f) inability to draw conclusions or inferences from material read; and
(g) use of general knowledge as background information rather than of information from a particular story to answer questions about a story read.

In later childhood and in adult life, it is common for spelling difficulties to be more profound than the reading deficits. It is characteristic that the spelling difficulties often involve phonetic errors, and it seems that both the reading and spelling problems may derive in part from an impairment in phonological analysis. Little is known about the nature or frequency of spelling errors in children who have to read non-phonetic languages, and little is known about the types of error in non-alphabetic scripts.

Specific developmental disorders of reading are commonly preceded by a history of disorders in speech or language development. In other cases, children may pass language milestones at the normal age but have difficulties in auditory processing as shown by problems in sound categorization, in rhyming, and possibly by deficits in speech sound discrimination, auditory sequential memory, and auditory association. In some cases, too, there may be problems in visual processing (such as in letter discrimination); however, these are common among children who are just beginning to learn to read and hence are probably not directly causally related to the poor reading. Difficulties in attention, often associated with overactivity and impulsivity, are also common. The precise pattern of developmental difficulties in the preschool period varies considerably from child to child, as does their severity; nevertheless such difficulties are usually (but not invariably) present.

Associated emotional and/or behavioural disturbances are also common during the school-age period. Emotional problems are more common during the early school years, but conduct disorders and hyperactivity syndromes are most likely to be present in later childhood and adolescence. Low self-esteem is common and problems in school adjustment and in peer relationships are also frequent.

Includes: "backward reading"
developmental dyslexia
specific reading retardation
spelling difficulties associated with a reading disorder

Excludes: acquired alexia and dyslexia (R48.0)
acquired reading difficulties secondary to emotional disturbance (F93. –)
spelling disorder not associated with reading difficulties (F81.1)

F81.1 Specific spelling disorder

The main feature of this disorder is a specific and significant impairment in the development of spelling skills in the *absence* of a history of specific reading disorder, which is not solely accounted for by low mental age, visual acuity problems, or inadequate schooling. The ability to spell orally and to write out words correctly are both affected. Children whose problem is solely one of handwriting should not be included, but in some cases spelling difficulties may be associated with problems in writing. Unlike the usual pattern of specific reading disorder, the spelling errors tend to be predominantly phonetically accurate.

Diagnostic guidelines

The child's spelling performance should be significantly below the level expected on the basis of his or her age, general intelligence, and school placement, and is best assessed by means of an individually administered, standardized test of spelling. The child's reading skills (with respect to both accuracy and comprehension) should be within the normal range and there should be no history of previous significant reading difficulties. The difficulties in spelling should not be mainly due to grossly inadequate teaching or to the direct effects of deficits of visual, hearing, or neurological function, and should not have been acquired as a result of any neurological, psychiatric, or other disorder.

Although it is known that a "pure" spelling disorder differs from reading disorders associated with spelling difficulties, little is known of the antecedents, course, correlates, or outcome of specific spelling disorders.

Includes: specific spelling retardation (without reading disorder)

Excludes: acquired spelling disorder (R48.8)
spelling difficulties associated with a reading disorder (F81.0)
spelling difficulties mainly attributable to inadequate teaching (Z55.8)

F81.2   Specific disorder of arithmetical skills

This disorder involves a specific impairment in arithmetical skills, which is not solely explicable on the basis of general mental retardation or of grossly inadequate schooling. The deficit concerns mastery of basic computational skills of addition, subtraction, multiplication, and division (rather than of the more abstract mathematical skills involved in algebra, trigonometry, geometry, or calculus).

Diagnostic guidelines

The child's arithmetical performance should be significantly below the level expected on the basis of his or her age, general intelligence, and school placement, and is best assessed by means of an individually administered, standardized test of arithmetic. Reading and spelling skills should be within the normal range expected for the child's mental age, preferably as assessed on individually administered, appropriately standardized tests. The difficulties in arithmetic should not be mainly due to grossly inadequate teaching, or to the direct effects of defects of visual, hearing, or neurological function, and should not have been acquired as a result of any neurological, psychiatric, or other disorder.

Arithmetical disorders have been studied less than reading disorders, and knowledge of antecedents, course, correlates, and outcome is quite limited. However, it seems that children with these disorders tend to have auditory-perceptual and verbal skills within the normal range, but impaired visuo-spatial and visual-perceptual skills; this is in contrast to many children with reading disorders. Some children have associated socio-emotional-behavioural problems but little is known about their characteristics or frequency. It has been suggested that difficulties in social interactions may be particularly common.

The arithmetical difficulties that occur are various but may include: failure to understand the concepts underlying particular arithmetical operations; lack of understanding of mathematical terms or signs; failure to recognize numerical symbols; difficulty in carrying out standard arithmetical manipulations; difficulty in understanding which numbers are relevant to the arithmetical problem being considered; difficulty in properly aligning numbers or in inserting decimal points or symbols during calculations; poor spatial organization of arithmetical calculations; and inability to learn multiplication tables satisfactorily.

Includes: developmental acalculia
developmental arithmetical disorder
developmental Gerstmann syndrome

Excludes: acquired arithmetical disorder (acalculia) (R48.8)
arithmetical difficulties associated with a reading or spelling disorder (F81.1)
arithmetical difficulties mainly attributable to inadequate teaching (Z55.8)

F81.3 Mixed disorder of scholastic skills

This is an ill-defined, inadequately conceptualized (but necessary) residual category of disorders in which both arithmetical and reading or spelling skills are significantly impaired, but in which the disorder is not solely explicable in terms of general mental retardation or inadequate schooling. It should be used for disorders meeting the criteria for F81.2 and either F81.0 or F81.1.

Excludes: specific disorder of arithmetical skills (F81.2)
specific reading disorder (F81.0)
specific spelling disorder (F81.1)

F81.8   Other developmental disorders of scholastic skills

Includes: developmental expressive writing disorder

F81.9   Developmental disorder of scholastic skills, unspecified

This category should be avoided as far as possible and should be
used only for unspecified disorders in which there is a significant
disability of learning that cannot be solely accounted for by mental
retardation, visual acuity problems, or inadequate schooling.

Includes: knowledge acquisition disability NOS
learning disability NOS
learning disorder NOS

F82   Specific developmental disorder of motor function

The main feature of this disorder is a serious impairment in the
development of motor coordination that is not solely explicable in
terms of general intellectual retardation or of any specific congenital
or acquired neurological disorder (other than the one that may
be implicit in the coordination abnormality). It is usual for the
motor clumsiness to be associated with some degree of impaired
performance on visuo-spatial cognitive tasks.

Diagnostic guidelines

The child's motor coordination, on fine or gross motor tasks, should
be significantly below the level expected on the basis of his or her
age and general intelligence. This is best assessed on the basis of
an individually administered, standardized test of fine and gross motor
coordination. The difficulties in co-ordination should have been
present since early in development (i.e. they should not constitute
an acquired deficit), and they should not be a direct result of any
defects of vision or hearing or of any diagnosable neurological
disorder.

The extent to which the disorder mainly involves fine or gross motor
coordination varies, and the particular pattern of motor disabilities

varies with age. Developmental motor milestones may be delayed and there may be some associated speech difficulties (especially involving articulation). The young child may be awkward in general gait, being slow to learn to run, hop, and go up and down stairs. There is likely to be difficulty learning to tie shoe laces, to fasten and unfasten buttons, and to throw and catch balls. The child may be generally clumsy in fine and/or gross movements – tending to drop things, to stumble, to bump into obstacles, and to have poor handwriting. Drawing skills are usually poor, and children with this disorder are often poor at jigsaw puzzles, using constructional toys, building models, ball games, and drawing and understanding maps.

In most cases a careful clinical examination shows marked neurodevelopmental immaturities such as choreiform movements of unsupported limbs, or mirror movements and other associated motor features, as well as signs of poor fine and gross motor coordination (generally described as "soft" neurological signs because of their normal occurrence in younger children and their lack of localizing value). Tendon reflexes may be increased or decreased bilaterally but will not be asymmetrical.

Scholastic difficulties occur in some children and may occasionally be severe; in some cases there are associated socio-emotional-behavioural problems, but little is known of their frequency or characteristics.

There is no diagnosable neurological disorder (such as cerebral palsy or muscular dystrophy). In some cases, however, there is a history of perinatal complications, such as very low birth weight or markedly premature birth.

The clumsy child syndrome has often been diagnosed as "minimal brain dysfunction", but this term is not recommended as it has so many different and contradictory meanings.

Includes: clumsy child syndrome
developmental coordination disorder
developmental dyspraxia

Excludes: abnormalities of gait and mobility (R26. –)
lack of coordination (R27. –) secondary to either mental

retardation (F70 – F79) or some specific diagnosable neurological disorder (G00 – G99)

F83 Mixed specific developmental disorders

This is an ill-defined, inadequately conceptualized (but necessary) residual category of disorders in which there is some admixture of specific developmental disorders of speech and language, of scholastic skills, and/or of motor function, but in which none predominates sufficiently to constitute the prime diagnosis. It is common for each of these specific developmental disorders to be associated with some degree of general impairment of cognitive functions, and this mixed category should be used only when there is a major overlap. Thus, the category should be used when there are dysfunctions meeting the criteria for two or more of F80. – , F81. – , and F82.

F84 Pervasive developmental disorders

This group of disorders is characterized by qualitative abnormalities in reciprocal social interactions and in patterns of communication, and by restricted, stereotyped, repetitive repertoire of interests and activities. These qualitative abnormalities are a pervasive feature of the individual's functioning in all situations, although they may vary in degree. In most cases, development is abnormal from infancy and, with only a few exceptions, the conditions become manifest during the first 5 years of life. It is usual, but not invariable, for there to be some degree of general cognitive impairment but the disorders are defined in terms of *behaviour* that is deviant in relation to mental age (whether the individual is retarded or not). There is some disagreement on the subdivision of this overall group of pervasive developmental disorders.

In some cases the disorders are associated with, and presumably due to, some medical condition, of which infantile spasms, congenital rubella, tuberous sclerosis, cerebral lipidosis, and the fragile X chromosome anomaly are among the most common. However, the disorder should be diagnosed on the basis of the behavioural features, irrespective of the presence or absence of any associated medical conditions; any such associated condition must, nevertheless, be separately coded. If mental retardation is present, it is important that it too should be separately coded, under F70 – F79, because it is not a universal feature of the pervasive developmental disorders.

F84.0 Childhood autism

A pervasive developmental disorder defined by the presence of abnormal and/or impaired development that is manifest before the age of 3 years, and by the characteristic type of abnormal functioning in all three areas of social interaction, communication, and restricted, repetitive behaviour. The disorder occurs in boys three to four times more often than in girls.

Diagnostic guidelines

Usually there is no prior period of unequivocally normal development but, if there is, abnormalities become apparent before the age of 3 years. There are always qualitative impairments in reciprocal social interaction. These take the form of an inadequate appreciation of socio-emotional cues, as shown by a lack of responses to other people's emotions and/or a lack of modulation of behaviour according to social context; poor use of social signals and a weak integration of social, emotional, and communicative behaviours; and, especially, a lack of socio-emotional reciprocity. Similarly, qualitative impairments in communications are universal. These take the form of a lack of social usage of whatever language skills are present; impairment in make-believe and social imitative play; poor synchrony and lack of reciprocity in conversational interchange; poor flexibility in language expression and a relative lack of creativity and fantasy in thought processes; lack of emotional response to other people's verbal and nonverbal overtures; impaired use of variations in cadence or emphasis to reflect communicative modulation; and a similar lack of accompanying gesture to provide emphasis or aid meaning in spoken communication.

The condition is also characterized by restricted, repetitive, and stereotyped patterns of behaviour, interests, and activities. These take the form of a tendency to impose rigidity and routine on a wide range of aspects of day-to day functioning; this usually applies to novel activities as well as to familiar habits and play patterns. In early childhood particularly, there may be specific attachment to unusual, typically non-soft objects. The children may insist on the performance of particular routines in rituals of a nonfunctional character; there may be stereotyped preoccupations with interests such as dates, routes or timetables; often there are motor stereotypies; a specific interest in nonfunctional elements of objects (such as their smell or feel) is common; and there may be a resistance to changes in routine or in details of the personal environment (such as the movement of ornaments or furniture in the family home).

In addition to these specific diagnostic features, it is frequent for children with autism to show a range of other nonspecific problems such as fear/phobias, sleeping and eating disturbances, temper tantrums, and aggression. Self-injury (e.g. by wrist-biting) is fairly common, especially when there is associated severe mental retardation. Most individuals with autism lack spontaneity, initiative, and creativity in the organization of their leisure time and have difficulty applying conceptualizations in decision-making in work (even when the tasks themselves are well within their capacity). The specific manifestation of deficits characteristic of autism change as the children grow older, but the deficits continue into and through adult life with a broadly similar pattern of problems in socialization, communication, and interest patterns. Developmental abnormalities must have been present in the first 3 years for the diagnosis to be made, but the syndrome can be diagnosed in all age groups.

All levels of IQ can occur in association with autism, but there is significant mental retardation in some three-quarters of cases.

Includes: autistic disorder
infantile autism
infantile psychosis
Kanner's syndrome

Differential diagnosis. Apart from the other varieties of pervasive developmental disorder it is important to consider: specific developmental disorder of receptive language (F80.2) with secondary socio-emotional problems; reactive attachment disorder (F94.1) or disinhibited attachment disorder (F94.2); mental retardation (F70 – F79) with some associated emotional/behavioural disorder; schizophrenia (F20. –) of unusually early onset; and Rett's syndrome (F84.2).

Excludes: autistic psychopathy (F84.5)

F84.1 Atypical autism

A pervasive developmental disorder that differs from autism in terms *either* of age of onset *or* of failure to fulfil all three sets of diagnostic criteria. Thus, abnormal and/or impaired development becomes manifest for the first time only after age 3 years; and/or there are insufficient demonstrable abnormalities in one or two of the three areas of psychopathology required for the diagnosis of autism (namely, reciprocal social interactions, communication, and restrictive, stereotyped, repetitive behaviour) in spite of characteristic abnormalities in the other area(s). Atypical autism arises most often in profoundly retarded individuals whose very low level of functioning provides little scope for exhibition of the specific deviant behaviours required for the diagnosis of autism; it also occurs in individuals with a severe specific developmental disorder of receptive language. Atypical autism thus constitutes a meaningfully separate condition from autism.

Includes: atypical childhood psychosis
mental retardation with autistic features

F84.2 Rett's syndrome

A condition of unknown cause, so far reported only in girls, which has been differentiated on the basis of a characteristic onset, course, and pattern of symptomatology. Typically, apparently normal or near-normal early development is followed by partial or complete loss of acquired hand skills and of speech, together with deceleration in head growth, usually with an onset between 7 and 24 months of age. Hand-wringing stereotypies, hyperventilation and loss of purposive hand movements are particularly characteristic. Social and play development are arrested in the first 2 or 3 years, but social interest tends to be maintained. During middle childhood, trunk ataxia and apraxia, associated with scoliosis or kyphoscoliosis tend to develop and sometimes there are choreoathetoid movements. Severe mental handicap invariably results. Fits frequently develop during early or middle childhood.

Diagnostic guidelines

In most cases onset is between 7 and 24 months of age. The most characteristic feature is a loss of purposive hand movements and acquired fine motor manipulative skills. This is accompanied by loss, partial loss or lack of development of language; distinctive stereotyped

255

tortuous wringing or "hand-washing" movements, with the arms flexed in front of the chest or chin; stereotypic wetting of the hands with saliva; lack of proper chewing of food; often episodes of hyperventilation; almost always a failure to gain bowel and bladder control; often excessive drooling and protrusion of the tongue; and a loss of social engagement. Typically, the children retain a kind of "social smile", looking at or "through" people, but not interacting socially with them in early childhood (although social interaction often develops later). The stance and gait tend to become broad-based, the muscles are hypotonic, trunk movements usually become poorly coordinated, and scoliosis or kyphoscoliosis usually develops. Spinal atrophies, with severe motor disability, develop in adolescence or adulthood in about half the cases. Later, rigid spasticity may become manifest, and is usually more pronounced in the lower than in the upper limbs. Epileptic fits, usually involving some type of minor attack, and with an onset generally before the age of 8 years, occur in the majority of cases. In contrast to autism, both deliberate self-injury and complex stereotyped preoccupations or routines are rare.

Differential diagnosis. Initially, Rett's syndrome is differentiated primarily on the basis of the lack of purposive hand movements, deceleration of head growth, ataxia, stereotypic "hand-washing" movements, and lack of proper chewing. The course of the disorder, in terms of progressive motor deterioration, confirms the diagnosis.

F84.3 Other childhood disintegrative disorder

A pervasive developmental disorder (other than Rett's syndrome) that is defined by a period of normal development before onset, and by a definite loss, over the course of a few months, of previously acquired skills in at least several areas of development, together with the onset of characteristic abnormalities of social, communicative, and behavioural functioning. Often there is a prodromic period of vague illness; the child becomes restive, irritable, anxious, and overactive. This is followed by impoverishment and then loss of speech and language, accompanied by behavioural disintegration. In some cases the loss of skills is persistently progressive (usually when the disorder is associated with a progressive diagnosable neurological condition), but more often the decline over a period of some months is followed by a plateau and then a limited improvement. The prognosis is usually very poor, and most individuals are left with severe mental retardation. There is uncertainty about the extent to which this condition differs from autism. In some cases the disorder can be shown to be due to some associated encephalopathy, but the diagnosis should be made on the behavioural features. Any associated neurological condition should be separately coded.

Diagnostic guidelines

Diagnosis is based on an apparently normal development up to the age of at least 2 years, followed by a definite loss of previously acquired skills; this is accompanied by qualitatively abnormal social functioning. It is usual for there to be a profound regression in, or loss of, language, a regression in the level of play, social skills, and adaptive behaviour, and often a loss of bowel or bladder control, sometimes with a deteriorating motor control. Typically, this is accompanied by a general loss of interest in the environment, by stereotyped, repetitive motor mannerisms, and by an autistic-like impairment of social interaction and communication. In some respects, the syndrome resembles dementia in adult life, but it differs in three key respects: there is usually no evidence of any identifiable organic disease or damage (although organic brain dysfunction of some type is usually inferred); the loss of skills may be followed by a degree of recovery; and the impairment in socialization and communication has deviant qualities typical of autism rather than of intellectual decline. For all these reasons the syndrome is included here rather than under F00 – F09.

Includes: dementia infantilis
disintegrative psychosis
Heller's syndrome
symbiotic psychosis

Excludes: acquired aphasia with epilepsy (F80.3)
elective mutism (F94.0)
Rett's syndrome (F84.2)
schizophrenia (F20. –)

F84.4 Overactive disorder associated with mental retardation and stereotyped movements

This is an ill-defined disorder of uncertain nosological validity. The category is included here because of the evidence that children with moderate to severe mental retardation (IQ below 50) who exhibit major problems in hyperactivity and inattention frequently show stereotyped behaviours; such children tend not to benefit from stimulant drugs (unlike those with an IQ in the normal range) and may exhibit a severe dysphoric reaction (sometimes with psychomotor retardation) when given stimulants; in adolescence the overactivity tends to be replaced by underactivity (a pattern that is *not* usual in hyperkinetic children with normal intelligence). It is also common for the syndrome to be associated with a variety of developmental delays, either specific or global.

The extent to which the behavioural pattern is a function of low IQ or of organic brain damage is not known, neither is it clear whether the disorders in children with mild mental retardation who show the hyperkinetic syndrome would be better classified here or under F90. – ; at present they are included in F90 – .

Diagnostic guidelines

Diagnosis depends on the combination of developmentally inappropriate severe overactivity, motor stereotypies, and moderate to severe mental retardation; all three must be present for the diagnosis. If the diagnostic criteria for F84.0, F84.1 or F84.2 are met, that condition should be diagnosed instead.

F84.5 Asperger's syndrome

A disorder of uncertain nosological validity, characterized by the same kind of qualitative abnormalities of reciprocal social interaction that typify autism, together with a restricted, stereotyped, repetitive repertoire of interests and activities. The disorder differs from autism primarily in that there is no general delay or retardation in language or in cognitive development. Most individuals are of normal general intelligence but it is common for them to be markedly clumsy; the condition occurs predominantly in boys (in a ratio of about eight boys to one girl). It seems highly likely that at least some cases represent mild varieties of autism, but it is uncertain whether or not that is so for all. There is a strong tendency for the abnormalities to persist into adolescence and adult life and it seems that they represent individual characteristics that are not greatly affected by environmental influences. Psychotic episodes occasionally occur in early adult life.

Diagnostic guidelines

Diagnosis is based on the combination of a lack of any clinically significant general delay in language or cognitive development plus, as with autism, the presence of qualitative deficiencies in reciprocal social interaction and restricted, repetitive, stereotyped patterns of behaviour, interests, and activities. There may or may not be problems in communication similar to those associated with autism, but significant language retardation would rule out the diagnosis.

Includes: autistic psychopathy
schizoid disorder of childhood

Excludes: anankastic personality disorder (F60.5)
attachment disorders of childhood (F94.1, F94.2)
obsessive – compulsive disorder (F42. –)
schizotypal disorder (F21)
simple schizophrenia (F20.6)

F84.8 Other pervasive developmental disorders

F84.9 Pervasive developmental disorder, unspecified

This is a residual diagnostic category that should be used for disorders which fit the general description for pervasive developmental disorders but in which a lack of adequate information, or contradictory findings, means that the criteria for any of the other F84 codes cannot be met.

F88 Other disorders of psychological development

Includes: developmental agnosia

F89 Unspecified disorder of psychological development

Includes: developmental disorder NOS

F90 – F98
Behavioural and emotional disorders with onset usually occurring in childhood and adolescence

F99 Unspecified mental disorder

Overview of this section

F90 Hyperkinetic disorders
F90.0 Disturbance of activity and attention
F90.1 Hyperkinetic conduct disorder
F90.8 Other hyperkinetic disorders
F90.9 Hyperkinetic disorder, unspecified

F91 Conduct disorders
F91.0 Conduct disorder confined to the family context
F91.1 Unsocialized conduct disorder
F91.2 Socialized conduct disorder
F91.3 Oppositional defiant disorder
F91.8 Other conduct disorders
F91.9 Conduct disorder, unspecified

F92 Mixed disorders of conduct and emotions
F92.0 Depressive conduct disorder
F92.8 Other mixed disorders of conduct and emotions
F92.9 Mixed disorder of conduct and emotions, unspecified

F93 Emotional disorders with onset specific to childhood
F93.0 Separation anxiety disorder of childhood
F93.1 Phobic anxiety disorder of childhood
F93.2 Social anxiety disorder of childhood
F93.3 Sibling rivalry disorder
F93.8 Other childhood emotional disorders
F93.9 Childhood emotional disorder, unspecified

F94 Disorders of social functioning with onset specific to childhood and adolescence
F94.0 Elective mutism
F94.1 Reactive attachment disorder of childhood

F94.2 Disinhibited attachment disorder of childhood

F94.8 Other childhood disorders of social functioning

F94.9 Childhood disorder of social functioning, unspecified

F95 Tic disorders

F95.0 Transient tic disorder

F95.1 Chronic motor or vocal tic disorder

F95.2 Combined vocal and multiple motor tic disorder [de la Tourette's syndrome]

F95.8 Other tic disorders

F95.9 Tic disorder, unspecified

F98 Other behavioural and emotional disorders with onset usually occurring in childhood and adolescence

F98.0 Nonorganic enuresis

F98.1 Nonorganic encopresis

F98.2 Feeding disorder of infancy and childhood

F98.3 Pica of infancy and childhood

F98.4 Stereotyped movement disorders

F98.5 Stuttering [stammering]

F98.6 Cluttering

F98.8 Other specified behavioural and emotional disorders with onset usually occurring in childhood and adolescence

F98.9 Unspecified behavioural and emotional disorders with onset usually occurring in childhood and adolescence

F99 Mental disorder, not otherwise specified

F90 Hyperkinetic disorders

This group of disorders is characterized by: early onset; a combination of overactive, poorly modulated behaviour with marked inattention and lack of persistent task involvement; and pervasiveness over situations and persistence over time of these behavioural characteristics.

It is widely thought that constitutional abnormalities play a crucial role in the genesis of these disorders, but knowledge on specific etiology is lacking at present. In recent years the use of the diagnostic term "attention deficit disorder" for these syndromes has been promoted. It has not been used here because it implies a knowledge of psychological processes that is not yet available, and it suggests the inclusion of anxious, preoccupied, or "dreamy" apathetic children whose problems are probably different. However, it is clear that, from the point of view of behaviour, problems of inattention constitute a central feature of these hyperkinetic syndromes.

Hyperkinetic disorders always arise early in development (usually in the first 5 years of life). Their chief characteristics are lack of persistence in activities that require cognitive involvement, and a tendency to move from one activity to another without completing any one, together with disorganized, ill-regulated, and excessive activity. These problems usually persist through school years and even into adult life, but many affected individuals show a gradual improvement in activity and attention.

Several other abnormalities may be associated with these disorders. Hyperkinetic children are often reckless and impulsive, prone to accidents, and find themselves in disciplinary trouble because of unthinking (rather than deliberately defiant) breaches of rules. Their relationships with adults are often socially disinhibited, with a lack of normal caution and reserve; they are unpopular with other children and may become isolated. Cognitive impairment is common, and specific delays in motor and language development are disproportionately frequent.

Secondary complications include dissocial behaviour and low self-esteem. There is accordingly considerable overlap between hyperkinesis and other patterns of disruptive behaviour such as

262

"unsocialized conduct disorder". Nevertheless, current evidence favours the separation of a group in which hyperkinesis is the main problem.

Hyperkinetic disorders are several times more frequent in boys than in girls. Associated reading difficulties (and/or other scholastic problems) are common.

Diagnostic guidelines

The cardinal features are impaired attention and overactivity: both are necessary for the diagnosis and should be evident in more than one situation (e.g. home, classroom, clinic).

Impaired attention is manifested by prematurely breaking off from tasks and leaving activities unfinished. The children change frequently from one activity to another, seemingly losing interest in one task because they become diverted to another (although laboratory studies do not generally show an unusual degree of sensory or perceptual distractibility). These deficits in persistence and attention should be diagnosed only if they are excessive for the child's age and IQ.

Overactivity implies excessive restlessness, especially in situations requiring relative calm. It may, depending upon the situation, involve the child running and jumping around, getting up from a seat when he or she was supposed to remain seated, excessive talkativeness and noisiness, or fidgeting and wriggling. The standard for judgement should be that the activity is excessive in the context of what is expected in the situation and by comparison with other children of the same age and IQ. This behavioural feature is most evident in structured, organized situations that require a high degree of behavioural self-control.

The associated features are not sufficient for the diagnosis or even necessary, but help to sustain it. Disinhibition in social relationships, recklessness in situations involving some danger, and impulsive flouting of social rules (as shown by intruding on or interrupting others' activities, prematurely answering questions before they have been completed, or difficulty in waiting turns) are all characteristic of children with this disorder.

Learning disorders and motor clumsiness occur with undue frequency, and should be noted separately (under F80 – F89) when present; they should not, however, be part of the actual diagnosis of hyperkinetic disorder.

Symptoms of conduct disorder are neither exclusion nor inclusion criteria for the main diagnosis, but their presence or absence constitutes the basis for the main subdivision of the disorder (see below).

The characteristic behaviour problems should be of early onset (before age 6 years) and long duration. However, before the age of school entry, hyperactivity is difficult to recognize because of the wide normal variation: only extreme levels should lead to a diagnosis in preschool children.

Diagnosis of hyperkinetic disorder can still be made in adult life. The grounds are the same, but attention and activity must be judged with reference to developmentally appropriate norms. When hyperkinesis was present in childhood, but has disappeared and been succeeded by another condition, such as dissocial personality disorder or substance abuse, the current condition rather than the earlier one is coded.

Differential diagnosis. Mixed disorders are common, and pervasive developmental disorders take precedence when they are present. The major problems in diagnosis lie in differentiation from conduct disorder: when its criteria are met, hyperkinetic disorder is diagnosed with priority over conduct disorder. However, milder degrees of overactivity and inattention are common in conduct disorder. When features of both hyperactivity and conduct disorder are present, and the hyperactivity is pervasive and severe, "hyperkinetic conduct disorder" (F90.1) should be the diagnosis.

A further problem stems from the fact that overactivity and inattention, of a rather different kind from that which is characteristic of a hyperkinetic disorder, may arise as a symptom of anxiety or depressive disorders. Thus, the restlessness that is typically part of an agitated depressive disorder should not lead to a diagnosis of a hyperkinetic disorder. Equally, the restlessness that is often part of severe anxiety should not lead to the diagnosis of a hyperkinetic disorder. If the criteria for one of the anxiety disorders (F40. –, F41. –, F43. –, or F93. –) are met, this should take precedence over hyperkinetic disorder unless there is evidence, apart from the restlessness associated with anxiety, for the additional presence of a hyperkinetic disorder. Similarly, if the criteria for a mood disorder (F30 – F39) are met, hyperkinetic disorder should not be diagnosed in addition simply because concentration is impaired and there is psychomotor agitation. The double diagnosis should be made only when symptoms that are not simply part of the mood disturbance clearly indicate the separate presence of a hyperkinetic disorder.

Acute onset of hyperactive behaviour in a child of school age is more probably due to some type of reactive disorder (psychogenic or organic), manic state, schizophrenia, or neurological disease (e.g. rheumatic fever).

Excludes: anxiety disorders (F41. – or F93.0)
mood [affective] disorders (F30 – F39)
pervasive developmental disorders (F84. –)
schizophrenia (F20. –)

F90.0 Disturbance of activity and attention

There is continuing uncertainty over the most satisfactory subdivision of hyperkinetic disorders. However, follow-up studies show that the outcome in adolescence and adult life is much influenced by whether or not there is associated aggression, delinquency, or dissocial behaviour. Accordingly, the main subdivision is made according to the presence or absence of these associated features. The code used should be F90.0 when the overall criteria for hyperkinetic disorder (F90. –) are met but those for F91. – (conduct disorders) are not.

Includes: attention deficit disorder or syndrome with hyperactivity
attention deficit hyperactivity disorder

Excludes: hyperkinetic disorder associated with conduct disorder
(F90.1)

F90.1 Hyperkinetic conduct disorder

This coding should be used when both the overall criteria for hyperkinetic disorders (F90. –) *and* the overall criteria for conduct disorders (F91. –) are met.

F90.8   Other hyperkinetic disorders

F90.9   Hyperkinetic disorder, unspecified

This residual category is not recommended and should be used only when there is a lack of differentiation between F90.0 and F90.1 but the overall criteria for F90. – are fulfilled.

Includes: hyperkinetic reaction or syndrome of childhood or adolescence NOS

F91   Conduct disorders

Conduct disorders are characterized by a repetitive and persistent pattern of dissocial, aggressive, or defiant conduct. Such behaviour, when at its most extreme for the individual, should amount to major violations of age-appropriate social expectations, and is therefore more severe than ordinary childish mischief or adolescent rebelliousness. Isolated dissocial or criminal acts are not in themselves grounds for the diagnosis, which implies an enduring pattern of behaviour.

Features of conduct disorder can also be symptomatic of other psychiatric conditions, in which case the underlying diagnosis should be coded.

Disorders of conduct may in some cases proceed to dissocial personality disorder (F60.2). Conduct disorder is frequently associated with adverse psychosocial environments, including unsatisfactory family relationships and failure at school, and is more commonly noted in boys. Its distinction from emotional disorder is well validated; its separation from hyperactivity is less clear and there is often overlap.

Diagnostic guidelines

Judgements concerning the presence of conduct disorder should take into account the child's developmental level. Temper tantrums, for example, are a normal part of a 3-year-old's development and their mere presence would not be grounds for diagnosis. Equally, the violation of other people's civic rights (as by violent crime) is not within the capacity of most 7-year-olds and so is not a necessary diagnostic criterion for that age group.

Examples of the behaviours on which the diagnosis is based include the following: excessive levels of fighting or bullying; cruelty to animals or other people; severe destructiveness to property; fire-setting; stealing; repeated lying; truancy from school and running away from home; unusually frequent and severe temper tantrums; defiant provocative behaviour; and persistent severe disobedience. Any one of these categories, if marked, is sufficient for the diagnosis, but isolated dissocial acts are not.

Exclusion criteria include uncommon but serious underlying conditions such as schizophrenia, mania, pervasive developmental disorder, hyperkinetic disorder, and depression.

This diagnosis is not recommended unless the duration of the behaviour described above has been 6 months or longer.

Differential diagnosis. Conduct disorder overlaps with other conditions. The coexistence of emotional disorders of childhood (F93. –) should lead to a diagnosis of mixed disorder of conduct and emotions (F92. –). If a case also meets the criteria for hyperkinetic disorder (F90. –), that condition should be diagnosed instead. However, milder or more situation-specific levels of overactivity and inattentiveness are common in children with conduct disorder, as are low self-esteem and minor emotional upsets; neither excludes the diagnosis.

Excludes: conduct disorders associated with emotional disorders
(F92. –) or hyperkinetic disorders (F90. –)
mood [affective] disorders (F30 – F39)
pervasive developmental disorders (F84. –)
schizophrenia (F20. –)

F91.0 Conduct disorder confined to the family context

This category comprises conduct disorders involving dissocial or aggressive behaviour (and not merely oppositional, defiant, disruptive behaviour) in which the abnormal behaviour is entirely, or almost entirely, confined to the home and/or to interactions with members of the nuclear family or immediate household. The disorder requires that the overall criteria for F91 be met; even severely disturbed parent – child relationships are not of themselves sufficient for diagnosis. There may be stealing from the home, often specifically focused on the money or possessions of one or two particular individuals. This may be accompanied by deliberately destructive behaviour, again often focused on specific family members — such as breaking of toys or ornaments, tearing of clothes, carving on furniture, or destruction of prized possessions. Violence against family members (but not others) and deliberate fire-setting confined to the home are also grounds for the diagnosis.

Diagnostic guidelines

Diagnosis requires that there be no significant conduct disturbance outside the family setting *and* that the child's social relationships outside the family be within the normal range.

In most cases these family-specific conduct disorders will have arisen in the context of some form of marked disturbance in the child's relationship with one or more members of the nuclear family. In some cases, for example, the disorder may have arisen in relation to conflict with a newly arrived step-parent. The nosological validity of this category remains uncertain, but it is possible that these highly situation-specific conduct disorders do not carry the generally poor prognosis associated with pervasive conduct disturbances.

F91.1 Unsocialized conduct disorder

This type of conduct disorder is characterized by the combination of persistent dissocial or aggressive behaviour (meeting the overall criteria for F91 and not merely comprising oppositional, defiant, disruptive behaviour), with a significant pervasive abnormality in the individual's relationships with other children.

Diagnostic guidelines

The lack of effective integration into a peer group constitutes the key distinction from "socialized" conduct disorders and this has precedence over all other differentiations. Disturbed peer relationships are evidenced chiefly by isolation from and/or rejection by or unpopularity with other children, and by a lack of close friends or of lasting empathic, reciprocal relationships with others in the same age group. Relationships with adults tend to be marked by discord, hostility, and resentment. Good relationships with adults can occur (although usually they lack a close, confiding quality) and, if present, do *not* rule out the diagnosis. Frequently, but not always, there is some associated emotional disturbance (but, if this is of a degree sufficient to meet the criteria of a mixed disorder, the code F92. – should be used).

Offending is characteristically (but not necessarily) solitary. Typical behaviours comprise: bullying, excessive fighting, and (in older children) extortion or violent assault; excessive levels of disobedience, rudeness, uncooperativeness, and resistance to authority; severe temper tantrums and uncontrolled rages; destructiveness to property, fire-setting, and cruelty to animals and other children. Some isolated children, however, become involved in group offending. The nature of the offence is therefore less important in making the diagnosis than the quality of personal relationships.

The disorder is usually pervasive across situations but it may be most evident at school; specificity to situations other than the home is compatible with the diagnosis.

Includes: conduct disorder, solitary aggressive type
unsocialized aggressive disorder

F91.2 Socialized conduct disorder

This category applies to conduct disorders involving persistent dissocial or aggressive behaviour (meeting the overall criteria for F91 and not merely comprising oppositional, defiant, disruptive behaviour) occurring in individuals who are generally well integrated into their peer group.

Diagnostic guidelines

The key differentiating feature is the presence of adequate, lasting friendships with others of roughly the same age. Often, but not always, the peer group will consist of other youngsters involved in delinquent or dissocial activities (in which case the child's socially unacceptable conduct may well be approved by the peer group and regulated by the subculture to which it belongs). However, this is not a necessary requirement for the diagnosis: the child may form part of a non-delinquent peer group with his or her dissocial behaviour taking place outside this context. If the dissocial behaviour involves bullying in particular, there may be disturbed relationships with victims or some other children. Again, this does not invalidate the diagnosis provided that the child has some peer group to which he or she is loyal and which involves lasting friendships.

Relationships with adults in authority tend to be poor but there may be good relationships with others. Emotional disturbances are usually minimal. The conduct disturbance may or may not include the family setting but if it is confined to the home the diagnosis is excluded. Often the disorder is most evident outside the family context and specificity to the school (or other extrafamilial setting) is compatible with the diagnosis.

Includes: conduct disorder, group type
group delinquency
offences in the context of gang membership
stealing in company with others
truancy from school

Excludes: gang activity without manifest psychiatric disorder (Z03.2)

F91.3 Oppositional defiant disorder

This type of conduct disorder is characteristically seen in children below the age of 9 or 10 years. It is defined by the *presence* of markedly defiant, disobedient, provocative behaviour and by the *absence* of more severe dissocial or aggressive acts that violate the law or the rights of others. The disorder requires that the overall criteria for F91 be met: even severely mischievous or naughty behaviour is not in itself sufficient for diagnosis. Many authorities consider that oppositional defiant patterns of behaviour represent a less severe type of conduct disorder, rather than a qualitatively distinct type. Research evidence is lacking on whether the distinction is qualitative or quantitative. However, findings suggest that, in so far as it is distinctive, this is true mainly or only in younger children. Caution should be employed in using this category, especially in the case of older children. Clinically significant conduct disorders in older children are usually accompanied by dissocial or aggressive behaviour that go beyond defiance, disobedience, or disruptiveness, although, not infrequently, they are preceded by oppositional defiant disorders at an earlier age. The category is included to reflect common diagnostic practice and to facilitate the classification of disorders occurring in young children.

Diagnostic guidelines

The essential feature of this disorder is a pattern of persistently negativistic, hostile, defiant, provocative, and disruptive behaviour, which is clearly outside the normal range of behaviour for a child of the same age in the same sociocultural context, and which does not include the more serious violations of the rights of others as reflected in the aggressive and dissocial behaviour specified for categories F91.0 and F91.2. Children with this disorder tend frequently and actively to defy adult requests or rules and deliberately to annoy other people. Usually they tend to be angry, resentful, and easily annoyed by other people whom they blame for their own mistakes or difficulties. They generally have a low frustration tolerance and readily lose their temper. Typically, their defiance has a provocative quality, so that they initiate confrontations and generally exhibit excessive levels of rudeness, uncooperativeness, and resistance to authority.

Frequently, this behaviour is most evident in interactions with adults or peers whom the child knows well, and signs of the disorder may not be evident during a clinical interview.

The key distinction from other types of conduct disorder is the *absence* of behaviour that violates the law and the basic rights of others, such as theft, cruelty, bullying, assault, and destructiveness. The definite presence of any of the above would exclude the diagnosis. However, oppositional defiant behaviour, as outlined in the paragraph above, is often found in other types of conduct disorder. If another type (F91.0 – F91.2) is present, it should be coded in preference to oppositional defiant disorder.

Excludes: conduct disorders including overtly dissocial or aggressive behaviour (F91.0 – F91.2)

F91.8   Other conduct disorders

F91.9   Conduct disorder, unspecified

This residual category is not recommended and should be used only for disorders that meet the general criteria for F91 but that have not been specified as to subtype or that do not fulfil the criteria for any of the specified subtypes.

Includes: childhood behavioural disorder NOS
childhood conduct disorder NOS

F92 Mixed disorders of conduct and emotions

This group of disorders is characterized by the combination of persistently aggressive, dissocial, or defiant behaviour with overt and marked symptoms of depression, anxiety, or other emotional upsets.

Diagnostic guidelines

The severity should be sufficient that the criteria for both conduct disorders of childhood (F91. –) and emotional disorders of childhood (F93. –), or for an adult-type neurotic disorder (F40 – 49) or mood disorder (F30 – 39) are met.

Insufficient research has been carried out to be confident that this category should indeed be separate from conduct disorders of childhood. It is included here for its potential etiological and therapeutic importance and its contribution to reliability of classification.

F92.0 Depressive conduct disorder

This category requires the combination of conduct disorder of childhood (F91. –) with persistent and marked depression of mood, as evidenced by symptoms such as excessive misery, loss of interest and pleasure in usual activities, self-blame, and hopelessness. Disturbances of sleep or appetite may also be present.

Includes: conduct disorder (F91. –) associated with depressive disorder (F30 – F39)

F92.8 Other mixed disorders of conduct and emotions

This category requires the combination of conduct disorder of childhood (F91. –) with persistent and marked emotional symptoms such as anxiety, fearfulness, obsessions or compulsions, depersonalization or derealization, phobias, or hypochondriasis. Anger and resentment are features of conduct disorder rather than of emotional disorder; they neither contradict nor support the diagnosis.

Includes: conduct disorder (F91. –) associated with emotional disorder (F93. –) or neurotic disorder (F40 – F48)

F92.9 Mixed disorder of conduct and emotions, unspecified

F93 Emotional disorders with onset specific to childhood

In child psychiatry a differentiation has traditionally been made between emotional disorders specific to childhood and adolescence and adult-type neurotic disorders. There have been four main justifications for this differentiation. First, research findings have been consistent in showing that the majority of children with emotional disorders go on to become normal adults: only a minority show neurotic disorders in adult life. Conversely, many adult neurotic disorders appear to have an onset in adult life without significant psychopathological precursors in childhood. Hence there is considerable discontinuity between emotional disorders occurring in these two age periods. Second, many emotional disorders in childhood seem to constitute exaggerations of normal developmental trends rather than phenomena that are qualitatively abnormal in themselves. Third, related to the last consideration, there has often been the theoretical assumption that the mental mechanisms involved in emotional disorders of childhood may not be the same as for adult neuroses. Fourth, the emotional disorders of childhood are less clearly demarcated into supposedly specific entities such as phobic disorders or obsessional disorders.

The third of these points lacks empirical validation, and epidemiological data suggest that, if the fourth is correct, it is a matter of degree only (with poorly differentiated emotional disorders quite common in both childhood and adult life). Accordingly, the second feature (i.e. developmental appropriateness) is used as the key diagnostic feature in defining the difference between the emotional disorders with an onset specific to childhood (F93. –) and the neurotic disorders (F40 – F49). The validity of this distinction is uncertain, but there is some empirical evidence to suggest that the developmentally appropriate emotional disorders of childhood have a better prognosis.

F93.0 Separation anxiety disorder of childhood
It is normal for toddlers and preschool children to show a degree of anxiety over real or threatened separation from people to whom they are attached. Separation anxiety disorder should be diagnosed only when fear over separation constitutes the focus of the anxiety and when such anxiety arises during the early years. It is differentiated from normal separation anxiety when it is of such

severity that is statistically unusual (including an abnormal persistence beyond the usual age period) and when it is associated with significant problems in social functioning. In addition, the diagnosis requires that there should be no generalized disturbance of personality development of functioning; if such a disturbance is present, a code from F40 – F49 should be considered. Separation anxiety that arises at a developmentally inappropriate age (such as during adolescence) should not be coded here unless it constitutes an abnormal continuation of developmentally appropriate separation anxiety.

Diagnostic guidelines

The key diagnostic feature is a focused excessive anxiety concerning separation from those individuals to whom the child is attached (usually parents or other family members), that is not merely part of a generalized anxiety about multiple situations. The anxiety may take the form of:

(a) an unrealistic, preoccupying worry about possible harm befalling major attachment figures or a fear that they will leave and not return;

(b) an unrealistic, preoccupying worry that some untoward event, such as the child being lost, kidnapped, admitted to hospital, or killed, will separate him or her from a major attachment figure;

(c) persistent reluctance or refusal to go to school because of fear about separation (rather than for other reasons such as fear about events at school);

(d) persistent reluctance or refusal to go to sleep without being near or next to a major attachment figure;

(e) persistent inappropriate fear of being alone, or otherwise without the major attachment figure, at home during the day;

(f) repeated nightmares about separation;

(g) repeated occurrence of physical symptoms (nausea, stomachache, headache, vomiting, etc.) on occasions that involve separation from a major attachment figure, such as leaving home to go to school;

(h) excessive, recurrent distress (as shown by anxiety, crying, tantrums, misery, apathy, or social withdrawal) in anticipation of, during, or immediately following separation from a major attachment figure.

Many situations that involve separation also involve other potential stressors or sources of anxiety. The diagnosis rests on the demonstration that the common element giving rise to anxiety in the various situations is the circumstance of separation from a major attachment figure. This arises most commonly, perhaps, in relation to school refusal (or "phobia"). Often, this does represent separation anxiety but sometimes (especially in adolescence) it does not. School refusal arising for the first time in adolescence should not be coded here unless it is primarily a function of separation anxiety, and that anxiety was first evident to an abnormal degree during the preschool years. Unless those criteria are met, the syndrome should be coded in one of the other categories in F93 or under F40 – F48.

Excludes: mood [affective] disorders (F30 – F39)
neurotic disorders (F40 – F48)
phobic anxiety disorder of childhood (F93.1)
social anxiety disorder of childhood (F93.2)

F93.1 Phobic anxiety disorder of childhood

Children, like adults, can develop fear that is focused on a wide range of objects or situations. Some of these fears (or phobias), for example agoraphobia, are not a normal part of psychosocial development. When such fears occur in childhood they should be coded under the appropriate category in F40 – F48. However, some fears show a marked developmental phase specificity and arise (in some degree) in a majority of children; this would be true, for example, of fear of animals in the preschool period.

Diagnostic guidelines

This category should be used only for developmental phase-specific fears when they meet the additional criteria that apply to all disorders in F93, namely that:

(a) the onset is during the developmentally appropriate age period;
(b) the degree of anxiety is clinically abnormal; and
(c) the anxiety does not form part of a more generalized disorder.

Excludes: generalized anxiety disorder (F41.1)

F93.2 Social anxiety disorder of childhood

A wariness of strangers is a normal phenomenon in the second half of the first year of life and a degree of social apprehension or anxiety is normal during early childhood when children encounter new, strange, or socially threatening situations. This category should therefore be used only for disorders that arise before the age of 6 years, that are both unusual in degree and accompanied by problems in social functioning, and that are not part of some more generalized emotional disturbance.

Diagnostic guidelines

Children with this disorder show a persistent or recurrent fear and/or avoidance of strangers; such fear may occur mainly with adults, mainly with peers, or with both. The fear is associated with a normal degree of selective attachment to parents or to other familiar persons. The avoidance or fear of social encounters is of a degree that is outside the normal limits for the child's age and is associated with clinically significant problems in social functioning.

Includes: avoidant disorder of childhood or adolescence

F93.3   Sibling rivalry disorder

A high proportion, or even a majority, of young children show some degree of emotional disturbance following the birth of a younger (usually immediately younger) sibling. In most cases the disturbance is mild, but the rivalry or jealousy set up during the period after the birth may be remarkably persistent.

Diagnostic guidelines

The disorder is characterized by the combination of:

(a) evidence of sibling rivalry and/or jealousy;
(b) onset during the months following the birth of the younger (usually immediately younger) sibling;
(c) emotional disturbance that is abnormal in degree and/or persistence and associated with psychosocial problems.

Sibling rivalry/jealousy may be shown by marked competition with siblings for the attention and affection of parents; for this to be regarded as abnormal, it should be associated with an unusual degree of negative feelings. In severe cases this may be accompanied by overt hostility, physical trauma and/or maliciousness towards, and undermining of, the sibling. In lesser cases, it may be shown by a strong reluctance to share, a lack of positive regard, and a paucity of friendly interactions.

The emotional disturbance may take any of several forms, often including some regression with loss of previously acquired skills (such as bowel or bladder control) and a tendency to babyish behaviour. Frequently, too, the child wants to copy the baby in activities that provide for parental attention, such as feeding. There is usually an increase in confrontational or oppositional behaviour with the parents, temper tantrums, and dysphoria exhibited in the form of anxiety, misery, or social withdrawal. Sleep may become disturbed and there is frequently increased pressure for parental attention, such as at bedtime.

Includes: sibling jealousy

Excludes: peer rivalries (non-sibling) (F93.8)

F93.8 Other childhood emotional disorders

Includes: identity disorder
overanxious disorder
peer rivalries (non-sibling)

Excludes: gender identity disorder of childhood (F64.2)

F93.9 Childhood emotional disorder, unspecified

Includes: childhood emotional disorder NOS

F94 Disorders of social functioning with onset specific to childhood and adolescence

This is a somewhat heterogeneous group of disorders, which have in common abnormalities in social functioning that begin during the developmental period, but that (unlike the pervasive developmental disorders) are not primarily characterized by an apparently constitutional social incapacity or deficit that pervades all areas of functioning. Serious environmental distortions or privations are commonly associated and are thought to play a crucial etiological role in many instances. There is no marked sex differential. The existence of this group of disorders of social functioning is well recognized, but there is uncertainty regarding the defining diagnostic criteria, and also disagreement regarding the most appropriate subdivision and classification.

F94.0 Elective mutism

The condition is characterized by a marked, emotionally determined selectivity in speaking, such that the child demonstrates his or her language competence in some situations but fails to speak in other (definable) situations. Most frequently, the disorder is first manifest in early childhood; it occurs with approximately the same frequency in the two sexes, and it is usual for the mutism to be associated with marked personality features involving social anxiety, withdrawal, sensitivity, or resistance. Typically, the child speaks at home or with close friends and is mute at school or with strangers, but other patterns (including the converse) can occur.

Diagnostic guidelines

The diagnosis presupposes:

(a) a normal, or near-normal, level of language comprehension;
(b) a level of competence in language expression that is sufficient for social communication;
(c) demonstrable evidence that the individual can and does speak normally or almost normally in some situations.

However, a substantial minority of children with elective mutism have a history of either some speech delay or articulation problems. The diagnosis may be made in the presence of such problems provided that there is adequate language for effective communication and a *gross* disparity in language usage according to the social context, such that the child speaks fluently in some situations but is mute or near-mute in others. There should also be demonstrable failure to speak in some social situations but not in others. The diagnosis requires that the failure to speak is persistent over time and that there is a consistency and predictability with respect to the situations in which speech does and does not occur.

Other socio-emotional disturbances are present in the great majority of cases but they do not constitute part of the necessary features for diagnosis. Such disturbances do not follow a consistent pattern, but abnormal temperamental features (especially social sensitivity, social anxiety, and social withdrawal) are usual and oppositional behaviour is common.

Includes: selective mutism

Excludes: pervasive developmental disorders (F84. –)
schizophrenia (F20. –)
specific developmental disorders of speech and language
(F80. –)
transient mutism as part of separation anxiety in young
children (F93.0)

F94.1 Reactive attachment disorder of childhood

This disorder, occurring in infants and young children, is characterized
by persistent abnormalities in the child's pattern of social relationships,
which are associated with emotional disturbance and reactive
to changes in environmental circumstances. Fearfulness and
hypervigilance that do not respond to comforting are characteristic,
poor social interaction with peers is typical, aggression towards the
self and others is very frequent, misery is usual, and growth failure
occurs in some cases. The syndrome probably occurs as a direct result
of severe parental neglect, abuse, or serious mishandling. The
existence of this behavioural pattern is well recognized and accepted,
but there is continuing uncertainty regarding the diagnostic criteria
to be applied, the boundaries of the syndrome, and whether the
syndrome constitutes a valid nosological entity. However, the category
is included here because of the public health importance of the
syndrome, because there is no doubt of its existence, and because
the behavioural pattern clearly does not fit the criteria of other
diagnostic categories.

Diagnostic guidelines

The key feature is an abnormal pattern of relationships with care-
givers that developed before the age of 5 years, that involves
maladaptive features not ordinarily seen in normal children, and that
is persistent yet reactive to sufficiently marked changes in patterns
of rearing.

Young children with this syndrome show strongly contradictory or
ambivalent social responses that may be most evident at times of
partings and reunions. Thus, infants may approach with averted look,
gaze strongly away while being held, or respond to care-givers with
a mixture of approach, avoidance, and resistance to comforting. The
emotional disturbance may be evident in apparent misery, a lack
of emotional responsiveness, withdrawal reactions such as huddling
on the floor, and/or aggressive responses to their own or others'

distress. Fearfulness and hypervigilance (sometimes described as "frozen watchfulness") that are unresponsive to comforting occur in some cases. In most cases, the children show interest in peer interactions but social play is impeded by negative emotional responses. The attachment disorder may also be accompanied by a failure to thrive physically and by impaired physical growth (which should be coded according to the appropriate somatic category (R62)).

Many normal children show insecurity in the pattern of their selective attachment to one or other parent, but this should not be confused with the reactive attachment disorder which differs in several crucial respects. The disorder is characterized by an abnormal type of insecurity shown in markedly contradictory social responses not ordinarily seen in normal children. The abnormal responses extend across different social situations and are not confined to a dyadic relationship with a particular care-giver; there is a lack of responsiveness to comforting; and there is associated emotional disturbance in the form of apathy, misery, or fearfulness.

Five main features differentiate this condition from pervasive developmental disorders. First, children with a reactive attachment disorder have a normal capacity for social reciprocity and responsiveness, whereas those with a pervasive developmental disorder do not. Second, although the abnormal patterns of social responses in a reactive attachment disorder are initially a general feature of the child's behaviour in a variety of situations, they remit to a major degree if the child is placed in a normal rearing environment that provides continuity in responsive care-giving. This does not occur with pervasive developmental disorders. Third, although children with reactive attachment disorders may show impaired language development (of the type described under F80.1), they do not exhibit the abnormal qualities of communication characteristic of autism. Fourth, unlike autism, reactive attachment disorder is not associated with persistent and severe cognitive deficits that do not respond appreciably to environmental change. Fifth, persistently restricted, repetitive, and stereotyped patterns of behaviour, interests and activities are not a feature of reactive attachment disorders.

Reactive attachment disorders nearly always arise in relation to grossly inadequate child care. This may take the form of psychological abuse or neglect (as evidenced by harsh punishment, persistent failure to respond to the child's overtures, or grossly inept parenting), or of physical abuse or neglect (as evidenced by persistent disregard of the child's basic physical needs, repeated deliberate injury, or inadequate provision of nutrition). Because there is insufficient knowledge of the consistency of association between inadequate child care and the disorder, the presence of environmental privation and distortion is not a diagnostic requirement. However, there should be caution in making the diagnosis in the absence of evidence of abuse or neglect. Conversely, the diagnosis should not be made automatically on the basis of abuse or neglect: not all abused or neglected children manifest the disorder.

Excludes: Asperger's syndrome (F84.5)
disinhibited attachment disorder of childhood (F94.2)
maltreatment syndromes, resulting in physical problems (T74)
normal variation in pattern of selective attachment
sexual or physical abuse in childhood, resulting in psychosocial problems (Z61.4 – Z61.6)

F94.2   Disinhibited attachment disorder of childhood

A particular pattern of abnormal social functioning that arises during the first 5 years of life and that, having become established, shows a tendency to persist despite marked changes in environmental circumstances. At age about 2 years it is usually manifest by clinging and diffuse, non-selectively focused attachment behaviour. By age 4 years, diffuse attachments remain but clinging tends to be replaced by attention-seeking and indiscriminately friendly behaviour. In middle and later childhood, individuals may or may not have developed selective attachments but attention-seeking behaviour often persists, and poorly modulated peer interactions are usual; depending on circumstances, there may also be associated emotional or behavioural disturbance. The syndrome has been most clearly identified in children reared in institutions from infancy but it also occurs in other situations; it is thought to be due in part to a persistent failure of opportunity to develop selective attachments as a consequence of extremely frequent changes in care-givers. The conceptual unity of the syndrome depends on the early onset of diffuse attachments, continuing poor social interactions, and lack of situation-specificity.

Diagnostic guidelines

Diagnosis should be based on evidence that the child showed an unusual degree of diffuseness in selective attachments during the first 5 years *and* that this was associated with generally clinging behaviour in infancy and/or indiscriminately friendly, attention-seeking behaviour in early or middle childhood. Usually there is difficulty in forming close, confiding relationships with peers. There may or may not be associated emotional or behavioural disturbance (depending in part on the child's current circumstances). In most cases there will be a clear history of rearing in the first years that involved marked discontinuities in care-givers or multiple changes in family placements (as with multiple foster family placements).

Includes: affectionless psychopathy
institutional syndrome

Excludes: Asperger's syndrome (F84.5)
hospitalism in children (F43.2)
hyperkinetic or attention deficit disorder (F90. –)
reactive attachment disorder of childhood (F94.1)

F94.8   Other childhood disorders of social functioning

Includes: disorders of social functioning with withdrawal and shyness due to social competence deficiencies

F94.9   Childhood disorder of social functioning, unspecified

F95   Tic disorders

The predominant manifestation in these syndromes is some form of tic. A tic is an involuntary, rapid, recurrent, non-rhythmic motor movement (usually involving circumscribed muscle groups), or vocal production, that is of sudden onset and serves no apparent purpose. Tics tend to be experienced as irresistible but they can usually be suppressed for varying periods of time. Both motor and vocal tics may be classified as either simple or complex, although the boundaries are not well defined. Common simple motor tics include eye-blinking, neck-jerking, shoulder-shrugging, and facial grimacing. Common simple vocal tics include throat-clearing, barking, sniffing, and hissing. Common complex tics include hitting one's self, jumping, and hopping. Common complex vocal tics include the repetition of particular words, and sometimes the use of socially unacceptable (often obscene) words (coprolalia), and the repetition of one's own sounds or words (palilalia).

There is immense variation in the severity of tics. At the one extreme the phenomenon is near-normal, with perhaps 1 in 5 to 1 in 10 children showing transient tics at some time. At the other extreme, Tourette's syndrome is an uncommon, chronic, incapacitating disorder. There is uncertainty about whether these extremes represent different conditions or are opposite ends of the same continuum; many authorities regard the latter as more likely. Tic disorders are substantially more frequent in boys than in girls and a family history of tics is common.

Diagnostic guidelines

The major features distinguishing tics from other motor disorders are the sudden, rapid, transient, and circumscribed nature of the movements, together with the lack of evidence of underlying neurological disorder; their repetitiveness; (usually) their disappearance during sleep; and the ease with which they may be voluntarily reproduced or suppressed. The lack of rhythmicity differentiates tics from the stereotyped repetitive movements seen in some cases of autism or of mental retardation. Manneristic motor activities seen in the same disorders tend to comprise more complex and variable movements than those usually seen with tics. Obsessive – compulsive activities sometimes resemble complex tics but differ in that their form tends to be defined by their purpose (such as touching some object or turning a number of times) rather than by the muscle groups involved; however, the differentiation is sometimes difficult.

Tics often occur as an isolated phenomenon but not infrequently they are associated with a wide variety of emotional disturbances, especially, perhaps, obsessional and hypochondriacal phenomena. However, specific developmental delays are also associated with tics.

There is no clear dividing line between tic disorder with some associated emotional disturbance and an emotional disorder with some associated tics. However, the diagnosis should represent the major type of abnormality.

F95.0   Transient tic disorder

Meets the general criteria for a tic disorder, but tics do not persist for longer than 12 months. This is the commonest form of tic and is most frequent about the age of 4 or 5 years; the tics usually take the form of eye-blinking, facial grimacing, or head-jerking. In some cases the tics occur as a single episode but in other cases there are remissions and relapses over a period of months.

F95.1   Chronic motor or vocal tic disorder

Meets the general criteria for a tic disorder, in which there are motor or vocal tics (but not both); tics may be either single or multiple (but usually multiple), and last for more than a year.

F95.2   Combined vocal and multiple motor tic disorder [de la Tourette's syndrome]

A form of tic disorder in which there are, or have been, multiple motor tics and one or more vocal tics, although these need not have occurred concurrently. Onset is almost always in childhood or adolescence. A history of motor tics before development of vocal tics is common; the symptoms frequently worsen during adolescence, and it is common for the disorder to persist into adult life.

The vocal tics are often multiple with explosive repetitive vocalizations, throat-clearing, and grunting, and there may be the use of obscene words or phrases. Sometimes there is associated gestural echopraxia, which also may be of an obscene nature (copropraxia). As with motor tics, the vocal tics may be voluntarily suppressed for short periods, be exacerbated by stress, and disappear during sleep.

F95.8   Other tic disorders

F95.9   Tic disorder, unspecified

A non-recommended residual category for a disorder that fulfils the general criteria for a tic disorder but in which the specific subcategory is not specified or in which the features do not fulfil the criteria for F95.0, F95.1 or F95.2.

F98 Other behavioural and emotional disorders with onset usually occurring in childhood and adolescence

This rubric comprises a heterogeneous group of disorders that share the characteristic of onset in childhood but otherwise differ in many respects. Some of the conditions represent well defined syndromes, but others are no more than symptom complexes which lack nosological validity, but which are included because of their frequency and association with psychosocial problems, and because they cannot be incorporated into other syndromes.

Excludes: breath-holding attacks (R06.8)
gender identity disorder of childhood (F64.2)
hypersomnolence and megaphagia (Kleine – Levin syndrome) (G47.8)
obsessive – compulsive disorder (F42. –)
sleep disorders (F51. –)

F98.0 Nonorganic enuresis

A disorder characterized by involuntary voiding of urine, by day and/or by night, which is abnormal in relation to the individual's mental age and which is not a consequence of a lack of bladder control due to any neurological disorder, to epileptic attacks, or to any structural abnormality of the urinary tract. The enuresis may have been present from birth (i.e. an abnormal extension of the normal infantile incontinence) or it may have arisen following a period of acquired bladder control. The later onset (or secondary) variety usually begins about the age of 5 to 7 years. The enuresis may constitute a monosymptomatic condition or it may be associated with a more widespread emotional or behavioural disorder. In the latter case there is uncertainty over the mechanisms involved in the association. Emotional problems may arise as a secondary consequence of the distress or stigma that results from enuresis, the enuresis may form part of some other psychiatric disorder, or both the enuresis and the emotional/behavioural disturbance may arise in parallel from related etiological factors. There is no straightforward, unambiguous way of deciding between these alternatives in the individual case, and the diagnosis should be made on the basis of which type of disturbance (i.e. enuresis or emotional/behavioural disorder) constitutes the main problem.

Diagnostic guidelines

There is no clear-cut demarcation between an enuresis disorder and the normal variations in the age of acquisition of bladder control. However, enuresis would not ordinarily be diagnosed in a child under the age of 5 years or with a mental age under 4 years. If the enuresis is associated with some (other) emotional or behavioural disorder, enuresis would normally constitute the primary diagnosis only if the involuntary voiding of urine occurred at least several times per week and if the other symptoms showed some temporal covariation with the enuresis. Enuresis sometimes occurs in conjunction with encopresis; when this is the case, encopresis should be diagnosed.

Occasionally, children develop transient enuresis as a result of cystitis or polyuria (as from diabetes). However, these do not constitute a sufficient explanation for enuresis that persists after the infection has been cured or after the polyuria has been brought under control. Not infrequently, the cystitis may be secondary to an enuresis that has arisen by ascending infection up the urinary tract as a result of persistent wetness (especially in girls).

Includes: enuresis (primary) (secondary) of nonorganic origin
functional or psychogenic enuresis
urinary incontinence of nonorganic origin

Excludes: enuresis NOS (R32)

F98.1 Nonorganic encopresis

Repeated voluntary or involuntary passage of faeces, usually of normal or near-normal consistency, in places not appropriate for that purpose in the individual's own sociocultural setting. The condition may represent an abnormal continuation of normal infantile incontinence, it may involve a loss of continence following the acquisition of bowel control, or it may involve the deliberate deposition of faeces in inappropriate places in spite of normal physiological bowel control. The condition may occur as a monosymptomatic disorder, or it may form part of a wider disorder, especially an emotional disorder (F93. –) or a conduct disorder (F91. –).

Diagnostic guidelines

The crucial diagnostic feature is the inappropriate placement of faeces. The condition may arise in several different ways. First, it may represent a lack of adequate toilet-training or of adequate response to training, with the history being one of continuous failure ever to acquire adequate bowel control. Second, it may reflect a psychologically determined disorder in which there is normal physiological control over defecation but, for some reason, a reluctance, resistance, or failure to conform to social norms in defecating in acceptable places. Third, it may stem from physiological retention, involving impaction of faeces, with secondary overflow and deposition of faeces in inappropriate places. Such retention may arise from parent/child battles over bowel-training, from withholding of faeces because of painful defecation (e.g. as a consequence of anal fissure), or for other reasons.

In some instances, the encopresis may be accompanied by smearing of faeces over the body or over the external environment and, less commonly, there may be anal fingering or masturbation. There is usually some degree of associated emotional/behavioural disturbance. There is no clear-cut demarcation between encopresis with associated emotional/behavioural disturbance and some other psychiatric disorder which includes encopresis as a subsidiary symptom. The recommended guideline is to code encopresis if that is the predominant phenomenon and the other disorder if it is not (or if the frequency of the encopresis is less than once a month). Encopresis and enuresis are not infrequently associated and, when this is the case, the coding of encopresis should have precedence. Encopresis may sometimes follow an organic condition such as anal fissure or a gastrointestinal infection; the organic condition should be the sole coding if it constitutes a sufficient explanation for the faecal soiling but, if it serves as precipitant but not a sufficient cause, encopresis should be coded (in addition to the somatic condition).

Differential diagnosis. It is important to consider the following:

(a) encopresis due to organic disease such as aganglionic megacolon (Q43.1) or spina bifida (Q05. –) (note, however, that encopresis may accompany or follow conditions such as anal fissure or gastrointestinal infection);

(b) constipation involving faecal blockage resulting in "overflow" faecal soiling of liquid or semiliquid faeces (K59.0); if, as happens in some cases, encopresis and constipation coexist, encopresis should be coded (with an additional code, if appropriate, to identify the cause of the constipation).

F98.2 Feeding disorder of infancy and childhood

A feeding disorder of varying manifestations, usually specific to infancy and early childhood. It generally involves refusal of food and extreme faddiness in the presence of an adequate food supply and a reasonably competent care-giver, and the absence of organic disease. There may or may not be associated rumination (repeated regurgitation without nausea or gastrointestinal illness).

Diagnostic guidelines

Minor difficulties in eating are very common in infancy and childhood (in the form of faddiness, supposed undereating, or supposed overeating). In themselves, these should not be considered as indicative of disorder. Disorder should be diagnosed only if the difficulties are clearly beyond the normal range, if the nature of the eating problem is qualitatively abnormal in character, or if the child fails to gain weight or loses weight over a period of at least 1 month.

Includes: rumination disorder of infancy

Differential diagnosis. It is important to differentiate this disorder from:

(a) conditions where the child readily takes food from adults other than the usual care-giver;
(b) organic disease sufficient to explain the food refusal;
(c) anorexia nervosa and other eating disorders (F50. –);
(d) broader psychiatric disorder;
(e) pica (F98.3);
(f) feeding difficulties and mismanagement (R63.3).

F98.3 Pica of infancy and childhood

Persistent eating of non-nutritive substances (soil, paint chippings, etc.). Pica may occur as one of many symptoms of a more widespread psychiatric disorder (such as autism), or as a relatively isolated psychopathological behaviour; *only* in the latter case should this code be used. The phenomenon is most common in mentally retarded children; if mental retardation is also present, it should be coded

(F70 – 79). However, pica may also occur in children (usually young children) of normal intelligence.

F98.4 Stereotyped movement disorders

Voluntary, repetitive, stereotyped, nonfunctional (and often rhythmic) movements that do not form part of any recognized psychiatric or neurological condition. When such movements occur as symptoms of some other disorder, only the overall disorder should be coded (i.e. F98.4 should not be used). The movements that are noninjurious include: body-rocking, head-rocking, hair-plucking, hair-twisting, finger-flicking mannerisms, and hand-flapping. (Nail-biting, thumb-sucking, and nose-picking should not be included as they are not good indicators of psychopathology, and are not of sufficient public health importance to warrant classification.) Stereotyped self-injurious behaviour includes repetitive head-banging, face-slapping, eye-poking, and biting of hands, lips or other body parts. All the stereotyped movement disorders occur most frequently in association with mental retardation; when this is the case, *both* disorders should be coded.

Eye-poking is particularly common in children with visual impairment. However, the visual disability does not constitute a sufficient explanation, and when both eye-poking and blindness (or partial blindness) occur, both should be coded: eye-poking under F98.4 and the visual condition under the appropriate somatic disorder code.

Excludes: abnormal involuntary movements (R25. –)
movement disorders of organic origin (G20 – G26)
nail-biting, nose-picking, thumb-sucking (F98.8)
obsessive – compulsive disorder (F42. –)
stereotypies that are part of a broader psychiatric condition
(such as pervasive developmental disorder)
tic disorders (F95. –)
trichotillomania (F63.3)

F98.5 Stuttering [stammering]

Speech that is characterized by frequent repetition or prolongation of sounds or syllables or words, or by frequent hesitations or pauses that disrupt the rhythmic flow of speech. Minor dysrhythmias of this type are quite common as a transient phase in early childhood, or as a minor but persistent speech feature in later childhood and adult life. They should be classified as a disorder only if their severity is such as markedly to disturb the fluency of speech. There may be associated movements of the face and/or other parts of the body that coincide in time with the repetitions, prolongations, or pauses in speech flow. Stuttering should be differentiated from cluttering (see below) and from tics. In some cases there may be an associated developmental disorder of speech or language, in which case this should be separately coded under F80. – .

Excludes: cluttering (F98.6)

neurological disorder giving rise to speech dysrhythmias (Chapter VI of ICD-10)

obsessive – compulsive disorder (F42. –)

tic disorders (F95. –)

F98.6 Cluttering

A rapid rate of speech with breakdown in fluency, but no repetitions or hesitations, of a severity to give rise to reduced speech intelligibility. Speech is erratic and dysrhythmic, with rapid, jerky spurts that usually involve faulty phrasing patterns (e.g. alternating pauses and bursts of speech, producing groups of words unrelated to the grammatical structure of the sentence).

Excludes: neurological disorder giving rise to speech dysrhythmias (Chapter VI of ICD-10)

obsessive – compulsive disorder (F42. –)

stuttering (F98.5)

tic disorders (F95. –)

F98.8 Other specified behavioural and emotional disorders with onset usually occurring in childhood and adolescence

Includes: attention deficit disorder without hyperactivity

(excessive) masturbation

nail-biting

nose-picking

thumb-sucking

F98.9 Unspecified behavioural and emotional disorders with onset usually occurring in childhood and adolescence

F99 Mental disorder, not otherwise specified

Non-recommended residual category, when no other code from F00 – F98 can be used.

ANNEX

Other conditions from ICD-10 often associated with mental and behavioural disorders

This appendix contains a list of conditions in other chapters of ICD-10 that are often found in association with the disorders in Chapter V(F) itself. They are provided here so that psychiatrists recording diagnoses by means of the Clinical Descriptions and Diagnostic Guidelines have immediately to hand the ICD terms and codes that cover the associated diagnoses most likely to be encountered in ordinary clinical practice. The majority of the conditions covered are given only at the three-character level, but four-character codes are given for a selection of those diagnoses that will be used most frequently.

Chapter I
Certain infectious and parasitic diseases (A00 – B99)

A50 **Congenital syphilis**
A50.4 Late congenital neurosyphilis [juvenile neurosyphilis]

A52 **Late syphilis**
A52.1 Symptomatic neurosyphilis

Includes: tabes dorsalis

A81 **Slow virus infections of central nervous system**
A81.0 Creutzfeldt – Jakob disease
A81.1 Subacute sclerosing panencephalitis
A81.2 Progressive multifocal leukoencephalopathy

B22 **Human immunodeficiency virus (HIV) disease resulting in other specified diseases**
B22.0 HIV disease resulting in encephalopathy

Includes: HIV dementia

Chapter II
Neoplasms (C00 – D48)

C70. –   Malignant neoplasm of meninges

C71. –   Malignant neoplasm of brain

C72. –   Malignant neoplasm of spinal cord, cranial nerves and other parts of central nervous system

D33. –   Benign neoplasm of brain and other parts of central nervous system

D42. –   Neoplasm of uncertain and unknown behaviour of meninges

D43. –   Neoplasm of uncertain and unknown behaviour of brain and central nervous system

Chapter IV
Endocrine, nutritional and metabolic diseases (E00 – E90)

E00. –   Congenital iodine-deficiency syndrome

E01. –   Iodine-deficiency-related thyroid disorders and allied conditions

E02   Subclinical iodine-deficiency hypothyroidism

E03   Other hypothyroidism
    E03.2 Hypothyroidism due to medicaments and other exogenous substances
    E03.5 Myxoedema coma

E05. –   Thyrotoxicosis [hyperthyroidism]

E15   Nondiabetic hypoglycaemic coma

E22   Hyperfunction of pituitary gland
    E22.0 Acromegaly and pituitary gigantism
    E22.1 Hyperprolactinaemia

    Includes: drug-induced hyperprolactinaemia

E23. – Hypofunction and other disorders of pituitary gland

E24. – Cushing's syndrome

E30 Disorders of puberty, not elsewhere classified
E30.0 Delayed puberty
E30.1 Precocious puberty

E34 Other endocrine disorders
E34.3 Short stature, not elsewhere classified

E51 Thiamine deficiency
E51.2 Wernicke's encephalopathy

E64. – Sequelae of malnutrition and other nutritional deficiencies

E66. – Obesity

E70 Disorders of aromatic amino-acid metabolism
E70.0 Classical phenylketonuria

E71 Disorders of branched-chain amino-acid metabolism and fatty-acid metabolism
E71.0 Maple-syrup-urine disease

E74. – Other disorders of carbohydrate metabolism

E80. – Disorders of porphyrin and bilirubin metabolism

Chapter VI
Diseases of the nervous system (G00 – G99)

G00. – Bacterial meningitis, not elsewhere classified

Includes: haemophilus, pneumococcal, streptococcal, staphylococcal and other bacterial meningitis

G02. – Meningitis in other infectious and parasitic diseases classified elsewhere

G03. – Meningitis due to other and unspecified causes

G04. –   **Encephalitis, myelitis and encephalomyelitis**

G06   **Intracranial and intraspinal abscess and granuloma**
G06.2 Extradural and subdural abscess, unspecified

G10   **Huntington's disease**

G11. –   **Hereditary ataxia**

G20   **Parkinson's disease**

G21   **Secondary parkinsonism**
G21.0 Malignant neuroleptic syndrome
G21.1 Other drug-induced secondary parkinsonism
G21.2 Secondary parkinsonism due to other external agents
G21.3 Postencephalitic parkinsonism

G24   **Dystonia**

Includes: dyskinesia

G24.0 Drug-induced dystonia
G24.3 Spasmodic torticollis
G24.8 Other dystonia

Includes: tardive dyskinesia

G25. –   **Other extrapyramidal and movement disorders**

Includes: restless legs syndrome, drug-induced tremor, myoclonus, chorea, tics

G30   **Alzheimer's disease**
G30.0 Alzheimer's disease with early onset
G30.1 Alzheimer's disease with late onset
G30.8 Other Alzheimer's disease
G30.9 Alzheimer's disease, unspecified

G31   **Other degenerative diseases of nervous system, not elsewhere classified**
G31.0 Circumscribed brain atrophy

Includes: Pick's disease

G31.1 Senile degeneration of brain, not elsewhere classified

G31.2 Degeneration of nervous system due to alcohol

Includes: alcoholic cerebellar ataxia and degeneration, cerebral degeneration and encephalopathy; dysfunction of the autonomic nervous system due to alcohol

G31.8 Other specified degenerative diseases of the nervous system

Includes: Subacute necrotizing encephalopathy [Leigh] grey-matter degeneration [Alpers]

G31.9 Degenerative disease of nervous system, unspecified

G32. – Other degenerative disorders of nervous system in diseases classified elsewhere

G35 Multiple sclerosis

G37 Other demyelinating diseases of central nervous system

G37.0 Diffuse sclerosis

Includes: periaxial encephalitis; Schilder's disease

G40 Epilepsy

G40.0 Localization-related (focal) (partial) idiopathic epilepsy and epileptic syndromes with seizures of localized onset

Includes: benign childhood epilepsy with centrotemporal EEG spikes or occipital EEG paroxysms

G40.1 Localization-related (focal) (partial) symptomatic epilepsy and epileptic syndromes with simple partial seizures

Includes: attacks without alteration of consciousness

G40.2 Localization-related (focal) (partial) symptomatic epilepsy and epileptic syndromes with complex partial seizures

Includes: attacks with alteration of consciousness, often with automatisms

G40.3 Generalized idiopathic epilepsy and epileptic syndromes

G40.4 Other generalized epilepsy and epileptic syndromes

Includes: salaam attacks

G40.5 Special epileptic syndromes

Includes: epileptic seizures related to alcohol, drugs and sleep deprivation

G40.6 Grand mal seizures, unspecified (with or without petit mal)
G40.7 Petit mal, unspecified, without grand mal seizures

G41. – **Status epilepticus**

G43. – **Migraine**

G44. – **Other headache syndromes**

G45. – **Transient cerebral ischaemic attacks and related syndromes**

G47 **Sleep disorders**
G47.2 Disorders of the sleep – wake schedule
G47.3 Sleep apnoea
G47.4 Narcolepsy and cataplexy

G70 **Myasthenia gravis and other myoneural disorders**
G70.0 Myasthenia gravis

G91. – **Hydrocephalus**

G92 **Toxic encephalopathy**

G93 **Other disorders of brain**
G93.1 Anoxic brain damage, not elsewhere classified
G93.3 Postviral fatigue syndrome

Includes: benign myalgic encephomyelitis

G93.4 Encephalopathy, unspecified

G97 **Postprocedural disorders of nervous system, not elsewhere classified**
G97.0 Cerebrospinal fluid leak from spinal puncture

Chapter VII
Diseases of the eye and adnexa (H00 – H59)

H40   **Glaucoma**
H40.6 Glaucoma secondary to drugs

Chapter VIII
Diseases of the ear and mastoid process (H60 – H95)

H93   **Other disorders of ear, not elsewhere classified**
H93.1 Tinnitus

Chapter IX
Diseases of the circulatory system (I00 – I99)

I10   **Essential (primary) hypertension**

I60. –   **Subarachnoid haemorrhage**

I61. –   **Intracerebral haemorrhage**

I62   **Other nontraumatic intracranial haemorrhage**
I62.0 Subdural haemorrhage (acute) (nontraumatic)
I62.1 Nontraumatic extradural haemorrhage

I63. –   **Cerebral infarction**

I64   **Stroke, not specified as haemorrhage or infarction**

I65. –   **Occlusion and stenosis of precerebral arteries, not resulting in cerebral infarction**

I66. –   **Occlusion and stenosis of cerebral arteries, not resulting in cerebral infarction**

I67   **Other cerebrovascular diseases**
I67.2 Cerebral atherosclerosis
I67.3 Progressive vascular leukoencephalopathy

Includes: Binswanger's disease

I67.4   Hypertensive encephalopathy

I69. –   Sequelae of cerebrovascular disease

I95   Hypotension
I95.2   Hypotension due to drugs

Chapter X
Diseases of the respiratory system (J00 – J99)

J10   Influenza due to identified influenza virus
J10.8   Influenza with other manifestations, influenza virus identified

J11   Influenza, virus not identified
J11.8   Influenza with other manifestations, virus not identified

J42   Unspecified chronic bronchitis

J43. –   Emphysema

J45. –   Asthma

Chapter XI
Diseases of the digestive system (K00 – K93)

K25   Gastric ulcer

K26   Duodenal ulcer

K27   Peptic ulcer, site unspecified

K29   Gastritis and duodenitis
K29.2   Alcoholic gastritis

K30   Dyspepsia

K58. –   Irritable bowel syndrome

K59. –   Other functional intestinal disorders

K70. –   Alcoholic liver disease

K71. –   Toxic liver disease

Includes: drug-induced liver disease

K86   Other diseases of pancreas

K86.0 Alcohol-induced chronic pancreatitis

Chapter XII
Diseases of the skin and subcutaneous tissue (L00 – L99)

L20. –   Atopic dermatitis

L98   Other disorders of skin and subcutaneous tissue, not elsewhere classified

L98.1 Factitial dermatitis

Includes: neurotic excoriation

Chapter XIII
Diseases of the musculoskeletal system and connective tissue (M00 – M99)

M32. –   Systemic lupus erythematosus

M54. –   Dorsalgia

Chapter XIV
Diseases of the genitourinary system (N00 – N99)

N48   Other disorders of penis

N48.3 Priapism

N48.4 Impotence of organic origin

N91. –   Absent, scanty and rare menstruation

N94 **Pain and other conditions associated with female genital organs and menstrual cycle**
N94.3 Premenstrual tension syndrome
N94.4 Primary dysmenorrhoea
N94.5 Secondary dysmenorrhoea
N94.6 Dysmenorrhoea, unspecified

N95 **Menopausal and other perimenopausal disorders**
N95.1 Menopausal and female climacteric states
N95.3 States associated with artificial menopause

Chapter XV
Pregnancy, childbirth and the puerperium (O00 – O99)

O04 **Medical abortion**

O35 **Maternal care for known or suspected fetal abnormality and damage**
O35.4 Maternal care for (suspected) damage to fetus from alcohol
O35.5 Maternal care for (suspected) damage to fetus by drugs

O99 **Other maternal diseases classifiable elsewhere but complicating pregnancy, childbirth and puerperium**
O99.3 Mental disorders and diseases of the nervous system complicating pregnancy, childbirth and the puerperium

Includes: conditions in F00 – F99 and G00 – G99

Chapter XVII
Congenital malformations, deformations, and chromosomal abnormalities (Q00 – Q99)

Q02 **Microcephaly**

Q03. – **Congenital hydrocephalus**

Q04. – **Other congenital malformations of brain**

Q05. – **Spina bifida**

Q75. – **Other congenital malformations of skull and face bones**

Q85   **Phakomatoses, not elsewhere classified**
Q85.0 Neurofibromatosis (nonmalignant)
Q85.1 Tuberous sclerosis

Q86   **Congenital malformation syndromes due to known exogenous causes, not elsewhere classified**
Q86.0 Fetal alcohol syndrome (dysmorphic)

Q90   **Down's syndrome**
Q90.0 Trisomy 21, meiotic nondisjunction
Q90.1 Trisomy 21, mosaicism (mitotic nondisjunction)
Q90.2 Trisomy 21, translocation
Q90.9 Down's syndrome, unspecified

Q91. –   **Edwards' syndrome and Patau's syndrome**

Q93   **Monosomies and deletions from the autosomes, not elsewhere classified**
Q93.4 Deletion of short arm of chromosome 5

Includes: cri-du-chat syndrome

Q96. –   **Turner's syndrome**

Q97. –   **Other sex chromosome abnormalities, female phenotype, not elsewhere classified**

Q98   **Other sex chromosome abnormalities, male phenotype, not elsewhere classified**
Q98.0 Klinefelter's syndrome karyotype 47,XXY
Q98.1 Klinefelter's syndrome, male with more than two
         X chromosomes
Q98.2 Klinefelter's syndrome, male with 46,XX karyotype
Q98.4 Klinefelter's syndrome, unspecified

Q99. –   **Other chromosome abnormalities, not elsewhere classified**

Chapter XVIII
Symptoms, signs and abnormal clinical and laboratory findings, not elsewhere classified (R00 – R99)

R55 **Syncope and collapse**
R56 **Convulsions, not elsewhere classified**
R56.0 Febrile convulsions
R56.8 Other and unspecified convulsions

R62 **Lack of expected normal physiological development**
R62.0 Delayed milestone
R62.8 Other lack of expected normal physiological development
R62.9 Lack of expected normal physiological development, unspecified

R63 **Symptoms and signs concerning food and fluid intake**
R63.0 Anorexia
R63.1 Polydipsia
R63.4 Abnormal weight loss
R63.5 Abnormal weight gain

R78. – **Findings of drugs and other substances, normally not found in blood**

Includes: alcohol (R78.0); opiate drug (R78.1); cocaine (R78.2); hallucinogen (R78.3); other drugs of addictive potential (R78.4); psychotropic drug (R78.5); abnormal level of lithium (R78.8)

R83 **Abnormal findings in cerebrospinal fluid**

R90. – **Abnormal findings on diagnostic imaging of central nervous system**

R94 **Abnormal results of function studies**
R94.0 Abnormal results of function studies of central nervous system

Includes: abnormal electroencephalogram [EEG]

Chapter XIX
Injury, poisoning and certain other consequences
of external causes (S00 – T98)

S06   **Intracranial injury**

    S06.0 Concussion

    S06.1 Traumatic cerebral oedema

    S06.2 Diffuse brain injury

    S06.3 Focal brain injury

    S06.4 Epidural haemorrhage

    S06.5 Traumatic subdural heaemorrhage

    S06.6 Traumatic subarachnoid haemorrhage

    S06.7 Intracranial injury with prolonged coma

Chapter XX
External causes of morbidity and mortality (V0I – Y98)

Intentional self-harm (X60 – X84)

> *Includes:* purposely self-inflicted poisoning or injury; suicide

X60   **Intentional self-poisoning by and exposure to nonopioid analgesics, antipyretics and antirheumatics**

X61   **Intentional self-poisoning by and exposure to antiepileptic, sedative – hypnotic, antiparkinsonism and psychotropic drugs, not elsewhere classified**

> *Includes:* antidepressants, barbiturates, neuroleptics, psychostimulants

X62   **Intentional self-poisoning by and exposure to narcotics and psychodysleptics [hallucinogens], not elsewhere classified**

> *Includes:* cannabis (derivatives), cocaine, codeine, heroin, lysergide
> [LSD], mescaline, methadone, morphine, opium (alkaloids)

X63   **Intentional self-poisoning by and exposure to other drugs acting on the autonomic nervous systems**

X64   **Intentional self-poisoning by and exposure to other and unspecified drugs and biological substances**

X65   **Intentional self-poisoning by and exposure to alcohol**

X66   **Intentional self-poisoning by and exposure to organic solvents and halogenated hydrocarbons and their vapours**

X67   **Intentional self-poisoning by and exposure to other gases and vapours**

Includes: carbon monoxide; utility gas

X68   **Intentional self-poisoning by and exposure to pesticides**

X69   **Intentional self-poisoning by and exposure to other and unspecified chemicals and noxious substances**

Includes: corrosive aromatics, acids and caustic alkalis

X70   **Intentional self-harm by hanging, strangulation and suffocation**

X71   **Intentional self-harm by drowning and submersion**

X72   **Intentional self-harm by handgun discharge**

X73   **Intentional self-harm by rifle, shotgun and larger firearm discharge**

X74   **Intentional self-harm by other and unspecified firearm discharge**

X75   **Intentional self-harm by explosive material**

X76   **Intentional self-harm by fire and flames**

X77   **Intentional self-harm by steam, hot vapours and hot objects**

X78   **Intentional self-harm by sharp object**

X79   **Intentional self-harm by blunt object**

X80   **Intentional self-harm by jumping from a high place**

X81   **Intentional self-harm by jumping or lying before moving object**

X82   **Intentional self-harm by crashing of motor vehicle**

X83   **Intentional self-harm by other specified means**

Includes: crashing of aircraft, electrocution, caustic substances (except poisoning)

X84   **Intentional self-harm by unspecified means**

Assault (X85 – Y09)

Includes: homicide; injuries inflicted by another person with intent to injure or kill, by any means

X93   **Assault by handgun discharge**

X99   **Assault by sharp object**

Y00   **Assault by blunt object**

Y04   **Assault by bodily force**

Y05   **Sexual assault by bodily force**

Y06. –   **Neglect and abandonment**

Y07. –   **Other maltreatment syndromes**

Includes: mental cruelty; physical abuse; sexual abuse; torture

Drugs, medicaments and biological substances causing adverse effects in therapeutic use (Y40 – Y59)

Y46   **Antiepileptics and antiparkinsonism drugs**
Y46.7 Antiparkinsonism drugs

Y47. –   **Sedatives, hypnotics and antianxiety drugs**

Y49   **Psychotropic drugs, not elsewhere classified**
Y49.0 Tricyclic and tetracyclic antidepressants
Y49.1 Monoamine-oxidase-inhibitor antidepressants
Y49.2 Other and unspecified antidepressants
Y49.3 Phenothiazine antipsychotics and neuroleptics

Y49.4 Butyrophenone and thioxanthene neuroleptics

Y49.5 Other antipsychotics and neuroleptics

Y49.6 Psychodysleptics [hallucinogens]

Y49.7 Psychostimulants with abuse potential

Y49.8 Other psychotropic drugs, not elsewhere classified

Y49.9 Psychotropic drug, unspecified

Y50. – Central nervous system stimulants, not elsewhere classified

Y51. – Drugs primarily affecting the autonomic nervous system

Y57. – Other and unspecified drugs and medicaments

Chapter XXI
Factors influencing health status and contact with health services (Z00 – Z99)

Z00   **General examination and investigation of persons without complaint and reported diagnosis**

Z00.4 General psychiatric examination, not elsewhere classified

Z02   **Examination and encounter for administrative purposes**

Z02.3 Examination for recruitment to armed forces

Z02.4 Examination for driving licence

Z02.6 Examination for insurance purposes

Z02.7 Issue of medical certificate

Z03   **Medical observation and evaluation for suspected diseases and conditions**

Z03.2 Observation for suspected mental and behavioural disorders

Includes: observation for dissocial behaviour, fire-setting, gang activity, and shoplifting, without manifest psychiatric disorder

Z04   **Examination and observation for other reasons**

Includes: examination for medicolegal reasons

Z04.6 General psychiatric examination, requested by authority

Z50 **Care involving use of rehabilitation procedures**
Z50.2 Alcohol rehabilitation
Z50.3 Drug rehabilitation
Z50.4 Psychotherapy, not elsewhere classified
Z50.7 Occupational therapy and vocational rehabilitation, not elsewhere classified
Z50.8 Care involving use of other specified rehabilitation procedures

Includes: tobacco abuse rehabilitation
training in activities of daily living [ADL]

Z54 **Convalescence**
Z54.3 Convalescence following psychotherapy

Z55. – **Problems related to education and literacy**

Z56. – **Problems related to employment and unemployment**

Z59. – **Problems related to housing and economic circumstances**

Z60 **Problems related to social environment**
Z60.0 Problems of adjustment to life-cycle transitions
Z60.1 Atypical parenting situation
Z60.2 Living alone
Z60.3 Acculturation difficulty
Z60.4 Social exclusion and rejection
Z60.5 Target of perceived adverse discrimination and persecution
Z60.8 Other specified problems related to social environment

Z61 **Problems related to negative life events in childhood**
Z61.0 Loss of love relationship in childhood
Z61.1 Removal from home in childhood
Z61.2 Altered pattern of family relationships in childhood
Z61.3 Events resulting in loss of self-esteem in childhood
Z61.4 Problems related to alleged sexual abuse of child by person within primary support group
Z61.5 Problems related to alleged sexual abuse of child by person outside primary support group
Z61.6 Problems related to alleged physical abuse of child
Z61.7 Personal frightening experience in childhood
Z61.8 Other negative life events in childhood

Z62	**Other problems related to upbringing**
	Z62.0 Inadequate parental supervision and control
	Z62.1 Parental overprotection
	Z62.2 Institutional upbringing
	Z62.3 Hostility towards and scapegoating of child
	Z62.4 Emotional neglect of child
	Z62.5 Other problems related to neglect in upbringing
	Z62.6 Inappropriate parental pressure and other abnormal qualities of upbringing
	Z62.8 Other specified problems related to upbringing

Z62 **Other problems related to upbringing**

Z62.0 Inadequate parental supervision and control
Z62.1 Parental overprotection
Z62.2 Institutional upbringing
Z62.3 Hostility towards and scapegoating of child
Z62.4 Emotional neglect of child
Z62.5 Other problems related to neglect in upbringing
Z62.6 Inappropriate parental pressure and other abnormal qualities of upbringing
Z62.8 Other specified problems related to upbringing

Z63 **Other problems related to primary support group, including family circumstances**

Z63.0 Problems in relationship with spouse or partner
Z63.1 Problems in relationship with parents and in-laws
Z63.2 Inadequate family support
Z63.3 Absence of family member
Z63.4 Disappearance and death of family member
Z63.5 Disruption of family by separation and divorce
Z63.6 Dependent relative needing care at home
Z63.7 Other stressful life events affecting family and household
Z63.8 Other specified problems related to primary support group

Z64 **Problems related to certain psychosocial circumstances**

Z64.0 Problems related to unwanted pregnancy
Z64.2 Seeking and accepting physical, nutritional and chemical interventions known to be hazardous and harmful
Z64.3 Seeking and accepting behavioural and psychological interventions known to be hazardous and harmful
Z64.4 Discord with counsellors

Includes: probation officer; social worker

Z65 **Problems related to other psychosocial circumstances**

Z65.0 Conviction in civil and criminal proceedings without imprisonment
Z65.1 Imprisonment and other incarceration
Z65.2 Problems related to release from prison
Z65.3 Problems related to other legal circumstances

Includes: arrest
child custody or support proceedings

Z65.4 Victim of crime and terrorism (including torture)

Z65.5 Exposure to disaster, war and other hostilities

Z70. – **Counselling related to sexual attitude, behaviour and orientation**

Z71 **Persons encountering health services for other counselling and medical advice, not elsewhere classified**

Z71.4 Alcohol abuse counselling and surveillance

Z71.5 Drug abuse counselling and surveillance

Z71.6 Tobacco abuse counselling

Z72 **Problems relating to lifestyle**

Z72.0 Tobacco use

Z72.1 Alcohol use

Z72.2 Drug use

Z72.3 Lack of physical exercise

Z72.4 Inappropriate diet and eating habits

Z72.5 High-risk sexual behaviour

Z72.6 Gambling and betting

Z72.8 Other problems related to lifestyle

Includes: self-damaging behaviour

Z73 **Problems related to life-management difficulty**

Z73.0 Burn-out

Z73.1 Accentuation of personality traits

Includes: type A behaviour pattern

Z73.2 Lack of relaxation or leisure

Z73.3 Stress, not elsewhere classified

Z73.4 Inadequate social skills, not elsewhere classified

Z73.5 Social role conflict, not elsewhere classified

Z75 **Problems related to medical facilities and other health care**

Z75.1 Person awaiting admission to adequate facility elsewhere

Z75.2 Other waiting period for an investigation and treatment

Z75.5 Holiday relief care

Z76   **Persons encountering health services in other circumstances**
Z76.0 Issue of repeat prescription
Z76.5 Malingerer [conscious simulation]

Includes: persons feigning illness with obvious motivation

Z81   **Family history of mental and behavioural disorders**
Z81.0 Family history of mental retardation
Z81.1 Family history of alcohol abuse
Z81.3 Family history of other psychoactive substance abuse
Z81.8 Family history of other mental and behavioural disorders

Z82   **Family history of certain disabilities and chronic diseases leading to disablement**
Z82.0 Family history of epilepsy and other diseases of the nervous system

Z85. – **Personal history of malignant neoplasm**

Z86   **Personal history of certain other diseases**
Z86.0 Personal history of other neoplasms
Z86.4 Personal history of psychoactive substance abuse
Z86.5 Personal history of other mental and behavioural disorders
Z86.6 Personal history of diseases of the nervous system and sense organs

Z87   **Personal history of other diseases and conditions**
Z87.7 Personal history of congenital malformations, deformations and chromosomal abnormalities

Z91   **Personal history of risk-factors, not elsewhere classified**
Z91.1 Personal history of noncompliance with medical treatment and regimen
Z91.4 Personal history of psychological trauma, not elsewhere classified
Z91.5 Personal history of self-harm

Includes: parasuicide; self-poisoning; suicide attempt

List of principal investigators

Field trials of the ICD-10 proposals involved researchers and clinicians in some 110 institutes in 40 countries. Their efforts and comments were of great importance for the successive revisions of the first draft of the classification and the clinical descriptions and diagnostic guidelines. All principal investigators are named below. The individuals who produced the initial drafts of the classification and guidelines are marked with an asterisk.

Australia

Dr P.J.V. Beumont (Sydney)
Dr E. Blackmore (Nedlands)
Dr R. Davidson (Nedlands)
Ms C.R. Dossetor (Melbourne)
Dr G.A. German (Nedlands)
*Dr A.S. Henderson (Canberra)
Dr H.E. Herrman (Melbourne)
Dr G. Johnson (Perth)
Dr A.F. Jorm (Canberra)
Dr S.D. Joshua (Melbourne)
Dr S. Kisely (Perth)
Dr T. Lambert (Nedlands)
Dr P.D. McGorry (Melbourne)
Dr I. Pilowski (Adelaide)
Dr J. Saunders (Camperdown)
Dr B. Singh (Melbourne)

Austria

Dr P. Berner (Vienna)
Dr H. Katschnig (Vienna)
Dr G. Koinig (Vienna)
Dr K. Meszaros (Vienna)
Dr P. Schuster (Vienna)
*Dr H. Strotzka (Vienna)

Bahrain

Dr M.K. Al-Haddad
Dr C.A. Kamel
Dr M.A. Mawgoud

Belgium

Dr D. Bobon (Liège)
Dr C. Mormont (Liège)
Dr W. Vandereyken (Louvain)

Brazil

Dr P.B. Abreu (Porto Alegre)
Dr N. Bezerra (Porto Alegre)
Dr M. Bugallo (Pelotas)
Dr E. Busnello (Porto Alegre)
Dr D. Caetano (Campinas)
Dr C. Castellarin (Porto Alegre)
Dr M.L.F. Chaves (Porto Alegre)
Dr D. Coniberti (Pelotas)
Dr V. Damiani (Pelotas)
Dr M.P.A. Fleck (Porto Alegre)
Dr M.K. Gehlen (Porto Alegre)
Dr D. Hilton Post (Pelotas)
Dr L. Knijnik (Porto Alegre)
Dr M. Knobel (Campinas)

Dr P.S.P. Lima (Porto Alegre)
Dr S. Olivé Leite (Pelotas)
Dr C.M.S. Osorio (Porto Alegre)
Dr F. Resmini (Pelotas)
Dr G. Soares (Porto Alegre)
Dr A.P. Santin (Porto Alegre)
Dr S.B. Zimmer (Porto Alegre)

Bulgaria

Dr M. Boyadjieva (Sofia)
Dr A. Jablensky (Sofia)
Dr K. Kirov (Sofia)
Dr V. Milanova (Sofia)
Dr V. Nikolov (Sofia)
Dr I. Temkov (Sofia)
Dr K. Zaimov (Sofia)

Canada

Dr J. Beitchman (London)
Dr D. Bendjilali (Baie-Comeau)
Dr D. Berube (Baie-Comeau)
Dr D. Bloom (Verdun)
Dr D. Boisvert (Baie-Comeau)
Dr R. Cooke (London)
Dr A.J. Cooper (St Thomas)
Dr J.J. Curtin (London)
Dr J.L. Deinum (London)
Dr M.L.D. Fernando (St Thomas)
Dr P. Flor-Henry (Edmonton)
Dr L. Gaborit (Baie-Comeau)
Dr P.D. Gatfield (London)
Dr A. Gordon (Edmonton)
Dr J.A. Hamilton (Toronto)
Dr G.P. Harnois (Verdun)
Dr G. Hasey (London)
Dr W.-T. Hwang (Toronto)
Dr H. Iskandar (Verdun)
Dr B. Jean (Verdun)
Dr W. Jilek (Vancouver)
Dr D.L. Keshav (London)

Dr M. Koilpillai (Edmonton)
Dr M. Konstantareas (London)
Dr T. Lawrence (Toronto)
Dr M. Lalinec (Verdun)
Dr G. Lefebvre (Edmonton)
Dr H. Lehmann (Montreal)
*Dr Z. Lipowski (Toronto)
Dr B.L. Malhotra (London)
Dr R. Manchanda (St Thomas)
Dr H. Merskey (London)
Dr J. Morin (Verdun)
Dr N.P.V. Nair (Verdun)
Dr J. Peachey (Toronto)
Dr B. Pedersen (Toronto)
Dr E. Persad (London)
Dr G. Remington (London)
Dr P. Roper (Verdun)
Dr C. Ross (Winnipeg)
Dr S.S. Sandhu (St Thomas)
Dr M. Sharma (Verdun)
Dr M. Subak (Verdun)
Dr R.S. Swaminath (St Thomas)
Dr G.N. Swamy (St Thomas)
Dr V.R. Velamoor (St Thomas)
Dr K. Zukowska (Baie-Comeau)

China

Dr He Wei (Chengdu)
Dr Huang Zong-mei (Shanghai)
Dr Liu Pei-yi (Chengdu)
Dr Liu Xie-he (Chengdu)
*Dr Shen Yu-cun (Beijing)
Dr Song Wei-sheng (Chengdu)
Dr Xu Tao-yuan (Shanghai)
Dr Xu Yi-feng (Shanghai)
*Dr Xu You-xin (Beijing)
Dr Yang De-sen (Changsha)
Dr Yang Quan (Chengdu)
Dr Zhang Lian-di (Shanghai)

Colombia

Dr A. Acosta (Cali)
Dr W. Arevalo (Cali)
Dr A. Calvo (Cali)
Dr E. Castrillon (Cali)
Dr C.E. Climent (Cali)
Dr L.V. de Aragon (Cali)
Dr M.V. de Arango (Cali)
Dr G. Escobar (Cali)
Dr L.F. Gaviria (Cali)
Dr C.H. Gonzalez (Cali)
Dr C.A. Léon (Cali)
Dr S. Martinez (Cali)
Dr R. Perdomo (Cali)
Dr E. Zambrano (Cali)

Costa Rica

Dr E. Madrigal-Segura (San José)

Côte d'Ivoire

Dr B. Claver (Abidjan)

Cuba

Dr C. Acosta Nodal (Havana)
Dr C. Acosta Rabassa (Manzanillo)
Dr O. Ares Freijo (Havana)
Dr A. Castro Gonzalez (Manzanillo)
Dr J. Cueria Basulto (Manzanillo)
Dr C. Dominguez Abreu (Havana)
Dr F. Duarte Castaneda (Havana)
Dr O.A. Freijo (Havana)
Dr F. Galan Rubi (Havana)
Dr A.C. Gonzalez (Manzanillo)
Dr R. Gonzalez Menendez (Havana)
Dr M. Guevara Machado (Havana)
Dr H. Hernandez Elias (Pinar del Rio)
Dr R. Hernandez Rios (Havana)
Dr M. Leyva Concepcion (Havana)
Dr M. Ochoa Cortina (Havana)

Dr A. Otero Ojeda (Havana)
Dr L. de la Parte Perez (Havana)
Dr V. Ravelo Perez (Havana)
Dr M. Ravelo Salazar (Havana)
Dr R.H. Rios (Havana)
Dr J. Rodriguez Garcia (Havana)
Dr T. Rodriguez Lopez (Pinar del Rio)
Dr E. Sabas Moraleda (Havana)
Dr M.R. Salazar (Havana)
Dr H. Suarez Ramos (Havana)
Dr I. Valdes Hidalgo (Havana)
Dr C. Vasallo Mantilla (Havana)

Czechoslovakia

Dr P. Baudis (Prague)
Dr V. Filip (Prague)
Dr D. Seifertova (Prague)
Dr D. Taussigova (Prague)

Denmark

Dr J. Aagaard (Aarhus)
Dr J. Achton (Aarhus)
Dr E. Andersen (Odense)
Dr T. Arngrim (Aarhus)
Dr E. Bach Jensen (Aarhus)
Dr U. Bartels (Aarhus)
Dr P. Bech (Hillerod)
Dr A. Bertelsen (Aarhus)
Dr B. Butler (Hillerod)
Dr L. Clemmesen (Hillerod)
Dr H. Faber (Aarhus)
Dr O. Falk Madsen (Aarhus)
Dr T. Fjord-Larsen (Aalborg)
Dr F. Gerholt (Odense)
Dr J. Hoffmeyer (Odense)
Dr S. Jensen (Aarhus)
Dr. P.W. Jepsen (Hillerod)
Dr P. Jorgensen (Aarhus)
Dr M. Kastrup (Hillerod)
Dr P. Kleist (Aarhus)

Dr A. Korner (Copenhagen)
Dr P. Kragh-Sorensen (Odense)
Dr K. Kristensen (Odense)
Dr I. Kyst (Aarhus)
Dr M. Lajer (Aarhus)
Dr J.K. Larsen (Copenhagen)
Dr P. Liisberg (Aarhus)
Dr H. Lund (Aarhus)
Dr J. Lund (Aarhus)
Dr S. Moller-Madsen (Copenhagen)
Dr I. Moulvad (Aarhus)
Dr B. Nielsen (Odense)
Dr B.M. Nielsen (Copenhagen)
Dr C. Norregard (Copenhagen)
Dr P. Pedersen (Odense)
Dr L. Poulsen (Odense)
Dr K. Raben Pedersen (Aarhus)
Dr P. Rask (Odense)
Dr N. Reisby (Aarhus)
Dr K. Retboll (Aarhus)
Dr F. Schulsinger (Copenhagen)
Dr C. Simonsen (Aarhus)
Dr E. Simonsen (Copenhagen)
Dr H. Stockmar (Aarhus)
Dr S.E. Straarup (Aarhus)
*Dr E. Strömgren (Aarhus)
Dr L.S. Strömgren (Aarhus)
Dr J.S. Thomsen (Aalborg)
Dr P. Vestergaard (Aarhus)
Dr T. Videbech (Aarhus)
Dr T. Vilmar (Hillerod)
Dr A. Weeke (Aarhus)

Egypt

Dr M. Sami Abdel-Gawad (Cairo)
Dr A.S. Eldawla (Cairo)
Dr K. El Fawal (Alexandria)
Dr A.H. Khalil (Cairo)
Dr S.S. Nicolas (Alexandria)
Dr A. Okasha (Cairo)
Dr M.A. Shohdy (Cairo)

Dr H. El Shoubashi (Alexandria)
Dr M.I. Soueif (Cairo)
Dr N.N. Wig (Alexandria)

Germany

Dr M. Albus (Munich)
Dr H. Amorosa (Munich)
Dr O. Benkert (Mainz)
Dr M. Berger (Freiburg)
Dr B. Blanz (Mannheim)
Dr M. von Bose (Munich)
Dr B. Cooper (Mannheim)
Dr. M. von Cranach (Kaufbeuren)
Mr T. Degener (Essen)
Dr H. Dilling (Lübeck)
Dr R.R. Engel (Munich)
Dr K. Foerster (Tübingen)
Dr H. Freyberger (Lübeck)
Dr G. Fuchs (Ottobrunn)
Dr M. Gastpar (Essen)
*Dr J. Glatzel (Mainz)
Dr H. Gutzmann (Berlin)
Dr H. Häfner (Mannheim)
Dr H. Helmchen (Berlin)
Dr S. Herdemerten (Essen)
Dr W. Hiller (Munich)
Dr A. Hillig (Mannheim)
Dr H. Hippius (Munich)
Dr P. Hoff (Munich)
Dr S.O. Hoffmann (Mainz)
Dr K. Koehler (Bonn)
Dr R. Kuhlmann (Essen)
*Dr G.-E. Kühne (Jena)
Dr E. Lomb (Essen)
Dr W. Maier (Mainz)
Dr E. Markwort (Lübeck)
Dr K. Maurer (Mannheim)
Dr J. Mittelhammer (Munich)
Dr H.-J. Moller (Bonn)
Dr W. Mombour (Munich)
Dr J. Niemeyer (Mannheim)

Dr R. Olbrich (Mannheim)
Dr M. Philipp (Mainz)
Dr K. Quaschner (Mannheim)
Dr H. Remschmidt (Marburg)
Dr G. Rother (Essen)
Dr R. Rummler (Munich)
Dr H. Sass (Aachen)
Mr H.W. Schaffert (Essen)
Dr H. Schepank (Mannheim)
Dr M.H. Schmidt (Mannheim)
Dr R.-D. Stieglitz (Berlin)
Dr M. Strockens (Essen)
Dr W. Trabert (Homburg)
Dr W. Tress (Mannheim)
Dr H.-U. Wittchen (Munich)
Dr M. Zaudig (Munich)

France

Dr J. F. Allilaire (Paris)
Dr J.M. Azorin (Marseilles)
Dr Baier (Strasbourg)
Dr M. Bouvard (Paris)
Dr C. Bursztejn (Strasbourg)
Dr P.F. Chanoit (Paris)
Dr M.-A. Crocq (Rouffach)
Dr J.M. Danion (Strasbourg)
Dr A. Des Lauriers (Paris)
Dr M. Dugas (Paris)
Dr B. Favre (Paris)
Dr C. Gerard (Paris)
Dr S. Giudicelli (Marseilles)
Dr J.D. Guelfi (Paris)
Dr M.F. Le Heuzey (Paris)
Dr V. Kapsambelis (Paris)
Dr Koriche (Strasbourg)
Dr S. Lebovici (Bobigny)
Dr J.P. Lepine (Paris)
Dr C. Lermuzeaux (Paris)
*Dr R. Misès (Paris)
Dr J. Oules (Montauban)
Dr P. Pichot (Paris)

Dr. D. Roume (Paris)
Dr L. Singer (Strasbourg)
Dr M. Triantafyllou (Paris)
Dr D. Widlocher (Paris)

Greece

*Dr C.R. Soldatos (Athens)
Dr C. Stefanis (Athens)

Hungary

Dr J. Szilard (Szeged)

India

Dr A.K. Agarwal (Lucknow)
Dr N. Ahuja (New Delhi)
Dr A. Avasthi (Chandigarh)
Dr G. Bandopaday (Calcutta)
Dr P.B. Behere (Varanasi)
Dr P.K. Chaturvedi (Lucknow)
Dr H.M. Chawla (New Delhi)
Dr H.M. Chowla (New Delhi)
Dr P.K. Dalal (Lucknow)
Dr P. Das (New Delhi)
Dr R. Gupta (Ludhiana)
Dr S.K. Khandelwal (New Delhi)
Dr S. Kumar (Lucknow)
Dr N. Lal (Lucknow)
Dr S. Malhotra (Chandigarh)
Dr D. Mohan (New Delhi)
Dr S. Murthy (Bangalore)
Dr P.S. Nandi (Calcutta)
Dr R.L. Narang (Ludhiana)
Dr J. Paul (Vellore)
Dr M. Prasad (Lucknow)
Dr R. Raghuram (Bangalore)
Dr G.N.N. Reddy (Bangalore)
Dr S. Saxena (New Delhi)
Dr B. Sen (Calcutta)
Dr C. Shamasundar (Bangalore)
Dr H. Singh (Lucknow)
Dr P. Sitholey (Lucknow)

Dr S.C. Tiwari (Lucknow)
Dr B.M. Tripathi (Varanasi)
Dr J.K. Trivedi (Lucknow)
Dr V.K. Varma (Chandigarh)
Dr A. Venkoba Rao (Madurai)
Dr A. Verghese (Vellore)
Dr K.R. Verma (Varanasi)

Indonesia

Dr R. Kusumanto Setyonegoro
  (Jakarta)
Dr D.B. Lubis (Jakarta)
Dr L. Mangendaan (Jakarta)
Dr W.M. Roan (Jakarta)
Dr K.B. Tun (Jakarta)

Islamic Republic of Iran

Dr H. Davidian (Tehran)

Ireland

Dr A. O'Grady-Walshe (Dublin)
Dr D. Walsh (Dublin)

Israel

Dr R. Blumensohn (Petach-Tikua)
Dr H. Hermesh (Petach-Tikua)
Dr H. Munitz (Petach-Tikua)
Dr S. Tyano (Petach-Tikua)

Italy

Dr M.G. Ariano (Naples)
Dr F. Catapano (Naples)
Dr A. Cerreta (Naples)
Dr S. Galderisi (Naples)
Dr M. Guazzelli (Pisa)
Dr D. Kemali (Naples)
Dr S. Lobrace (Naples)
Dr C. Maggini (Pisa)
Dr M. Maj (Naples)

Dr A. Mucci (Naples)
Dr M. Mauri (Pisa)
Dr P. Sarteschi (Pisa)
Dr M.R. Solla (Naples)
Dr F. Veltro (Naples)

Japan

Dr Y. Atsumi (Tokyo)
Dr T. Chiba (Sapporo)
Dr T. Doi (Tokyo)
Dr F. Fukamauchi (Tokyo)
Dr J. Fukushima (Sapporo)
Dr T. Gotohda (Sapporo)
Dr R. Hayashi (Ichikawa)
Dr I. Hironaka (Nagasaki)
Dr H. Hotta (Fukuoka)
Dr J. Ichikawa (Sapporo)
Dr T. Inoue (Sapporo)
Dr K. Kadota (Fukuoka)
Dr R. Kanena (Tokyo)
Dr T. Kasahara (Sapporo)
Dr M. Kato (Tokyo)
Dr D. Kawatani (Fukuoka)
Dr R. Kobayashi (Fukuoka)
Dr M. Kohsaka (Sapporo)
Dr T. Kojima (Tokyo)
Dr M. Komiyama (Tokyo)
Dr T. Koyama (Sapporo)
Dr A. Kuroda (Tokyo)
Dr H. Machizawa (Ichikawa)
Dr R. Masui (Fukuoka)
Dr R. Matsubara (Sapporo)
Dr M. Matsumori (Ichikawa)
Dr E. Matsushima (Tokyo)
Dr M. Matsuura (Tokyo)
Dr M. S. Michituji (Nagasaki)
Dr H. Mori (Sapporo)
Dr N. Morita (Sapporo)
Dr I. Nakama (Nagasaki)
Dr Y. Nakane (Nagasaki)
Dr M. Nakayama (Sapporo)

Dr M. Nankai (Tokyo)
Dr R. Nishimura (Fukuoka)
Dr M. Nishizono (Fukuoka)
Dr Y. Nonaka (Fukuoka)
Dr T. Obara (Sapporo)
Dr Y. Odagaki (Sapporo)
Dr U.Y. Ohta (Nagasaki)
Dr K. Ohya (Tokyo)
Dr S. Okada (Ichikawa)
Dr Y. Okubo (Tokyo)
Dr J. Semba (Tokyo)
Dr H. Shibuya (Tokyo)
Dr N. Shinfuku (Tokyo)
Dr M. Shintani (Tokyo)
Dr K. Shoda (Tokyo)
Dr T. Sumi (Sapporo)
Dr R. Takahashi (Tokyo)
Dr T. Takahashi (Ichikawa)
Dr T. Takeuchi (Ichikawa)
Dr S. Tanaka (Sapporo)
Dr G. Tomiyama (Ichikawa)
Dr S. Tsutsumi (Fukuoka)
Dr J. Uchino (Nagasaki)
Dr H. Uesugi (Tokyo)
Dr S. Ushijima (Fukuoka)
Dr M. Wada (Sapporo)
Dr T. Watanabe (Tokyo)
Dr Y. Yamashita (Sapporo)
Dr N. Yamanouchi (Ichikawa)
Dr H. Yasuoka (Fukuoka)

Kuwait

Dr F. El-Islam (Kuwait)

Liberia

Dr B.L. Harris (Monrovia)

Luxembourg

Dr G. Chaillet (Luxembourg)

*Dr C.B. Pull (Luxembourg)
Dr M.C. Pull (Luxembourg)

Mexico

Dr S. Altamirano (Mexico D.F.)
Dr G. Barajas (Mexico D.F.)
Dr C. Berlanga (Mexico D.F.)
Dr J. Cravioto (Mexico D.F.)
Dr G. Enriquez (Mexico D.F.)
Dr R. de la Fuente (Mexico D.F.)
Dr G. Heinze (Mexico D.F.)
Dr J. Hernandez (Mexico D.F.)
Dr M. Hernandez (Mexico D.F.)
Dr M. Ruiz (Mexico D.F.)
Dr M. Solano (Mexico D.F.)
Dr A. Sosa (Mexico D.F.)
Dr D. Urdapileta (Mexico D.F.)
Dr L.E. de la Vega (Mexico D.F.)

Netherlands

Dr V.D. Bosch (Groningen)
Dr R.F.W. Diekstra (Leiden)
*Dr R. Giel (Groningen)
Dr O. Van der Hart (Amsterdam)
Dr W. Heuves (Leiden)
Dr Y. Poortinga (Tilburg)
Dr C. Slooff (Groningen)

New Zealand

Dr C.M. Braganza (Tokanui)
Dr J. Crawshaw (Wellington)
Dr P. Ellis (Wellington)
Dr P. Hay (Wellington)
Dr G. Mellsop (Wellington)
Dr J.R.B. Saxby (Tokanui)
Dr G.S. Ungvari (Tokanui)

Nigeria

*Dr R. Jegede (Ibadan)

Dr K. Ogunremi (Ilorin)
Dr J.U. Ohaeri (Ibadan)
Dr M. Olatawura (Ibadan)
Dr B.O. Osuntokun (Ibadan)

Norway

Dr M. Bergem (Oslo)
Dr A.A. Dahl (Oslo)
Dr L. Eitinger (Oslo)
Dr C. Guldberg (Oslo)
Dr H. Hansen (Oslo)
*Dr U. Malt (Oslo)

Pakistan

Dr S. Afgan (Rawalpindi)
Dr A.R. Ahmed (Rawalpindi)
Dr M.M. Ahmed (Rawalpindi)
Dr S.H. Ahmed (Karachi)
Dr M. Arif (Karachi)
Dr S. Baksh (Rawalpindi)
Dr T. Baluch (Karachi)
Dr K.Z. Hasan (Karachi)
Dr I. Haq (Karachi)
Dr S. Hussain (Rawalpindi)
Dr S. Kalamat (Rawalpindi)
Dr K. Lal (Karachi)
Dr F. Malik (Rawalpindi)
Dr M.H. Mubbashar (Rawalpindi)
Dr Q. Nazar (Rawalpindi)
Dr T. Qamar (Rawalpindi)
Dr T.Y. Saraf (Rawalpindi)
Dr Sirajuddin (Karachi)
Dr I.A.K. Tareen (Lahore)
Dr K. Tareen (Lahore)
Dr M.A. Zahid (Lahore)

Peru

Dr J. Marietegui (Lima)
Dr A. Perales (Lima)
Dr C. Sogi (Lima)

Dr D. Worton (Lima)
Dr H. Rotondo (Lima)

Poland

Dr M. Anczewska (Warsaw)
Dr E. Bogdanowicz (Warsaw)
Dr A. Chojnowska (Warsaw)
Dr K. Gren (Warsaw)
Dr J. Jaroszynski (Warsaw)
Dr A. Kiljan (Warsaw)
Dr E. Kobrzynska (Warsaw)
Dr L. Kowalski (Warsaw)
Dr S. Leder (Warsaw)
Dr E. Lutynska (Warsaw)
Dr B. Machowska (Warsaw)
Dr A. Piotrowski (Warsaw)
Dr S. Puzynski (Warsaw)
Dr M. Rzewuska (Warsaw)
Dr I. Stanikowska (Warsaw)
Dr K. Tarczynska (Warsaw)
Dr I. Wald (Warsaw)
Dr J. Wciorka (Warsaw)

Republic of Korea

Dr Young Ki Chung (Seoul)
Dr M.S. Kil (Seoul)
Dr B.W. Kim (Seoul)
Dr H.Y. Lee (Seoul)
Dr M.H. Lee (Seoul)
Dr S.K. Min (Seoul)
Dr B.H. Oh (Seoul)
Dr S.C. Shin (Seoul)

Romania

Dr M. Dehelean (Timisoara)
Dr P. Dehelean (Timisoara)
Dr M. Ienciu (Timisoara)
Dr M. Lazarescu (Timisoara)
Dr O. Nicoara (Timisoara)

Dr F. Romosan (Timisoara)
Dr D. Schrepler (Timisoara)

Russian Federation

Dr I. Anokhina (Moscow)
Dr V. Kovalev (Moscow)
Dr A. Lichko (St Petersburg)
*Dr R.A. Nadzharov (Moscow)
*Dr A.B. Smulevitch (Moscow)
Dr A.S. Tiganov (Moscow)
Dr V. Tsirkin (Moscow)
Dr M. Vartanian (Moscow)
Dr A.V. Vovin (St Petersburg)
Dr N.N. Zharikov (Moscow)

Saudi Arabia

Dr O.M. Al-Radi (Taif)
Dr H. Amin (Riyadh)
Dr W. Dodd (Riyadh)
Dr S.R.A. El Fadl (Riyadh)
Dr A.T. Ibrahim (Riyadh)
Dr M. Marasky (Riyadh)
Dr F.M.A. Rahim (Riyadh)

Spain

Dr A. Abrines (Madrid)
Dr J.L. Alcázar (Madrid)
Dr C. Alvarez (Bilbao)
Dr C. Ballús (Barcelona)
Dr P. Benjumea (Seville)
Dr V. Beramendi (Bilbao)
Dr M. Bernardo (Barcelona)
Dr J. Blanco (Seville)
Dr J.M. Blazquez (Salamanca)
Dr E. Bodega (Madrid)
Dr I. Boulandier (Bilbao)
Dr A. Cabero (Granada)
Dr M. Camacho (Seville)
Dr A. Candina (Bilbao)
Dr J.L. Carrasco (Madrid)

Dr N. Casas (Seville)
Dr C. Caso (Bilbao)
Dr A. Castaño (Madrid)
Dr M.L. Cerceño (Salamanca)
Dr V. Corcés (Madrid)
Dr D. Crespo (Madrid)
Dr O. Cuenca (Madrid)
Dr E. Ensunza (Bilbao)
Dr A. Fernández (Madrid)
Dr P. Fernández-Argüelles (Seville)
Dr E. Gallego (Bilbao)
Dr García (Madrid)
Dr E. Giles (Seville)
Dr J. Giner (Seville)
Dr J. González (Saragossa)
Dr A. González-Pinto (Bilbao)
Dr C. Guaza (Madrid)
Dr J. Guerrero (Seville)
Dr C. Hernández (Madrid)
Dr A. Higueras (Granada)
Dr D. Huertas (Madrid)
Dr J.A. Izquierdo (Salamanca)
Dr J.L. Jimenez (Granada)
Dr L. Jordá (Madrid)
Dr J. Laforgue (Bilbao)
Dr F. Lana (Madrid)
Dr A. Lobo (Saragossa)
Dr J.J. López-Ibor Jr (Madrid)
Dr J. López-Plaza (Saragossa)
Dr C. Maestre (Granada)
Dr F. Marquínez (Bilbao)
Dr M. Martin (Madrid)
Dr T. Monsalve (Madrid)
Dr P. Morales (Madrid)
Dr P.E. Muñoz (Madrid)
Dr A. Nieto (Bilbao)
Dr P. Oronoz (Bilbao)
Dr A. Otero (Barcelona)
Dr A. Ozamiz (Bilbao)
Dr J. Padierna (Bilbao)
Dr E. Palacios (Madrid)

Dr J. Pascual (Bilbao)
Dr M. Paz (Granada)
Dr J. Pérez de los Cobos (Madrid)
Dr J. Pérez-Arango (Madrid)
Dr A. Pérez-Torres (Granada)
Dr A. Pérez-Urdaniz (Salamanca)
Dr J. Perfecto (Salamanca)
Dr R. del Pino (Granada)
Dr J.M. Poveda (Madrid)
Dr A. Preciado (Salamanca)
Dr L. Prieto-Moreno (Madrid)
Dr J.L. Ramos (Salamanca)
Dr F. Rey (Salamanca)
Dr M.L. Rivera (Seville)
Dr P. Rodríguez (Madrid)
Dr P. Rodríguez-Sacristan (Seville)
Dr C. Rueda (Madrid)
Dr J. Ruiz (Granada)
Dr B. Salcedo (Bilbao)
Dr J. San Sebastián (Madrid)
Dr J. Sola (Granada)
Dr S. Tenorio (Madrid)
Dr R. Teruel (Bilbao)
Dr F. Torres (Granada)
Dr J. Vallejo (Barcelona)
Dr M. Vega (Madrid)
Dr B. Viar (Madrid)
Dr D. Vico (Granada)
Dr V. Zubeldia (Madrid)

Sudan

Dr M.B. Bashir (Khartoum)
Dr A.O. Sirag (Khartoum)

Sweden

Dr T. Bergmark (Danderyd)
Dr G. Dalfelt (Lund)
Dr G. Elofsson (Lund)
Dr E. Essen-Möller (Lysekil)
Dr L. Gustafson (Lund)

*Dr B. Hagberg (Gothenburg)
*Dr C. Perris (Umea)
Dr B. Wistedt (Danderyd)

Switzerland

Dr N. Aapro (Geneva)
Dr J. Angst (Zurich)
Dr L. Barrelet (Perreux)
Dr L. Ciompi (Bern)
Dr V. Dittman (Basel)
Dr P. Kielholz (Basel)
Dr E. Kolatti (Geneva)
Dr D. Ladewig (Basel)
Dr C. Müller (Prilly)
Dr J. Press (Geneva)
Dr C. Quinto (Basel)
Dr B. Reith (Geneva)
*Dr C. Scharfetter (Zurich)
Dr M. Sieber (Zurich)
Dr H.-C. Steinhausen (Zurich)
Mr. A. Tongue (Lausanne)

Thailand

Dr C. Krishna (Bangkok)
Dr S. Dejatiwongse (Bangkok)

Turkey

Dr I.F. Dereboy (Ankara)
Dr A. Gōğūş (Ankara)
Dr C. Gūleç (Ankara)
Dr O. Öztürk (Ankara)
Dr D.B. Uluğ (Ankara)
Dr N.A. Uluşahin (Ankara)
Dr T.B. Üstün (Ankara)

United Kingdom

Dr Adityanjee (London)
Dr P. Ainsworth (Manchester)
Dr T. Arie (Nottingham)
Dr J. Bancroft (Edinburgh)

Dr P. Bebbington (London)
Dr S. Benjamin (Manchester)
Dr I. Berg (Leeds)
Dr K. Bergman (London)
Dr I. Brockington (Birmingham)
Dr J. Brothwell (Nottingham)
Dr C. Burford (London)
Dr J. Carrick (London)
*Dr A. Clare (London)
Dr A.W. Clare (London)
Dr D. Clarke (Birmingham)
*Dr J.E. Cooper (Nottingham)
Dr P. Coorey (Liverpool)
Dr S.J. Cope (London)
Dr J. Copeland (Liverpool)
Dr A. Coppen (Epsom)
*Dr J.A. Corbett (London)
Dr T.K.J. Craig (London)
Dr C. Darling (Nottingham)
Dr C. Dean (Birmingham)
Dr R. Dolan (London)
*Dr J. Griffith Edwards (London)
Dr D.M. Eminson (Manchester)
Dr A. Farmer (Cardiff)
Dr K. Fitzpatrick (Nottingham)
Dr T. Fryers (Manchester)
*Dr M. Gelder (Oxford)
*Dr D. Goldberg (Manchester)
Dr I.M. Goodyer (Manchester)
*Dr M. Gossop (London)
*Dr P. Graham (London)
Dr T. Hale (London)
Dr M. Harper (Cardiff)
Dr A. Higgitt (London)
Dr J. Higgs (Manchester)
Dr N. Holden (Nottingham)
Dr P. Howlin (London)
Dr C. Hyde (Manchester)
Dr R. Jacoby (London)
Dr I. Janota (London)
Dr P. Jenkins (Cardiff)

Dr R. Jenkins (London)
Dr G. Jones (Cardiff)
*Dr R.E. Kendell (Edinburgh)
Dr N. Kreitman (Edinburgh)
Dr R. Kumar (London)
Dr M.H. Lader (London)
Dr R. Levy (London)
Dr J.E.B. Lindesay (London)
Dr W.A. Lishman (London)
Dr A. McBride (Cardiff)
Dr A.D.J. MacDonald (London)
Dr C. McDonald (London)
Dr P. McGuffin (Cardiff)
Dr M. McKenzie (Manchester)
Dr J. McLaughlin (Leeds)
Dr A.H. Mann (London)
Dr S. Mann (London)
*Dr I. Marks (London)
Dr D. Masters (London)
Dr M. Monaghan (Manchester)
Dr K.W. Moses (Manchester)
Dr J. Oswald (Edinburgh)
Dr E. Paykel (London)
Dr N. Richman (London)
Dr Sir Martin Roth (Cambridge)
*Dr G. Russell (London)
*Dr M. Rutter (London)
Dr N. Seivewright (Nottingham)
Dr D. Shaw (Cardiff)
*Dr M. Shepherd (London)
Dr A. Steptoe (London)
*Dr E. Taylor (London)
Dr D. Taylor (Manchester)
Dr R. Thomas (Cardiff)
Dr P. Tyrer (London)
*Dr D.J. West (Cambridge)
Dr P.D. White (London)
Dr A.O. Williams (Liverpool)
Dr P. Williams (London)
*Dr J. Wing (London)
*Dr L. Wing (London)

Dr S. Wolff (Edinburgh)
Dr S. Wood (London)
Dr W. Yule (London)

United Republic of Tanzania

*Dr J.S. Neki (Dar es Salaam)

United States of America

Dr T.M. Achenbach (Burlington)
Dr H.S. Akiskal (Memphis)
Dr N. Andreasen (Iowa City)
Dr T. Babor (Farmington)
Dr T. Ban (Nashville)
Dr G. Barker (Cincinnati)
Dr J. Bartko (Rockville)
Dr M. Bauer (Richmond)
Dr C. Beebe (Columbia)
Dr D. Beedle (Cambridge)
Dr B. Benson (Chicago)
*Dr F. Benson (Los Angeles)
Dr J. Blaine (Rockville)
Dr G. Boggs (Cincinnati)
Dr R. Boshes (Cambridge)
Dr J. Brown (Farmington)
Dr J. Burke (Rockville)
Dr J. Cain (Dallas)
Dr M. Campbell (New York)
*Dr D. Cantwell (Los Angeles)
Dr R.C. Casper (Chicago)
Dr A. Conder (Richmond)
Dr P. Coons (Indianapolis)
Mrs W. Davis (Washington, DC)
Dr J. Deltito (White Plains)
Dr M. Diaz (Farmington)
Dr M. Dumaine (Cincinnati)
Dr C. DuRand (Cambridge)
Dr M.H. Ebert (Nashville)
Dr J.I. Escobar (Farmington)
Dr R. Falk (Richmond)
Dr M. First (New York)

Dr M.F. Folstein (Baltimore)
Dr S. Foster (Philadelphia)
Dr A. Frances (New York)
Dr S. Frazier (Belmont)
Dr S. Freeman (Cambridge)
Dr H.E. Genaidy (Hastings)
Dr P.M. Gillig (Cincinnati)
Dr M. Ginsburg (Cincinnati)
Dr F. Goodwin (Rockville)
Dr E. Gordis (Rockville)
Dr I.I. Gottesman (Charlottesville)
Dr B. Grant (Rockville)
*Dr S. Guze (St Louis)
Dr R. Hales (San Francisco)
Dr D. Haller (Richmond)
Dr J. Harris (Baltimore)
Dr R. Hart (Richmond)
*Dr J. Helzer (St Louis)
Dr L. Hersov (Worcester)
Dr J.R. Hillard (Cincinnati)
Dr R.M.A. Hirschfeld (Rockville)
Dr C.E. Holzer (Galveston)
*Dr P. Holzman (Cambridge)
Dr M.J. Horowitz (San Francisco)
Dr T.R. Insel (Bethesda)
Dr L.F. Jarvik (Los Angeles)
Dr V. Jethanandani (Philadelphia)
Dr L. Judd (Rockville)
Dr C. Kaelber (Rockville)
Dr I. Katz (Philadelphia)
Dr B. Kaup (Baltimore)
Dr S.A. Kelt (Dallas)
Dr P. Keck (Belmont)
Dr K.S. Kendler (Richmond)
Dr D.F. Klein (New York)
*Dr A. Kleinman (Cambridge)
Dr G. Klerman (Boston)
Dr R. Kluft (Philadelphia)
Dr R.D. Kobes (Dallas)
Dr R. Kolodner (Dallas)
Dr J.S. Ku (Cincinnati)

*Dr D.J. Kupfer (Pittsburgh)
Dr M. Lambert (Dallas)
Dr M. Lebowitz (New York)
Dr B. Lee (Cambridge)
Dr L. Lettich (Cambridge)
Dr N. Liebowitz (Farmington)
Dr B.R. Lima (Baltimore)
Dr A.W. Loranger (New York)
Dr D. Mann (Cambridge)
Dr W.G. McPherson (Hastings)
Dr L. Meloy (Cincinnati)
Dr W. Mendel (Hastings)
Dr R. Meyer (Farmington)
*Dr J. Mezzich (Pittsburgh)
Dr C. Moran (Richmond)
Dr P. Nathan (Chicago)
Dr D. Neal (Ann Arbor)
Dr G. Nestadt (Baltimore)
Dr B. Orrok (Farmington)
Dr D. Orvin (Cambridge)
Dr H. Pardes (New York)
Dr J. Parks (Cincinnati)
Dr R. Pary (Pittsburgh)
Dr R. Peel (Washington, DC)
Dr M. Peszke (Farmington)
Dr R. Petry (Richmond)
Dr F. Petty (Dallas)
Dr R. Pickens (Rockville)
Dr H. Pincus (Washington, DC)
Dr M. Popkin (Long Lake)
Dr R. Poss Rosen (Bayside)
Dr H. van Praag (Bronx)
Mr D. Rae (Rockville)
Dr J. Rapoport (Bethesda)
Dr D. Regier (Rockville)
Dr R. Resnick (Richmond)
Dr R. Room (Berkeley)
Dr S. Rosenthal (Cambridge)
Dr B. Rounsaville (New Haven)
Dr A.J. Rush (Dallas)
Dr M. Sabshin (Washington, DC)

Dr R. Salomon (Farmington)
Dr B. Schoenberg (Bethesda)
Dr E. Schopler (Chicago)
Dr M.A. Schuckit (San Diego)
Dr R. Schuster (Rockville)
Dr M. Schwab-Stone (New Haven)
Dr S. Schwartz (Richmond)
Dr D. Shaffer (New York)
Dr T. Shapiro (New York)
*Dr R. Spitzer (New York)
Dr T.S. Stein (East Lansing)
Dr R. Stewart (Dallas)
Dr G. Tarnoff (New Haven)
Dr J.R. Thomas (Richmond)
Dr K. Towbin (New Haven)
Mr L. Towle (Rockville)
Dr M.T. Tsuang (Iowa City)
Dr J. Wade (Richmond)
Dr J. Walkup (New Haven)
Dr M. Weissmann (New Haven)
Dr J. Williams (New York)
Dr R.W.Winchel (New York)
Dr K. Winters (St Paul)
Dr T.K. Wolff (Dallas)
Dr W.C. Young (Littleton)

Uruguay

Dr R. Almada (Montevideo)
Dr P. Alterwain (Montevideo)
Dr L. Bolognin (Montevideo)
Dr P. Bustelo (Montevideo)
Dr U. Casarotti (Montevideo)
Dr E. Dorfman (Montevideo)
Dr F. Leite Gastal (Montevideo)
Dr A.J. Montoya (Montevideo)
Dr A. Nogueira (Montevideo)
Dr E. Probst (Montevideo)
Dr C. Valino (Montevideo)

Yugoslavia

Dr N. Bohacek (Zagreb)
Dr M. Kocmur (Ljubljana)
*Dr J. Lokar (Ljubljana)
Dr B. Milac (Ljubljana)
Dr M. Tomori (Ljubljana)

Index

Note: For those entries marked # see List of categories for additional fourth or fifth character. The letters NEC stand for "not elsewhere classified"; they are added after terms classified to residual categories, as a warning that specified forms of the conditions are classified differently.

Abuse (of) (*see also* **Use, harmful**)
- analgesics F55.2
- antacids F55.3
- antidepressants F55.0
- - tetracyclic F55.0
- - tricyclic F55.0
- aspirin F55.2
- diuretics F55.8
- hormones F55.5
- laxatives F55.1
- monamine oxidase inhibitors F55.0
- non-dependence-producing substances F55.9
- - specified NEC F55.8
- paracetamol F55.2
- phenacetin F55.2
- specific folk remedies F55.6
- specific herbal remedies F55.6
- steroids F55.5
- vitamins F55.4

Acalculia, developmental F81.2

Acrophobia F40.2

Addiction (*see* **Syndrome, dependence**)

Adjustment disorder (*see* **Disorder, adjustment**)

Aerophagy, psychogenic F45.31

Agnosia, developmental F88

Agoraphobia
− with panic disorder F40.01
− without panic disorder F40.00

AIDS-dementia complex F02.4 #

Alcohol
− amnesic syndrome F10.5
− dependence F10.2 #
− drunkenness, acute F10.0 #
− withdrawal state F10.3 #
− − with delirium F10.4 #

Alcoholic
− hallucinosis (acute) F10.5 #
− jealousy F10.5 #
− paranoia F10.5 #
− psychosis F10.5 #

Alcoholism
− chronic F10.2 #
− Korsakov's F10.6

Alzheimer's disease
− dementia in F00.9 #
− − atypical type F00.2 #
− − early onset F00.0 #
− − late onset F00.1 #
− − mixed type F00.2 #
− − presenile F00.0 #
− − senile F00.1 #
− type 1 F00.1 #
− type 2 F00.0 #

Amnesia, dissociative F44.0

Amnesic syndrome (*see* Syndrome, amnesic)

Anaesthesia and sensory loss, dissociative F44.6

Anhedonia (sexual) F52.11

Anorexia nervosa F50.0
– atypical F50.1

Anorgasmy, psychogenic F52.3

Anthropophobia F40.1

Anxiety
– depression F41.2
– dream F51.5
– episodic paroxysmal F41.0
– hysteria F41.8
– neurosis F41.1
– phobic, of childhood F93.1
– reaction F41.1
– separation, of childhood F93.0
– social, of childhood F93.2
– state F41.1

Anxiety disorder (*see* Disorder, anxiety)

Aphasia
– acquired, with epilepsy F80.3
– developmental
– – expressive type F80.1
– – receptive type F80.2
– – Wernicke's F80.2

Aphonia, psychogenic F44.4

Asperger's syndrome F84.5

Asthenia, neurocirculatory F45.30

Attachment disorder of childhood (*see* Disorder, attachment)

Attack, panic F41.0

Attention deficit
– hyperactivity disorder F90.0
– syndrome with hyperactivity F90.0
– without hyperactivity F98.8

Autism
- atypical F84.1
- childhood F84.0
- infantile F84.0

Autistic
- disorder F84.0
- psychopathy F84.5

Aversion, sexual F52.10

Backache, psychogenic F45.4

Bad trip (due to hallucinogens) F16.0 #

Behaviour disorder, childhood F91.9

Beziehungswahn, sensitiver F22.0

Bipolar affective disorder (*see* **Disorder, bipolar affective**)

Biting, stereotyped, self-injurious F98.4

Borderline personality (disorder) F60.31

Bouffée délirante
- with symptoms of schizophrenia F23.1
- - with acute stress F23.11
- - without acute stress F23.10
- without symptoms of schizophrenia F23.0
- - with acute stress F23.01
- - without acute stress F23.00

Briquet's disorder F45.0

Bulimia nervosa F50.2
- atypical F50.3

Circadian rhythm inversion, psychogenic F51.2

Claustrophobia F40.2

Clumsy child syndrome F82

Cluttering F98.6

Compulsive acts F42.1

Conduct disorder (*see* **Disorder, conduct**)

Confusion, psychogenic F44.88

Confusional state (nonalcoholic) F05. –
– subacute F05.8

Conversion
– disorder F44. –
– hysteria F44. –
– reaction F44. –

Convulsions, dissociative F44.5

Cough, psychogenic F45.33

Cramp, writer's F48.8

Creutzfeldt – Jakob disease F02.1 ⧧

Culture shock F43.28

Cyclothymia F34.0

Da Costa's syndrome F45.30

Deafness, psychogenic F44.6

Deficiency, mental (*see* **Retardation, mental**)

Delinquency (juvenile), group F91.2

Delirium (of) F05.9
– mixed origin F05.8
– not superimposed on dementia F05.0

Dementia (in) (*continued*)
- primary degenerative (*continued*)
- – Alzheimer's type F00.0 #
- senile F03 #
- – Alzheimer's type F00.1 #
- systemic lupus erthematosus F02.8 #
- trypanosomiasis F02.8 #
- vascular (of) F01.9 #
- – acute onset F01.0 #
- – mixed cortical and subcortical F01.3 #
- – specified NEC F01.8 #
- – subcortical F01.2 #
- vitamin B_{12} deficiency F02.8 #

Dependence (*see* **Syndrome, dependence**)

Depersonalization – derealization syndrome F48.1

Depression F32.9
- agitated, single episode F32.2
- anxiety
- – mild or not persistent F41.2
- – persistent (dysthymia) F34.1
- atypical F32.8
- endogenous F33. –
- major
- – single episode F32. –
- – recurrent F33. –
- masked F32.8
- monopolar F33.9
- neurotic (persistent) F34.1
- post-schizophrenic F20.4 #
- postnatal F53.0
- postpartum F53.0
- psychogenic F32. –
- psychotic F32.3
- reactive F32. –
- vital, without psychotic symptoms F32.2

Depressive
- disorder (*see* Disorder, depressive)
- episode (*see* Episode, depressive)

Derealization F48.1

Dermatozoenwahn F06.0

Desire, sexual, lack or loss F52.0

Developmental disorder (*see* **Disorder, developmental**)

Deviation, sexual F65.9

Dhat syndrome F48.8

Diarrhoea
- gas syndrome F45.32
- psychogenic F45.32

Dipsomania F10.2 #

Disability
- knowledge acquisition NOS F81.9
- learning NOS F81.9

Disease
- Alzheimer's F00. − #
- Creutzfeldt − Jakob F02.1 #
- Huntington's F02.2 #
- Parkinson's F02.3 #
- Pick's F02.0 #

Disorder (of)
- adjustment
- − anxiety and depressive reaction (mixed) F43.22
- − brief depressive reaction F43.20
- − prolonged depressive reaction F43.21
- − with mixed disturbance of emotions and conduct F43.25
- − with other specified predominant symptoms F43.28
- − with predominant disturbance of conduct F43.24
- − with predominant disturbance of other emotions F43.23
- affective (*see* Disorder, mood)
- anxiety F41.9
- − and depressive, mixed F41.2
- − generalized F41.1

Disorder (of) (*continued*)
- anxiety (*continued*)
- − mixed F41.3
- − phobic F40.9
- − − of childhood F93.1
- − separation, of childhood F93.0
- − social, of childhood F93.2
- − specified NEC F41.8
- arithmetical skills, specific F81.2
- articulation, functional F80.0
- attachment, of childhood
- − disinhibited F94.2
- − reactive F94.1
- attention deficit
- − with hyperactivity F90.0
- − without hyperactivity F98.8
- autistic F84.0
- avoidant, of childhood or adolescence F93.2
- behavioural (*see* Disorder, mental and behavioural)
- bipolar II F31.8
- bipolar (affective) F31.9
- − current episode
- − − hypomanic F31.0
- − − manic
- − − − with psychotic symptoms F31.2
- − − − without psychotic symptoms F31.1
- − − mild or moderate depression
- − − − with somatic syndrome F31.31
- − − − without somatic syndrome F31.30
- − − mixed F31.6
- − − severe depression
- − − − with psychotic symptoms F31.5
- − − − without psychotic symptoms F31.4
- − in remission (currently) F31.7
- − organic F06.31
- − single manic episode F30. −
- − specified NEC F31.8
- body dysmorphic F45.2
- Briquet's F48.8
- character F68.8
- childhood disintegrative, specified NEC F84.3

Disorder (of) (*continued*)
- developmental F89
- – arithmetical skills F81.2
- – articulation F80.0
- – coordination F82
- – expressive writing F81.8
- – language F80.9
- – – specified NEC F80.8
- – mixed, specific F83
- – motor function F82
- – pervasive F84. –
- – phonological F80.0
- – psychological F89
- – scholastic skills F81.9
- – – mixed F81.3
- – specified NEC F88
- – speech F80.9
- – – specified NEC F80.8
- dissociative F44.9
- – mixed F44.7
- – motor F44.4
- – organic F06.5
- – specified NEC F44.88
- – transient, in childhood and adolescence F44.82
- dream anxiety F51.5
- eating F50.9
- – specified NEC F50.8
- emotional, childhood onset F93.9
- – specified NEC F93.8
- expressive writing, developmental F81.8
- feeding, of infancy and childhood F98.2
- female sexual arousal F52.2
- gender identity or role F64.9
- – adolescence or adulthood, nontranssexual type F64.1
- – of childhood F64.2
- – specified NEC F64.8
- habit and impulse F63.9
- – specified NEC F63.8
- hyperkinetic F90.9
- – conduct F90.1
- – specified NEC F90.8
- identity, of childhood F93.8

Disorder (of) (*continued*)

− mental and behavioural (due to) (*continued*)

− − stimulant-induced F15.9

− − symptomatic F09

− − tobacco-induced F17.9

− − volatile solvent-induced F18.9

− mental, nonpsychotic F99

− mild cognitive F06.7

− mood [affective] F39

− − organic F06.3

− − persistent F34.9

− − − specified NEC F34.8

− − recurrent, specified NEC F38.1

− − single episode, specified NEC F38.0

− − specified NEC F38.8

− motor function, specific F82

− neurotic F48.9

− − specified NEC F48.8

− obsessive − compulsive F42.9

− − specified NEC F42.8

− oppositional defiant F93.3

− organic F09

− − anxiety F06.4

− − asthenic F06.6

− − bipolar F06.31

− − catatonic F06.1

− − delusional [schizophrenia-like] F06.2

− − depressive F06.32

− − dissociative F06.5

− − emotionally labile [asthenic] F06.6

− − manic F06.30

− − mental F09

− − mixed affective F06.33

− − mood [affective] F06.3

− − paranoid F06.2

− − personality F07.0

− − schizophrenia-like F06.2

− overactive, with mental retardation and stereotyped movements F84.4

− overanxious, of childhood F93.8

− pain, persistent somatoform F45.4

− panic F41.0

− − with agoraphobia F40.01

Disorder (of) (*continued*)
– personality (*continued*)
– – psychoinfantile F60.4
– – psychoneurotic F60.8
– – psychopathic F60.2
– – querulant F60.0
– – schizoid F60.1
– – schizotypal F21
– – self-defeating F60.7
– – sensitive paranoid F60.0
– – sociopathic F60.2
– – specified NEC F60.8
– pervasive developmental F84.9
– – specified NEC F84.8
– phobic anxiety F40.9
– – of childhood F93.1
– – specified NEC F40.8
– phonological, developmental F80.0
– possession F44.3
– post-traumatic stress F43.1
– psychosexual development F66.9 #
– – specified NEC F66.8 #
– psychosomatic
– – multiple F45.0
– – undifferentiated F45.1
– psychotic
– – acute
– – – polymorphic
– – – – with symptoms of schizophrenia F23.1
– – – – – with acute stress F23.11
– – – – – without acute stress F23.10
– – – – without symptoms of schizophrenia F23.0
– – – – – with acute stress F23.01
– – – – – without acute stress F23.00
– – – predominantly delusional F23.3
– – – – with acute stress F23.31
– – – – without acute stress F23.30
– – – schizophrenia-like
– – – – with acute stress F23.21
– – – – without acute stress F23.20
– – acute and transient F23.9

Disorder (of) (*continued*)
- schizoid
- - of childhood F84.5
- - personality F60.1
- schizophreniform F20.8 #
- - brief F23.23
- schizotypal personality F21
- scholastic skills, developmental F81.9
- - mixed F81.3
- - specified NEC F81.8
- seasonal affective F33. –
- sexual
- - desire, hypoactive F52.0
- - maturation F66.0 #
- - preference F65.9
- - - specified NEC F65.8
- - relationship F66.2 #
- sibling rivalry F93.3
- sleep
- - emotional F51.9
- - nonorganic F51.9
- - - specified NEC F51.8
- social functioning
- - specified NEC F94.8
- - withdrawal and shyness due to social competence deficiencies F94.8
- somatization F45.0
- somatoform F45.9
- - pain, persistent F45.4
- - specified NEC F45.8
- - undifferentiated F45.1
- spelling, specific F81.1
- stress, post-traumatic F43.1
- tic F95.9
- - chronic
- - - motor F95.1
- - - vocal F95.1
- - combined vocal and multiple motor F95.2
- - specified NEC F95.8
- - transient F95.0
- trance and possession F44.3
- unsocialized aggressive F91.1

Dissociative disorder (*see* **Disorder, dissociative**)

Disturbance (predominant) of
- activity and attention F90.0
- conduct in adjustment disorder F43.24
- emotions and conduct, mixed in adjustment disorder F43.25
- emotions, specified NEC in adjustment disorder F43.23

Dream anxiety disorder F51.5

Drunkenness, acute, in alcoholism F10.0 #

Dysfunction
- orgasmic F52.3
- sexual, not caused by organic disorder or disease F52.9
- – specified NEC F52.8
- somatoform autonomic (of) F45.3
- – genitourinary system F45.34
- – heart and cardiovascular system F45.30
- – lower gastrointestinal tract F45.32
- – respiratory system F45.33
- – specified organ NEC F45.38
- – upper gastrointestinal tract F45.31

Dyslalia (developmental) F80.0

Dyslexia, developmental F81.0

Dysmorphophobia (nondelusional) F45.2
- delusional F22.8

Dyspareunia, nonorganic F52.6

Dyspepsia, psychogenic F45.31

Dysphasia, developmental
- expressive type F80.1
- receptive type F80.2

Dysphonia, psychogenic F44.4

Dyspraxia, developmental F82

Dyssomnia F51. –

Dysthymia F34.1

Dysuria, psychogenic F45.34

Ejaculation, premature F52.4

Elaboration of physical symptoms for psychological reasons F68.0

Elective mutism F94.0

Encephalitis, subacute, HIV F02.4 #

Encephalopathy
– HIV F02.4 #
– postcontusional F07.2

Encopresis, nonorganic origin F98.1

Enuresis (primary) (secondary)
– functional F98.0
– nonorganic origin F98.0
– psychogenic F98.0

Episode
– depressive F32.9
– – mild F32.0
– – – with somatic symptoms F32.01
– – – without somatic symptoms F32.00
– – moderate F32.1
– – – with somatic symptoms F32.11
– – – without somatic symptoms F32.10
– – severe
– – – with psychotic symptoms F32.3
– – – without psychotic symptoms F32.2
– – specified NEC F32.8
– hypomanic F30.0

– manic F30.9
– – specified NEC F30.8
– – with psychotic symptoms F30.2
– – without psychotic symptoms F30.1
– mixed affective F38.00
– mood [affective], single, specified NEC F38.0

Exhibitionism F65.2

Eye-poking, stereotyped, self-injurious F98.4

Face-slapping, stereotyped, self-injurious F98.4

Factors, psychological and behavioural
– affecting physical conditions F54
– associated with disorders or diseases classified elsewhere F54

Failure of genital response F52.2

Fatigue
– combat F43.0
– syndrome F48.0

Feeble-mindedness (*see* Retardation, mental)

Feeding disorder of infancy and childhood F98.2

Feigning of symptoms or disabilities (physical) (psychological) F68.1

Fetishism F65.0
– transvestic F65.1

Fetishistic transvestism F65.1

Fire-setting, pathological F63.1

Flatulence, psychogenic F45.32

Folie à deux F24

Frigidity F52.0

Frontal lobe syndrome F07.0

Frotteurism F65.8

Fugue, dissociative F44.1

Gambling
– compulsive F63.0
– pathological F63.0

Ganser's syndrome F44.80

Gender identity or role disorder (*see* Disorder, gender identity or role)

Genital response, failure of F52.2

Gerstmann syndrome, developmental F81.2

Gilles de la Tourette's syndrome F95.2

Hair-plucking F98.4

Hallucinatory
– psychosis, chronic F28
– state, organic F06.0

Hallucinosis
– alcoholic F10.5
– organic F06.0

Harmful use (*see* Use, harmful)

Head-banging (repetitive) F98.4

Headache, psychogenic F45.4

Hebephrenia F20.1 #

Heller's syndrome F84.3

Hiccough, psychogenic F45.31

HIV
– encephalitis, subacute F02.4 #
– encephalopathy F02.4 #

Hospital hopper syndrome F68.1

Hospitalism in children F43.28

Huntington's chorea or disease F02.2 #

Hyperemesis gravidarum, psychogenic F50.5

Hyperkinetic disorder (*see* Disorder, hyperkinetic)

Hyperorexia nervosa F50.2

Hypersomnia, nonorganic F51.1

Hyperventilation, psychogenic F45.33

Hypochondriasis F45.2

Hypomania F30.0

Hysteria F44 #
– anxiety F41.8
– conversion F44 #

Idiocy F73 #

Imbecility F71 #

Imperception, congenital auditory F80.2

Impotence (sexual) (psychogenic) F52.2

Incontinence, nonorganic origin
– faeces F98.1
– urine F98.0

Insomnia, nonorganic F51.0

Institutional syndrome F94.2

Intoxication, acute (due to)
- alcohol F10.0#
- cannabinoids F12.0#
- cocaine F14.0#
- hallucinogens F16.0#
- hypnotics F13.0#
- multiple drugs F19.0#
- opioids F11.0#
- psychoactive substances NEC F19.0#
- sedatives F13.0#
- stimulants NEC F15.0#
- tobacco F17.0#
- volatile solvents F18.0#

Irritable bowel syndrome F45.32

Jealousy
- alcoholic F10.5
- sibling F93.3

Kanner's syndrome F84.0

Kleptomania F63.2

Koro F48.8

Lack of sexual
- desire F52.0
- enjoyment F52.11

Lalling F80.0

Landau – Kleffner syndrome F80.3

Language disorder, developmental F80.9

Latah F48.8

Limbic epilepsy personality syndrome F07.0

Lisping F80.8

Lobotomy syndrome F07.0

Loss of
− appetite, psychogenic F50.8
− sexual desire F52.0

Mania F30.9
− with psychotic symptoms F30.2
− without psychotic symptoms F30.1

Masochism F65.5

Masturbation, excessive F98.8

Melancholia F32.9

Mental retardation (*see* Retardation, mental)

Micturition, increased frequency, psychogenic F45.34

Moron F70 #

Munchhausen's syndrome F68.1

Mutism
− elective F94.0
− selective F94.0

Nail-biting F98.8

Necrophilia F65.8

Neurasthenia F48.0

Neurosis
− anankastic F42
− cardiac F45.30

Neurosis (*continued*)
- character F60.9
- compensation F68.0
- depressive F34.1
- gastric F45.31
- hypochondriacal F45.2
- obsessional F42. –
- obsessive – compulsive F42. –
- occupational F48.8
- psychasthenic F48.8
- social F40.1
- traumatic F43.1

Nightmare F51.5

Night terrors F51.4

Nose-picking F98.8

Nosophobia F45.2

Nymphomania F52.7

Nyctohemeral rhythm inversion, psychogenic F51.2

Obsessional
- neurosis F42. –
- rituals F42.1
- ruminations F42.0
- thoughts F42.0
- thoughts and acts, mixed F42.2

Obsessive – compulsive
- disorder F42.9
- – specified NEC F42.8
- neurosis F42. –

Oligophrenia (*see* **Retardation, mental**)

Oneirophrenia F23.2

Orgasm, inhibited (male) (female) F52.3

Orgasmic dysfunction F52.3

Orientation, sexual, egodystonic F66.1 #

Overeating (associated with)
- psychogenic F50.4
- psychological disturbances, specified NEC F50.4

Paedophilia F65.4

Pain disorder, somatoform, persistent F45.4

Panic
- attack F41.0
- disorder F41.0

Paralysis of limb(s)
- hysterical F44.4
- psychogenic F44.4

Paranoia F22.0
- alcoholic F10.5
- querulans F22.8

Paranoid
- personality F60.0
- psychosis F22.0
- schizophrenia F20.0 #
- state F22.0
- - involutional F22.8

Paraphilia F65.9

Paraphrenia (late) F22.0

Parasomnia F51. −

Parkinson's disease F02.3 #

Parkinsonism – dementia complex of Guam F02.8 #

Pathological
- fire-setting F63.1
- gambling F63.0
- stealing F63.2

Peregrinating patient F68.1

Persistent somatoform pain disorder F45.4

Personality
- change (not due to brain damage or disease), enduring (after) F62.9
- – bereavement F62.8
- – catastrophic experience F62.0
- – psychiatric illness F62.1
- – specified NEC F62.8
- disorder (*see* Disorder, personality)
- – troublesome F61.1
- syndrome, chronic pain F62.8

Phobia F40.9
- animal F40.2
- examination F40.2
- simple F40.2
- social F40.1
- specific (isolated) F40.2

Phobic
- anxiety (reaction) (disorder) F40.9
- – specified NEC F40.8
- states F40.9

Physical symptoms, elaboration of F68.0

Pica
- in adults, nonorganic origin F50.8
- of infancy or childhood F98.3

Pick's disease F02.0 #

Possession disorder F44.3

Postconcussional syndrome F07.2

Postcontusional
- encephalopathy F07.2
- syndrome F07.2

Postencephalitic syndrome F07.1

Postleukotomy syndrome F07.0

Post-schizophrenic depression F20.4 #

Post-traumatic brain syndrome, nonpsychotic F07.2

Psychalgia F45.4

Psychasthenia F48.8

Psychopathy
- affectionless (in childhood) F94.2
- autistic F84.5

Psychosis F29
- affective F39
- - specified NEC F38.8
- alcoholic F10.5
- childhood, atypical F84.1
- cycloid F23.0
- - with symptoms of schizophrenia F23.1
- - - with acute stress F23.11
- - - without acute stress F23.10
- - without symptoms of schizophrenia F23.0
- - - with acute stress F23.01
- - - without acute stress F23.00
- disintegrative (of childhood) F84.3
- epileptic F06.8
- hallucinatory, chronic F28

Psychosis (*continued*)
- hysterical F44.8
- induced F24
- infantile F84.0
- Korsakov's (due to) (*see also* Syndrome, amnesic)
- - nonalcoholic F04
- - psychoactive substances F19.6
- manic depressive F31. –
- mixed schizophrenic and affective F25.2
- nonorganic F29
- organic F09
- paranoid F22.0
- presenile F03 #
- psychogenic
- - depressive F32.3
- - paranoid F23.3 #
- puerperal F53.1
- reactive depressive F32.3
- schizoaffective (*see* Disorder, schizoaffective)
- schizophrenia-like, in epilepsy F06.2
- schizophreniform F20.8
- - and affective, mixed F25.2
- - brief F23.2
- - - with acute stress F23.21
- - - without acute stress F23.20
- - depressive type F25.1
- - manic type F25.0
- senile F03 #
- symbiotic F24
- - in childhood F84.3
- symptomatic F09

Psychosyndrome, organic F07.9

Pylorospasm, psychogenic F45.31

Pyromania F63.1

Reaction
- adjustment (*see* Disorder, adjustment)
- anxiety F41.1
- crisis, acute F43.0

- depressive
- - and anxiety, mixed F43.22
- - brief F43.20
- - prolonged F43.21
- grief F43.28
- hyperkinetic (of childhood or adolescence) F90.9
- paranoid F23.3 #
- schizophrenic F32.2 #
- severe stress F43.9
- - specified NEC F43.8
- stress, acute F43.0

Reading
- backward F81.0
- disorder, specific F81.0
- - with spelling difficulties F81.0
- retardation, specific F81.0

Restzustand, schizophrenic F20.5 #

Retardation
- mental F79 #
- - mild F70 #
- - moderate F71 #
- - profound F73 #
- - severe F72 #
- - specified NEC F78 #
- - with autistic features F84.1
- specific reading F81.0
- specific spelling
- - with reading disorder F81.0
- - without reading disorder F81.1

Rett's syndrome F84.2

Rivalry
- peer (non-sibling) F93.8
- sibling F93.3

Rumination
- disorder of infancy F98.2
- obsessional F42.0

Sadism (sexual) F65.5

Sadomasochism F65.5

Satyriasis F52.7

Schizoid
- disorder of childhood F84.5
- personality disorder F60.1

Schizotypal (personality) disorder F21

Schizophrenia F20.9 #
- acute, undifferentiated F23.2 #
- atypical F20.3 #
- borderline F21
- catatonic F20.2 #
- cenesthopathic F20.8 #
- chronic, undifferentiated F20.5 #
- cyclic F25.2
- disorganized F20.1 #
- hebephrenic F20.1 #
- latent F21
- paranoid F20.0 #
- paraphrenic F20.0 #
- prepsychotic F21
- prodromal F21
- pseudoneurotic F21
- pseudopsychopathic F21
- residual F20.5 #
- simple F20.6 #
- simplex F20.6 #
- specified NEC F20.8 #
- undifferentiated F20.3 #

Schizophrenia-like
- acute psychotic disorder (*see* Disorder, psychotic)
- disorder, organic F06.2

Schizophrenic
- catalepsy F20.2 #
- catatonia F20.2
- flexibilitas cerea F20.2
- reaction, latent F21
- Restzustand F20.5 #

Schizophreniform disorder F20.8 #
- brief F23.2

Selective mutism F94.0

Separation anxiety of childhood F93.0

Sexual
- aversion F52.10
- desire, lack or loss F52.0
- drive, excessive F52.7
- enjoyment, lack of F52.11
- maturation disorder F66.0 #
- orientation, egodystonic F66.1 #
- preference disorder F65.9
- − multiple F65.6
- − specified NEC F65.8
- relationship disorder F66.2 #

Shock
- culture F43.28
- psychic F43.0

Sleep
- disorder F51.9
- − specified NEC F51.8
- rhythm inversion, psychogenic F51.2
- terrors F51.4

Sleepwalking F51.3

Social phobia F40.1

Somatization disorder F45.0

Somatoform autonomic dysfunction (*see* Dysfunction, somatoform autonomic)

Somatoform disorder (*see* Disorder, somatoform)

Somnambulism F51.3

Specific disorder (of)
− arithmetical skills F81.2
− reading F81.0
− speech articulation F80.0
− spelling F81.1

Stammering F98.5

State
− anxiety F41.1
− crisis F43.0
− organic hallucinatory (nonalcoholic) F06.0
− panic F41.0
− paranoid F22.0
− − involutional F22.8
− − organic F06.2
− paranoid − hallucinatory F06.2
− twilight
− − dissociative F44.88
− − organic F06.5
− − psychogenic F44.88
− withdrawal
− − alcohol F10.3
− − − with delirium F10.4 #
− − caffeine F15.3 #
− − cannabinoids F12.3 #
− − cocaine F14.3 #
− − − with delirium F14.4 #
− − hallucinogens F16.3 #
− − − with delirium F16.4 #
− − hypnotics F13.3 #
− − − with delirium F13.4 #

Syncope, psychogenic F48.8

Syndrome
- alcohol withdrawal F10.3 #
- amnesic
- - alcohol-induced F10.6
- - cannabinoid-induced F12.6
- - hallucinogen-induced F16.6
- - hypnotic-induced F14.6
- - multiple drug-induced F19.6
- - opioid-induced F11.6
- - organic (nonalcoholic) F04
- - psychoactive substance-induced NEC F19.6
- - sedative-induced F13.6
- - stimulant-induced NEC F15.6
- - volatile solvent-induced F18.6
- Asperger's F84.5
- behavioural, associated with physiological disturbances and physical factors F59
- brain F05. –
- - post-traumatic F07.2
- chronic pain personality F62.8
- clumsy child F82
- Da Costa's F45.30
- dependence
- - alcohol F10.2 #
- - caffeine F15.2 #
- - cannabinoids F12.2 #
- - cocaine F14.2 #
- - hallucinogens F16.2 #
- - hypnotics F13.2 #
- - multiple drugs F19.2 #
- - opioids F11.2 #
- - psychoactive substances NEC F19.2 #
- - sedatives F13.2 #
- - stimulants NEC F15.2 #
- - tobacco F17.2 #
- - volatile solvents F18.2 #
- depersonalization – derealization F48.1
- Dhat F48.8
- diarrhoea gas F45.32

Trichotillomania F63.3

Truancy from school F91.2

Twilight state (*see* State, twilight)

Use, harmful (nondependent)
- alcohol F10.1
- caffeine F15.1
- cannabinoids F12.1
- cocaine F14.1
- hallucinogens F16.1
- hypnotics F13.1
- multiple drugs F19.1
- opioids F11.1
- psychoactive substances NEC F19.1
- sedatives F13.1
- stimulants NEC F15.1
- tobacco F17.1
- volatile solvents F18.1

Vaginismus, nonorganic F52.5

Vascular dementia (*see* Dementia, vascular)

Vomiting (associated with)
- psychogenic F50.5
- psychological disturbances, specified NEC F50.5

Voyeurism F65.3

Wernicke's aphasia, developmental F80.2

Withdrawal state (*see* State, withdrawal)

Word deafness F80.2

Zoophobia F40.2

The ICD–10 Classification of Mental and Behavioural Disorders

DIAGNOSTIC CRITERIA FOR RESEARCH

This book sets out internationally-agreed diagnostic criteria specifically designed for use when conducting research on mental and behavioural disorders. Deliberately restrictive, the criteria are intended to facilitate the selection of groups of individuals whose symptoms and other characteristics resemble each other in clearly stated ways, and thus to maximize the homogeneity of study groups and the comparability of findings in multicentre and international studies.

The book, which covers over 300 disorders, is derived from chapter V(F) of the Tenth Revision of the International Statistical Classification of Diseases and Related Health Problems (ICD-10). The research criteria were developed in collaboration with the world's leading experts and finalized after testing by researchers and clinicians in 32 countries, representing all the major traditions and schools of psychiatry. Descriptions of clinical concepts upon which the research criteria are based are contained in the companion volume, *Clinical Descriptions and Diagnostic Guidelines*, which is also available from WHO.

For each disorder, criteria are labelled with letters or numbers to indicate their place in a hierarchy of generality and importance. This hierarchy includes general criteria, which must be fulfilled by all members of a group of disorders, obligatory criteria for individual disorders, and further groups and sub-groups of characteristics, of which only some are required for the diagnosis. Where appropriate, the most commonly used exclusion clause is also listed.

A number of disorders of uncertain or provisional status are described in two annexes. The first covers affective disorders that have been the subject of recent research, together with certain personality disorders. The second provides descriptions of several disorders that seem to appear almost exclusively in particular cultures. These disorders are described with the aim of stimulating the research needed to clarify their diagnostic relevance and allow their more precise classification.

A list of the hundreds of experts involved in field trials of the research criteria, followed by a detailed index, concludes the book.

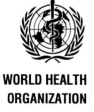

WORLD HEALTH ORGANIZATION

MARKETING AND DISSEMINATION
1211 GENEVA 27
SWITZERLAND

1993, xiii + 248 pages. ISBN 92 4 154455 4